fourth edition

APPLETON & LANGE REVIEW OF SURGERY

Simon Wapnick, MBChB, MD, FRCS(Eng), FACS
Director of Postgraduate Clinical Anatomy Courses
Department of Cell Biology and Anatomy
New York Medical College
Valhalla, New York

C. Gene Cayten, MD, FACS, MPH
Professor of Surgery
New York Medical College
Director of Surgery
Our Lady of Mercy Medical Center
Bronx, New York

Max Goldberg, MBBCh, MD, FRCSI, FACS
Department of Surgery
Long Beach Medical Center
Long Beach, New York

Nanakram Agarwal, MD, MPH, FACS
Professor of Surgery
New York Medical College
Chief of Surgical ICU
Our Lady of Mercy Medical Center
Bronx, New York

John A. Savino, MD
Professor and Chairman
Department of Surgery
New York Medical College
Valhalla, New York

Appleton & Lange Reviews/McGraw-Hill
Medical Publishing Division

New York   Chicago   San Francisco   Lisbon   London   Madrid   Mexico City   Milan
New Delhi   San Juan   Seoul   Singapore   Sydney   Toronto

Appleton & Lange Review of Surgery, Fourth Edition

1 2 3 4 5 6 7 8 9 0 CUS/CUS 0 9 8 7 6 5 4 3 2

ISBN 0-07-137814-6

Notice

Medicine is an ever-changing science. As new research and clinical experience broaden our knowledge, changes in treatment and drug therapy are required. The authors and the publisher of this work have checked with sources believed to be reliable in their efforts to provide information that is complete and generally in accord with the standards accepted at the time of publication. However, in view of the possibility of human error or changes in medical sciences, neither the authors nor the publisher nor any other party who has been involved in the preparation or publication of this work warrants that the information contained herein is in every respect accurate or complete, and they disclaim all responsibility for any errors or omissions or for the results obtained from use of such information contained in this work. Readers are encouraged to confirm the information contained herein with other sources. For example and in particular, readers are advised to check the product information sheet included in the package of each drug they plan to administer to be certain that the information contained in this work is accurate and that changes have not been made in the recommended dose or in the contraindications for administration. This recommendation is of particular importance in connection with new or infrequently used drugs.

This book was set in Palatino by Circle Graphics.
The editors were Catherine A. Johnson, Janene M. Oransky and John M. Morriss.
The production supervisor was Lisa Mendez.
The cover designer was Elizabeth Pisacreta.
Von Hoffmann Graphics was printer and binder.
This book is printed on acid-free paper.

Library of Congress Cataloging-in-Publication Data

Appleton & Lange review of surgery / Simon Wapnick. . . [et al.].—4th ed.
    p. cm.
  ISBN 0-07-137814-6 (alk. paper)
   1. Surgery—Examinations, questions, etc. I. Title: Appleton and Lange review of surgery. II. Title: Review of surgery. III. Wapnick, Simon.

RD37.2.W37 2003
617′.0076—dc21

                                                              2002067173

Contents

Contributors

Nanakram Agarwal, MD, MPH, FACS
Professor of Surgery
New York Medical College
Chief of Surgical Intensive Care Unit
Our Lady of Mercy Medical Center
Bronx, New York

Andrew Ashikari, MD
Assistant Professor of Surgery
New York Medical College
Our Lady of Mercy Medical Center
Bronx, New York

Khawaja Azimuddin, MD, FACS
Assistant Clinical Professor of Surgery
University of New Mexico
Espanola, New Mexico

Nicholas A. Balsano, MD
Clinical Associate Professor of Surgery
New York Medical College
Chief of Vascular Surgery
Our Lady of Mercy Medical Center
Bronx, New York

Alan Berkower, MD, PhD
Assistant Professor of Otorhinolaryngology
New York Medical College
Chief of Otolaryngology
Our Lady of Mercy Medical Center
Bronx, New York

Jaroslaw Bilaniuk, MD
Assistant Professor of Surgery
New York Medical College
Valhalla, New York

C. Gene Cayten, MD, FACS, MPH
Professor of Surgery
New York Medical College
Director of Surgery
Our Lady of Mercy Medical Center
Bronx, New York

Haroon H. Durrani
Department of Radiology
New York Medical College
Westchester Medical Center
Valhalla, New York

Kenneth A. Falvo, MD, FAAOS
Department of Surgery
Our Lady of Mercy Medical Center
Bronx, New York

Max Goldberg, MBBCh, MD, FRCSI, FACS
Professor of Surgery
New York Medical College
Valhalla, New York
Department of Surgery
Long Beach Medical Center
Long Beach, New York

Virany Huynh Hillard, MD
Department of Neurosurgery
New York Medical College
Valhalla, New York

Rao R. Ivatury, MD, FACS
Professor of Surgery
Director, Trauma/Critical Care Surgery
Medical College of Virginia
Virginia Commonwealth University
Richmond, Virginia

Zahi E. Nassoura, MD, FACS
San Fernando Valley Vascular Group
Tarzana, California

Mayank Patel, MD
Department of Surgery
Our Lady of Mercy Medical Center
Bronx, New York

John A. Savino, MD
Professor and Chairman
Department of Surgery
New York Medical College
Valhalla, New York

Jose A. Torres-Gluck, MD
Department of Neurosurgery
Our Lady of Mercy Medical Center
Bronx, New York

Simon Wapnick, MBChB, MD, FRCS(Eng), FACS
Director Postgraduate Clinical Anatomy Courses
Department of Cell Biology and Anatomy
New York Medical College
Valhalla, New York

Scott I. Zeitlin, MD, FACS
Assistant Professor Surgery
Department of Urology
University of California, Los Angeles
Los Angeles, California

Preface

The popularity of the previous editions of *Appleton & Lange Review of Surgery* has encouraged this revised fourth edition. The questions have been selected from the most current pertinent topics, facets, and principles of the wide range of general surgery and its specialities.

The main format of question presentation has been changed to coincide with that recommended by the USMLE guidelines. The material is presented in the form of clinical cases with appropriate answers to mirror the focus of the USMLE Step 2. *Appleton & Lange Review of Surgery*, Fourth Edition, will also help equip and familiarize students preparing for the Surgery Miniboard Examinations. Surgical residents have found both the questions and the annotated answers useful in preparation for various inservice examinations leading to the qualifying and certifying exams of the American Board of Surgery and equivalent examinations in other parts of the world. Surgeons in practice and those preparing for recertification in their specialty have found this book to be a useful addendum to their armamentarium of surgical knowledge.

The types of questions have been arranged into two major groupings: one best answer (usually out of four to five possible answers) and the selection of one or more possible answers (choose N) from a given list of seven or more items. These question types are explained further in the introduction.

The questions are divided into 11 chapters not including the practice test. The reader is encouraged to tackle each chapter in full before referring to the corresponding answer section. Each question should be completed in less than 1 minute. When correcting a chapter, the reader should review the answer and refer back to the question to consolidate knowledge gained during test preparation. Incorrect answers should be reviewed and attempted at a later date. If you have any comments as to the contents or usefulness of this book, e-mail **simon_wapnick@nymc.edu**.

ACKNOWLEDGMENTS

We would like to thank Professor Terence A. S. Matalon, Chairman and Professor of Radiology, New York Medical College and Westchester Medical Center, for permission to use the numerous radiological images included. Dr. H. Durrani participated in the preparation of these radiographs. Isabelle Wapnick made valuable contributions to editing this book.

Introduction

This book has been designed to help you review surgery for both examination and patient management. Here in one package is a comprehensive review with over 1,000 multiple-choice questions with paragraph-length discussions of each answer. The whole book has been designed to help you assess your areas of relative strength and weakness.

Appleton & Lange Review of Surgery is divided into 12 chapters. Eleven chapters provide a review of the major areas of surgery. The last chapter, a Practice Test, integrates diverse specialities into one simulated examination.

This introduction provides information on question types, question-taking strategies, various ways you can use this book, and specific information on the USMLE Step 2.

QUESTIONS

The USMLE Step 2 now contains only two different types of questions. In general, most of these are "one-best-answer–single-item" questions; whereas, the remainder require selection of a stated number of answers from a list of seven or more items (choose N). "Multiple true–false item" and "comparison–matching set" questions have been excluded. Questions that are negatively phrased ("All of the following are correct EXCEPT . . .") have been disposed of in accordance with current USMLE guidelines. In some cases (in both types of questions), a group of two or three questions may be related to a situational theme. Certain questions have illustrative material (diagrams and x-rays) that require understanding and interpretation on your part. Some illustrations, however, are included mainly for their instructive value in clinical surgical practice.

Questions are stratified into three levels of difficulty: (a) rote memory questions; (b) memory questions that require more understanding of the question; and (c) questions that require understanding and judgment. Because the NBME and other examination bodies are moving away from the rote memory questions, we have tried to emphasize judgment cases throughout this text.

One-Best-Answer–Single-Item Question

This type of question presents a problem or asks a question and is followed by five or more choices, only one of which is entirely correct. The directions preceding this type of question will generally appear as follows:

DIRECTIONS: (Questions 1 through 82): Each of the numbered items or incomplete statements in this section is followed by answers or by completions of the statements. Select the ONE lettered answer or completion that is BEST in each case.

An example for this item type follows:

1. An obese 21-year-old woman reports increased growth of coarse hair on her lip, chin, chest, and abdomen. She also notes menstrual irregularity, with periods of amenorrhea. What is the most likely cause is?

   (A) polycystic ovary disease
   (B) an ovarian tumor
   (C) an adrenal tumor
   (D) Cushing's disease
   (E) familial hirsutism

   In this type of question, choices other than the correct answer may be partially correct, but there can only be one *best* answer. In the question above the key word is "most." Although ovarian tumors, adrenal tumors, and Cushing's disease are causes of hirsutism (described in the stem of the question), polycystic ovary disease is a much more common cause. Familial hirsutism is not associated with the menstrual irregularities mentioned. Thus, the *most* likely cause of the manifestations described can only be "(A) polycystic ovary disease."

TABLE 1. STRATEGIES FOR ANSWERING ONE-BEST-ANSWER–SINGLE-ITEM QUESTIONS*

1. Remember that only one choice can be the correct answer.
2. Read the question carefully to be sure that you understand what is being asked.
3. Quickly read each choice for familiarity. (This important step is often not done by test takers.)
4. Go back and consider each choice individually.
5. If a choice is partially correct, tentatively consider it to be incorrect. (This step will help you lessen your choices and increase your odds of choosing the correct answer.)
6. Consider the remaining choices and select the one you think is the answer. At this point, you may want to quickly scan the stem to be sure you understand the question and your answer.
7. Select the appropriate answer. (Even if you do not know the answer, you should at least guess. Your score is based on the number of correct answers, so **do not skip any questions**.)

* Note that steps 2 through 7 should take an average of 50 seconds total. The actual examination is timed for an average of 60 seconds per question.

One (or More)-Best-Answer–Matching-Set Questions

These questions are usually accompanied by the following general directions.

DIRECTIONS: (Questions 83 through 100): Each set of matching questions in this section consists of a list of lettered options followed by several numbered items. For each numbered item, select the appropriate lettered options(s). Each lettered option may be selected once, more than once, or not at all. EACH ITEM WILL STATE THE NUMBER OF OPTIONS TO SELECT. SELECT EXACTLY THIS NUMBER.

An example for this item type is:

Questions 83 through 84

In each condition listed, select the most appropriate antibiotics.

(A) tetracycline
(B) chloramphenicol
(C) clindamycin
(D) ceftriaxone and doxycycline
(E) penicillin
(F) metronidazole
(G) ciprofloxacin
(H) chloroquine
(I) fluconazole

83. Bone marrow suppression. SELECT ONLY ONE.

Answer. (B)

84. A 34-year-old woman complains of lower abdominal pain and vaginal discharge due to gonorrhea. SELECT ONLY THREE.

Answer. (D), (E), (G). Each one of THE THREE DIFFERENT choices would be appropriate treatment of this condition.

TABLE 2. STRATEGIES FOR ANSWERING ONE (OR MORE)-BEST-ANSWER–MATCHING-SET QUESTIONS*

1. Remember that the lettered choices are *followed by the numbered questions*.
2. *Apply steps 2 through 7 in Table 1 but select EXACTLY ONLY ONE, TWO, THREE (OR MORE) ANSWER(S) as stated.*

* Remember, you only have an average of 60 seconds per question.

ANSWERS, EXPLANATIONS, AND REFERENCES

In each of the sections of *Appleton & Lange Review of Surgery, Fourth Edition*, the question sections are followed by a section containing the answers and explanations for the questions. This section: (a) tells you the answer to each question; and (b) gives you an explanation and review of why the answer is correct, background information on the subject matter, and/or why the other answers are incorrect. We encourage you to use this section as a basis for further study and understanding.

If you choose the correct answer to a question, you can then read the explanation: (a) for reinforcement; and (b) to add to your knowledge about the subject matter. **If you choose the wrong answer** to a question, you can read the explanation for an instructional review of the material in the question.

PRACTICE TEST

The 98-question Practice Test at the end of the book covers and reviews all the topics covered in Chapters 1 through 11. The questions are integrated according to question type (one-best-answer–single item, one (or more)-best-answer–matching sets.)

HOW TO USE THIS BOOK

There are two logical ways to get the most value from this book. We call them Plan A and Plan B.

In **Plan A,** you go straight to the Practice Test and complete it. Analyze your areas of strength and weakness. This will be a good indicator of your initial knowledge of the subject and will help to identify specific areas for preparation and review. You can now use the first 11 chapters of the book to help you improve your relative weak points.

In **Plan B,** you go through Chapters 1 through 11 checking off your answers, and then comparing your choices with the answers and discussions in the book. Once you have completed this process, you can take the Practice Test and see how well prepared you are. If you still have a major weakness, it should be apparent in time for you to take remedial action.

In Plan A, by taking the Practice Test first, you get quick feedback regarding your initial areas of strength and weakness. You may find that you have a good command of the material, indicating that perhaps only a cursory review of the first 11 chapters is necessary. This, of course, would be good to know early in your examination preparation. On the other hand, you may find that you have many areas of weakness. In this case, you could focus on these areas in your review–not just with this book, but also with textbooks.

However, it is unlikely that you will not do some studying before taking the USMLE (especially because you have this book). Therefore, it may be more realistic to take the Practice Test after you have

reviewed the first 11 chapters (as in Plan B). This will probably give you a more realistic type of testing situation, because very few of us sit down to a test without study. In this case, you will have done some reviewing (from superficial to in-depth), and your Practice Test will reflect this study time. If, after reviewing the first 11 chapters and then taking the Practice Test, you still have some weaknesses, you can then go back through chapters 1 through 11 and supplement your review with your texts.

SPECIFIC INFORMATION ON THE STEP 2 EXAMINATION

The official source of all information with respect to the USMLE is the National Board of Medical Examiners (NBME), 3750 Market Street, Philadelphia, PA 19104. Established in 1915, the NBME is a voluntary, nonprofit, independent organization whose sole function is the design, implementation, distribution, and processing of a vast bank of question items, certifying examinations, and evaluative services in the professional medical field.

To be eligible to sit for the USMLE Step 2, a person must be either officially enrolled in or a graduate of a US or Canadian medical school accredited by the LCME; officially enrolled in or a graduate of a US osteopathic medical school accredited by the AOA; or officially enrolled in or a graduate of a foreign medical school and eligible for examination by the ECFMG for its certificate. It is not necessary to complete any particular year of medical school in order to be a candidate for Step 2; neither is it required to take Step 1 before Step 2.

SCORING

Because there is no penalty for guessing, you should answer every question. Do not skip any questions. Each question answered correctly counts as one point, and partial credit may be given to partially correct answers.

Information on the USMLE is posted on the NBME's web page, **www.usmle.org.**

CHAPTER 1

Trauma
Questions

C. Gene Cayten, Kenneth A. Falvo, and Rao R. Ivatury

DIRECTIONS (Questions 1 through 85): Each of the numbered items or incomplete statements in this section is followed by answers or by completions of the statement. Select the ONE lettered answer or completion that is BEST in each case.

1. A 40-year-old man is involved in a car crash, presenting with blood pressure of 80 mmHg. The patient is found to have subdural hematoma and a supracondylar fracture of the left femur. He is taken to the operating room, where intra-abdominal bleeding is controlled, and the subdural hematoma is drained. The femur fracture (Figure 1–1) should be treated by which of the following?

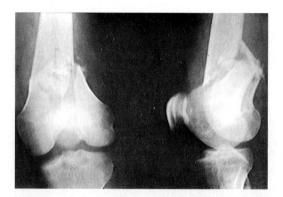

Figure 1–1. Comminuted fracture of the distal femur. (Reproduced, with permission, from Way, LW: Current Surgical Diagnosis & Treatment, 10th ed., Appleton & Lange, 1994.)

   (A) long leg cast
   (B) Steinmann pin insertion and traction
   (C) operative reduction and internal reduction
   (D) aspiration of knee joint
   (E) operative reduction with internal fixation

2. An 18-year-old man is brought to the emergency department with a stab wound just to the right of the sternum in the sixth intercostal space. His blood pressure is 80 mmHg. Faint heart sounds and pulsus paradoxus are noted. Auscultation of the right chest reveals decreased breath sounds. The *initial* management of this patient should be which of the following?

   (A) aspiration of the right chest cavity
   (B) aspiration of the pericardium
   (C) echocardiogram
   (D) pericardial window
   (E) insertion of central venous access line

3. A 60-year-old woman runs her car off the road and it hits a telephone pole. She presents to the emergency department with severe anterior chest pain and a blood pressure of 110/80. A chest x-ray shows a questionably widened mediastinum. The next step in management should be which of the following?

   (A) transthoracic echocardiogram
   (B) pericardiocentesis
   (C) aortogram
   (D) central venous access line
   (E) computed tomography (CT) of chest

4. An 18-year-old man presents to the emergency department with a gunshot wound to the left chest in the anterior axillary line in the seventh intercostal space. A rushing sound is audible during inspiration. Immediate management is which of the following?

   (A) exploratory laparotomy
   (B) exploratory thoracotomy
   (C) pleurocentesis
   (D) closure of the hole with sterile dressing
   (E) insertion of chest tube

5. A 25-year-old man is shot in the left lateral chest. In the emergency department, his blood pressure is 120/90, his pulse rate is 104 bpm, and his respiration rate is 36 breaths per minute. Chest x-ray shows air and fluid in the left pleural cavity. Nasogastric aspiration reveals blood-stained fluid. What is the best step to rule out esophageal injury?

   (A) insertion of chest tube
   (B) insertion of nasogastric tube
   (C) esophagogram with gastrografin
   (D) esophagoscopy
   (E) peritoneal lavage

6. A 32-year-old female falls from the 10th floor of her apartment building in an apparent suicide attempt. Upon presentation, the patient has obvious head and extremity injuries. Primary survey reveals that the patient is totally apneic. By which method is the immediate need for a definitive airway in this patient best provided?

   (A) orotracheal intubation
   (B) nasotracheal intubation
   (C) percutaneous cricothyroidotomy
   (D) intubation over a bronchoscope
   (E) needle cricothyroidotomy

7. A 17-year-old girl presents to the emergency department with a stab wound to the abdomen and a blow to the head that left her groggy. Her blood pressure is 80/0, her pulse is 120 bpm, and her respiration rate is 28. Her abdomen has a stab wound in the anterior axillary line at the right costal margin. Two large-bore intravenous lines, a nasogastric tube, and a Foley catheter are inserted. The blood pressure rises to 85 mmHg after 2 L of Ringer's lactate. The appropriate management is which of the following?

   (A) peritoneal lavage
   (B) ultrasound of the abdomen
   (C) laparoscopic assessment of the peritoneal cavity
   (D) exploratory laparotomy
   (E) CT of the head

8. A 22-year-old woman presents to the emergency department with a chief complaint of severe left upper quadrant (LUQ) pain after being punched by her husband. Her blood pressure is 110/70, her pulse is 100 bpm, and her respiration rate is 24 breaths per minute. The best means to establish a diagnosis is which of the following?

   (A) four-quadrant tap of the abdomen
   (B) physical examination
   (C) CT of the abdomen
   (D) peritoneal lavage
   (E) upper gastrointestinal (GI) series

9. A 60-year-old man is attacked with a baseball bat and sustains multiple blows to the abdomen. He presents to the emergency department in shock and is brought to the operating room (OR), where a laparotomy reveals massive hemoperitoneum and a stellate fracture of the right and left lobes of the liver. Which of the following techniques should be used immediately?

   (A) Pringle maneuver
   (B) packing the liver
   (C) suture ligation
   (D) ligation of the right hepatic artery
   (E) ligation of the proper hepatic artery

10. A 12-year-old girl presents to the emergency department following a skiing crash in which the left side of her midtorso hit a tree. She presents with left side lower chest and upper abdominal pain. She also complains of left shoulder pain. The most likely diagnosis is which of the following?

(A) rib fractures

(B) liver injury

(C) ruptured diaphragm

(D) splenic injury

(E) ruptured stomach

11. A 23-year-old man is shot with a handgun and found to have a through-and-through injury to the right transverse colon. There is little fecal contamination and no bowel devascularization. At operation, what does he require?

(A) right hemicolectomy with ileotransverse colon anastomosis

(B) right hemicolectomy with ileostomy and mucous fistula

(C) debridement and closure of wounds with exteriorization of colon

(D) debridement and closure of wounds

(E) segmental resection with primary anastomosis

12. A 20-year-old woman presents to the emergency department with a stab wound to the abdomen. There is minimal abdominal tenderness. Local wound exploration indicates that the knife penetrated the peritoneum. What is the ideal use of antibiotic administration?

(A) preoperatively

(B) intraoperatively, if a colon injury is found

(C) postoperatively, if the patient develops fever

(D) postoperatively, based on culture and sensitivity of fecal contamination found at the time of surgery

(E) intraoperatively, if any hollow viscus is found to be injured

13. A 70-year-old woman is hit by a car and injures her midabdomen. The best way to rule out a rupture of the second part of the duodenum is by which mode?

(A) repeated physical examinations

(B) ultrasound

(C) repeated amylase levels

(D) CT with oral and intravenous contrast

(E) peritoneal lavage

Questions 14 and 15

14. A 35-year-old woman was punched in the right side of the abdomen and chest. There was some right upper abdomen tenderness but no guarding or rebound. Results of a gastrografin upper GI study showed a coiled-spring (stack of coins) appearance of the second and third part of the duodenum. What is the most likely diagnosis?

(A) rupture of the duodenum

(B) contusion to the head of the pancreas

(C) intraluminal blood clot

(D) retroperitoneal hematoma

(E) duodenal hematoma

15. Which would be the appropriate management of the patient described above?

(A) exploratory laparotomy and drainage

(B) duodenal diverticularization

(C) pyloric exclusion

(D) repeat upper GI series at 5- to 7-day intervals

(E) CT-guided percutaneous drainage

16. A 15-year-old girl had an injury to the right retroperitoneum with duodenal contusion. What is the test required to exclude a rupture of the duodenum?

(A) serum amylase

(B) dimethyliminodiacetic acid (HIDA) scan

(C) gastrografin study

(D) intravenous pyelogram (IVP)

(E) endoscopic retrograde cholangiopancreatogram (ERCP)

17. A 33-year-old man presents to the emergency department with a gunshot injury to the abdomen. At laparotomy, a deep laceration is found in the pancreas just to the left of the vertebral column with severance of the pancreatic duct. What is the next step in management?

(A) intraoperative cholangiogram

(B) debridement and drainage of defect

(C) distal pancreatectomy

(D) closure of abdomen

(E) vagotomy

18. A 40-year-old man is hit by a car and sustains an injury to the pelvis. Which of the following is most indicative of a urethral injury?

    (A) hematuria
    (B) scrotal ecchymosis
    (C) oliguria
    (D) high-riding prostate on rectal examination
    (E) IVP showing dye extravasation in the pelvis

19. For the patient described in question 18, urine did not extend to the leg because the membranous layer (Scarpa's fascia) is fused inferiorly with which of the following?

    (A) femoral sheath
    (B) fascia lata
    (C) femoral fascia
    (D) deep inguinal ring
    (E) superficial inguinal ring

20. A 70-year-old man is brought to the emergency department following a car crash. X-rays revealed a fractured rib on the left and a fracture of the right femur. A CT scan of the abdomen showed a left-sided retroperitoneal hematoma adjacent to the left kidney and no evidence of urine extravasation. The hematoma should be managed by which of the following?

    (A) observation
    (B) exploratory laparotomy through a midline incision
    (C) CT scan-guided aspiration
    (D) surgical exploration through a left-flank retroperitoneal approach
    (E) Pneumatic antishock garment (PASG)

21. A 60-year-old man is hit by a pickup truck and brought to the emergency department with a blood pressure of 70/0 mmHg. Peritoneal lavage showed no blood in the abdomen. The blood pressure is elevated to 85 systolic following the administration of 2 L of Ringer's lactate. An x-ray showed a pelvic fracture. What is the next step in management?

    (A) exploratory laparotomy with packing of the pelvis

    (B) CT scan of the pelvis
    (C) external fixation of the pelvis
    (D) open reduction and internal fixation (ORIF) of the pelvis
    (E) exploratory laparotomy with bilateral ligation of the internal iliac arteries

22. An 18-year-old man is brought to the emergency department after falling down a flight of stairs and losing consciousness for 3 minutes. A cervical collar is in place. The cervical spine is considered to be free of serious injury following which procedure?

    (A) a physical examination revealing no pain or tenderness
    (B) a lateral cervical spine x-ray
    (C) completely negative findings on neurological examination
    (D) anteroposterior (AP), lateral, and odontoid views of the neck
    (E) flexion and extension views of the neck

23. A 16-year-old boy presents to the emergency department with a stab wound to the anterior midneck. On physical examination, it is difficult to determine if the plane of the platysma has been violated. However, subcutaneous emphysema is found on palpation. What is the next management step?

    (A) esophagogram
    (B) arteriography
    (C) surgical exploration
    (D) esophagoscopy
    (E) CT scan of the neck with oral and intravenous contrast

24. A 20-year-old woman presents to the emergency department after being hit in the face during a baseball game. On physical examination, the patient's blood pressure is 90 mmHg, and there is significant bleeding from the nose that cannot be controlled either by fracture reduction or by anterior and posterior nasopharyngeal packing. What is the next step in management?

    (A) external carotid artery ligation
    (B) bilateral internal maxillary artery ligation

(C) angiographic evaluation and embolization

(D) foley catheter balloon tamponade of bleeding

(E) insertion of nasogastric tube

25. A 65-year-old man is brought to the hospital after being hit by a car. His blood pressure is 150/90, and his pulse is 120 bpm. There is deformity just below the left knee and no distal pulses palpable in that leg. Plain films show proximal tibia and fibula fractures. What is the next step in management?

(A) operative intervention to restore flow with an arterial shunt

(B) angiography

(C) Doppler ultrasound

(D) operative reduction and internal fixation

(E) heparinization

26. A 70-year-old man is brought into the emergency department following his injury as a passenger in a car crash. He complains of right side chest pain. Physical examination reveals a respiratory rate of 42 breaths per minute and multiple broken ribs of a segment of the chest wall that moves paradoxically with respiration. What should the next step be?

(A) tube thoracostomy

(B) tracheostomy

(C) thoracentesis

(D) endotracheal intubation

(E) intercostal nerve blocks

27. A 30-year-old man is brought to the emergency department in respiratory distress following a shotgun wound to the face. There is a possible cervical spine injury. Which is the best way to gain rapid control of the airway?

(A) nasotracheal intubation

(B) percutaneous jet ventilation

(C) cricothyroidotomy

(D) endotracheal intubation

(E) aspiration of blood from pharynx and jaw thrust

28. A 14-year-old boy is hit in the right eye with a stick. There is extensive ecchymosis. On physical examination, upward gaze is found to be lost. The most likely diagnosis is injury to which of the following (Figure 1–2)?

(A) superior rectus muscle

(B) inferior rectus muscle

(C) superior oblique muscle

(D) levator palpebrae superioris muscle

(E) medial rectus muscle

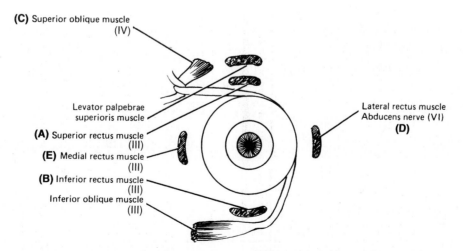

Figure 1–2. The muscles of extraocular movement. (Reproduced, with permission, from Lindner, HH: Clinical Anatomy, Appleton & Lange, 1989.)

29. Following a car crash in which her face hit the steering wheel, a 37-year-old woman presents to the emergency department with facial deformity. Facial x-rays showed a transverse fracture through the articulation of the maxillary and nasal bones with the frontal bone. The fracture also passed below the zygomatic bone. What is the diagnosis?

    (A) sphenoid wing fracture
    (B) LeFort II fracture
    (C) petrous temporal fracture
    (D) palatal split
    (E) mandibular disruption

30. A 43-year-old man is hit in the face with a baseball bat and presents to the emergency department with massive facial swelling, ecchymosis, and an elongated face. There is mobility of the middle third of the face on digital manipulation of the maxilla. What is the likely diagnosis?

    (A) lamdoid injury
    (B) odontoid fracture
    (C) LeFort III fracture
    (D) palatal split
    (E) mandibular disruption

31. A 26-year-old man is stabbed in the right intercostal space in the midclavicular line and presents to the emergency department. On examination, subcutaneous emphysema of the right chest wall, absent breath sounds, and a trachea shifted to the left are noted. What is the most likely serious diagnosis?

    (A) pneumothorax
    (B) tension pneumothorax
    (C) massive hemothorax
    (D) hemopneumothorax
    (E) chest wall laceration

Questions 32 and 33

32. A 31-year-old man is shot in the back of the left chest, and the bullet exits the left anterior chest. The patient's blood pressure is 130/90, his respiration rate is 28 breaths per minute, and his pulse is 110 bpm. A chest x-ray reveals hemothorax. A chest tube is inserted and yields 800 mL of blood; the 1st- and 2nd-hour drainage is 200 mL/h and 240 mL/h, respectively. Which is the next step in management?

    (A) place a second chest tube
    (B) collect the blood for autotransfusion
    (C) transfuse and observe drainage for another hour
    (D) insert a Swan–Ganz catheter
    (E) perform a left thoracotomy

33. The most likely cause of the bleeding in the patient described in Question 32 is injury to which of the following?

    (A) pulmonary artery
    (B) lung parenchyma
    (C) internal thoracic (mammary) and/or intercostals arteries
    (D) pulmonary vein
    (E) left atrium

34. A 60-year-old man crashes his car into a bridge abutment and is found slumped over his steering wheel. In the emergency department, the signs and symptoms of pericardial tamponade are evident. These findings are most likely attributable to which of the following?

    (A) coronary artery laceration
    (B) left atrial rupture
    (C) right atrial rupture
    (D) coronary vein laceration
    (E) intrapericardial vena cava injury

35. Following an injury to the shoulder joint, a New York Yankees catcher developed a "catcher's mitt hand" or shoulder and hand syndrome. There was swelling of the right upper extremity, skin atrophy, and vasomotor instability. He also complained of a burning sensation in the involved extremity. What would be the next step in management?

    (A) immobilization of right arm in cast
    (B) to avoid physical therapy for 3 months
    (C) forceful shoulder joint manipulation
    (D) prednisone for 2 weeks in resistant cases
    (E) surgical procedure on wrist joint

36. A 47-year-old woman involved in a skiing accident suffered a severe blow to the middle upper abdomen. Physical examination revealed diffuse tenderness, but there was no evidence of rebound tenderness or guarding. What test would be performed to rule out traumatic pancreatitis?

   (A) peritoneal lavage
   (B) serum amylase
   (C) CT scan with oral and intravenous contrast
   (D) upper GI study
   (E) ERCP

37. A 19-year-old man presents to the emergency department with a gunshot wound through the umbilicus. The systolic blood pressure is 70 mmHg on palpation, and his abdomen is tightly distended. Large-bore intravenous lines are placed, and Ringer's lactate is infused. What should be the next step?

   (A) peritoneal lavage
   (B) CT scan of the abdomen
   (C) exploratory laparotomy
   (D) transfusion of the patient until the systolic blood pressure reaches 90 mmHg
   (E) pneumatic antishock garment (PASG)

38. A 34-year-old man is brought into the emergency department with a large open knife wound to the left thigh. The patient's systolic blood pressure is 90 mmHg. Blood is spurting from the wound. What is the initial management step?

   (A) Clamp the bleeding artery with a vascular clamp.
   (B) Apply a tourniquet 7.5 cm above the wound.
   (C) Apply direct pressure with sterile gauze.
   (D) Apply PASG, and inflate both legs.
   (E) Insert central venous access line.

39. A 40-year-old construction worker is pulled from the rubble after a building collapses and pins his right lower leg. X-rays in the emergency department reveal a comminuted fracture of the right tibia and fibula. The dorsal pedis and posterior tibial pulses are palpable.

The patient complains of severe pain that is accentuated with dorsiflexion of the foot. The calf feels tense. What is the appropriate step?

   (A) Open reduction and internal fixation (ORIF) of fracture
   (B) ORIF of fracture plus three-compartment fasciotomy
   (C) closed reduction and observation
   (D) ORIF only if pulses become weak
   (E) arteriogram

40. An 18-year-old woman who is 8 months pregnant is brought into the emergency department. She was hit by a car and now complains of abdominal pain. Her blood pressure is 80/60, her pulse is 120 bpm, and her respiration rate is 30 breaths per minute. Large-bore intravenous lines are placed through the antecubital fossa. The fetal heart rate is 160 bpm. What is the next step?

   (A) Infuse 2000 mL of Ringer's lactate over 10–15 minutes.
   (B) Apply a PASG, inflating only the legs.
   (C) Displace the uterus to the left.
   (D) Order an ultrasound of abdomen and pelvis to rule out free blood.
   (E) Perform peritoneal lavage 2 cm above the umbilicus.

41. A 60-year-old man is a front-seat passenger in a car crash. He is found to have three fractured ribs on the right, rupture of the liver, pelvic fracture, right femoral fracture, and a left tibial fracture. The patient is given broad-spectrum antibiotics, and his injuries are managed by surgery, requiring 12 units of blood. The patient improves initially, but on the third postoperative day, he develops hypoxia (PaO_2 55 mmHg), with confusion, tachypnea, and petechia. What is the most likely diagnosis?

   (A) recurrent intra-abdominal hemorrhage from dilutional thrombocytopenia
   (B) transfusion reaction
   (C) antibiotic allergy
   (D) fat embolus
   (E) disseminated intravascular clotting (DIC)

42. A 43-year-old woman is thrown from a car following a car crash. She presents to the emergency department with a fracture of the pelvis (Figure 1–3). Her blood pressure is 80/60 mmHg, her pulse is 110 bpm, and her respiratory rate is 26 breaths per minute. Bright red blood is found on rectal examination and bony fragments can be palpated through the rectal wall. The patient remains hypotensive despite 3 L of Ringer's lactate and 2 units of type-specific blood. What is the most important step in management?

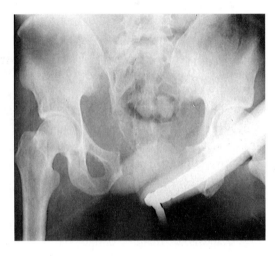

Figure 1–3. Pelvic injury demonstrating open book (symphysis diastasis and vertical displacement of the hemipelvis). (Reproduced, with permission, from Way, LW: Current Surgical Diagnosis & Treatment, 10th ed., Appleton & Lange, 1994.)

(A) exploratory laparotomy and colostomy
(B) external fixation of the pelvic fracture
(C) PASG
(D) fresh-frozen plasma
(E) wiring of symphysis pubis

43. With regard to neck injuries, which of the following is true?

(A) The internal jugular vein may be ligated unilaterally without unfavorable sequelae.
(B) Unilateral ligation of the common carotid artery results in a neurologic deficiency in 90% of cases.
(C) Esophageal injuries should be drained externally only when extensive devitalization is present.

(D) Tracheostomy is indicated in dealing with most laryngeal or tracheal injuries.
(E) Injuries to the trachea must be drained externally.

44. The injury most often missed by selective nonoperative management of abdominal stab wounds is to which of the following?

(A) colon
(B) spleen
(C) ureter
(D) diaphragm
(E) small bowel

45. A 40-year-old woman is brought to the emergency department following a car crash in which she was the driver. In the emergency department, her blood pressure is 80/60 mmHg, her pulse is 128 bpm, and her respiratory rate is 32 breaths per minute. She complains of right lower chest wall and severe right upper quadrant (RUQ) tenderness. Her breath sounds are questionably diminished. The immediate priority is to perform which of the following?

(A) peritoneal lavage
(B) chest x-ray
(C) CT scan of chest and abdomen
(D) thoracentesis with an 18-gauge needle
(E) endotracheal intubation

46. A 30-year-old woman is brought to the emergency department after she stepped on a rusty nail and sustained a puncture wound to the foot. The patient has been on a therapeutic dose of steroids for the past 5 years for ulcerative colitis. Her last tetanus toxoid booster was 8 years ago. Which should the patient receive?

(A) tetanus toxoid booster
(B) human immunoglobulin
(C) antibiotics with anaerobic coverage
(D) tetanus toxoid plus human immunoglobulin
(E) tetanus toxoid plus human immunoglobulin and antibiotics with aerobic and anaerobic coverage

47. A 24-year-old woman with blunt trauma to the head sustained in a car accident presents with a history of loss of consciousness for approximately 10 minutes at the scene of the accident. She is currently fully awake, oriented, and responsive. With regard to the appropriate care of this woman, which of the following statements is true?

   (A) In this setting, a fully awake patient who has a normal examination does not require hospital ad mission for observation.
   (B) If skull x-rays show no fracture, the likelihood of a significant intracranial injury is low, and hospital admission is unwarranted.
   (C) If fundoscopic examination of this patient shows no papilledema, elevated intracranial pressure can be ruled out.
   (D) The initial effects of elevated intracranial pressure are bradycardia and hypertension.
   (E) If this patient were to exhibit a sudden fall in blood pressure and alteration in mental status, spinal cord or brain stem injury would be most likely.

48. A 12-year-old girl is brought into the emergency department after an unprovoked attack and bite by a raccoon. The bite is on the left lower leg. Which treatment should be provided?

   (A) administration of human rabies immunoglobulin (HRIG) into the left gluteal area
   (B) administration of a five-dose course of human diploid cell rabies vaccine (HDCV)
   (C) administration of a 5-day course of HDCV and a 3-day course of HRIG
   (D) administration of a 5-day course of HDCV and a single dose of HRIG with up to half of the dose administered directly around the wound
   (E) administration of a 5-day course of HDCV and a single dose of HRIG administered into the gluteal area

49. An 18-year-old man is bitten on the leg by what appears to be a rattlesnake. A tourniquet has been placed above the wound, and the patient arrives at the emergency department 70 minutes after the injury. There are two fang marks with 15 cm of edema and erythema surrounding the wound. What should immediate treatment include?

   (A) suction applied through longitudinal incisions directly through the fang marks
   (B) suction applied through longitudinal incisions proximal to the bite
   (C) excision of the fang mark, including skin and subcutaneous tissues
   (D) administration of four ampules of antivenin
   (E) removal of tourniquet

50. A 20-year-old woman presents to the emergency department with a stab wound to the neck above the angle of the mandible. The patient's blood pressure is 110/80 mmHg, her pulse rate is 100 bpm, and her respiration rate is 24 breaths per minute. Between initial presentation and insertion of intravenous lines, the hematoma in the upper neck enlarges significantly. What should be the next step in the patient's management?

   (A) barium swallow
   (B) flexible endoscopy
   (C) operative exploration
   (D) doppler ultrasound
   (E) angiography

51. A 65-year-old man is brought into the emergency department with a gunshot wound to the neck. His blood pressure is 80/50 mmHg. The patient undergoes rapid resuscitation and is brought immediately to the OR, where a carotid artery injury is found in zone II (between the angle of mandible and cricoid) (Figure 1–4). The patient has no internal carotid flow; just before surgery, his neurological status deteriorates, and he becomes unresponsive. The operative management should be which of the following?

   (A) immediate intravascular bypass shunt
   (B) ligation of the internal carotid artery
   (C) primary anastomosis
   (D) interposition saphenous vein graft
   (E) patch vein graft

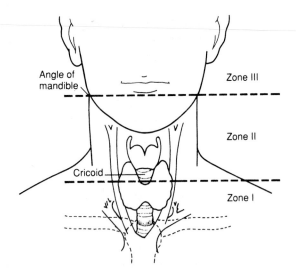

Figure 1–4. Classification neck injuries; zones of the neck. (Reproduced, with permission, from Way, LW: Current Surgical Diagnosis & Treatment, 10th ed., Appleton & Lange, 1994.)

52. A 19-year-old man is brought to the emergency department with a stab wound at the base of the neck (zone I) (Figure 1–4). The most important concern for patients with such injuries is which of the following?

(A) upper extremity ischemia
(B) cerebral infarction
(C) exsanguinating hemorrhage
(D) mediastinitis
(E) tracheal stenosis

53. A 42-year-old man is hit on the left side of his body by a car and is brought to the emergency department with fractures of the left 10th, 11th, and 12th ribs and left tibia and fibula fractures. The patient's blood pressure is 120/90 mmHg, his pulse rate is 100 bpm, and his respiration rate is 24 breaths per minute. He has hematuria and left flank pain. Intravenous lines are inserted. IVP shows no excretion from the left kidney but normal excretion from the right. Which would be the next step in management?

(A) exploratory laparotomy
(B) CT scan with intravenous contrast
(C) arteriography
(D) cystogram
(E) peritoneal lavage

54. A 26-year-old man is brought to the emergency department with a stab wound to the right side of the back just medial to the posterioraxillary line. His blood pressure is 120/80 mmHg, his pulse rate is 98 bpm, and his respiration rate is 22 breaths per minute. Physical examination reveals no abdominal tenderness, guarding, or neurologic changes. Local exploration of the stab wound is performed using local anesthesia. The track to the wound ends in the paraspinal muscles. What would be the next step in management?

(A) Admit the patient for 24 hours of observation.
(B) Perform peritoneal lavage.
(C) Perform CT scan with rectal and intravenous contrast.
(D) Discharge to outpatient clinic for follow-up monitoring.
(E) Perform ultrasound.

55. A 25-year-old woman is brought to the emergency department with multiple gunshot wounds to her abdomen. Her blood pressure is 70/0 mmHg. Her abdomen is massively distended. Large intravenous lines are placed, and a nasogastric tube and Foley catheter are inserted. The patient is brought immediately to the operating room. After 2 L of normal saline, her blood pressure is 75/0 mmHg, her pulse rate is 140 bpm, and her respiration rate is 30 breaths per minute. The next step in management should be which of the following?

(A) Open the abdomen and use a large Richardson retractor to compress the abdominal aorta against the vertebrae just below the diaphragm.
(B) Perform left thoracotomy, and cross clamp the descending aorta just above the diaphragm.
(C) Apply the PASG to elevate blood pressure before incision.
(D) Infuse four units of whole blood before incision.
(E) Perform exploratory laparotomy and pack obvious bleeding sites.

56. A 30-year-old woman involved in a car crash is brought into the emergency department. Her blood pressure is 90/60 mmHg, her pulse rate is 120 bpm, and her respiration rate is 18 breaths per minute. On peritoneal lavage, she is noted to have free blood in the peritoneal cavity. At the time of exploratory laparotomy, a liver laceration is noted, and there is a 2.5-cm-diameter contusion to an area of small bowel. How should the small-bowel contusion be treated?

(A) transillumination evaluation of hematoma with meticulous hemostasis

(B) resection of the bowel with single-layer anastomosis

(C) inversion of the area of contusion with a row of fine nonabsorbable mattress sutures

(D) resection of the bowel and ileostomy

(E) observation (no surgical therapy)

57. A 19-year-old man is brought into the emergency department with a gunshot wound that occurred 4 hours before admission. At exploratory laparotomy, an injury is noted in the transverse colon with extensive tissue destruction. There is a large amount of fecal contamination. Management of this injury should include which of the following?

(A) debridement and closure of wound with a proximal colostomy

(B) resection with proximal colostomy and distal mucous fistula

(C) resection of the injured colon with primary anastomosis and proximal colostomy

(D) resection of the wound with primary anastomosis and proximal cecostomy

(E) exteriorization of repaired colon

58. A 60-year-old man is brought into the emergency department after being hit by a car. His blood pressure is 70 mmHg palpable, and his abdomen is massively distended and tender. A large stellate fracture of the right lower liver is noted, and despite repeated attempts at suturing, bleeding persists. The anesthesiologist notes that the pH of arterial blood is 7.20 and

that the patient has become hypothermic. A total of eight units of blood have been transfused. Which is the next step in management?

(A) Insert an atriocaval shunt.

(B) Perform a right hepatic lobectomy.

(C) Pack the RUQ for 15–20 minutes while the anesthesiologist transfuses more blood.

(D) Perform a right hepatic artery ligation.

(E) Firmly pack the RUQ, close the abdomen, and plan to return to the OR within 36–72 hours.

59. A 40-year-old man sustained injuries to the liver, gallbladder, small intestine, and colon from gunshot wounds. At the time of surgery, a cholecystostomy was placed in the injured gallbladder to expedite operative management. Four weeks later, the patient is doing well. Which is the next step in management?

(A) Remove the cholecystostomy tube.

(B) Perform a cholangiogram through the cholecystostomy tube.

(C) Perform a cholecystectomy.

(D) Perform a choledochoduodenostomy.

(E) Perform a permanent cholecystostomy.

60. A 22-year-old man is found to have a complete transection of the common bile duct following a gunshot wound to the abdomen. There is also a through-and-through wound to the edge of the right lobe of the liver that is not bleeding at the time of surgery. How should the bile duct injury be managed?

(A) choledochojejunostomy and cholecystectomy

(B) Whipple operation

(C) primary repair with a cholecystostomy tube decompressing the gallbladder

(D) cholecystectomy alone

(E) choledochoileostomy

61. An 18-year-old man presents to the emergency department with a stab wound to the abdomen. His blood pressure is 80/50 mmHg. He is brought immediately to the OR, where an enlarged hemoperitoneum is found at laparotomy. Primary repair of the hepatic artery is performed, but because of ongoing blood loss resulting in an unstable hemodynamic situation, the portal vein injury is simply ligated. Bleeding is well controlled. The patient is brought to the recovery room, where his blood pressure drops to 80/60 mmHg and central venous pressure is 2 cm H_2O. What should be the next step in management?

    (A) transfusion of whole blood to elevate blood pressure
    (B) re-exploration to determine site of bleeding
    (C) re-exploration to repair portal vein
    (D) vasopressor to increase blood pressure
    (E) Ringer's lactate to increase blood pressure

62. A 25-year-old man presents to the emergency department with a gunshot wound to the abdomen. On exploratory laparotomy, he is found to have multiple small-bowel enterotomies, transverse colon enterotomy, and a partial injury just to the left of the midline of the pancreas. The pancreatic duct appears intact. What is the appropriate management of the pancreatic injury?

    (A) closed-suction drainage and lavage
    (B) drain with sump drains
    (C) distal pancreatectomy
    (D) operative pancreatogram followed by distal pancreatectomy if ductal injury is noted
    (E) transection of injured area of pancreas with Roux-en-Y (jejunal) anastomosis to the transected tail of the pancreas

63. A 29-year-old woman is brought to the emergency department with a gunshot wound to the abdomen. Her blood pressure is 80/60 mmHg, her pulse rate is 118 bpm, and her respiration rate is 24 breaths per minute. She is brought immediately to the OR, where a large amount of blood and clots are found within the abdomen. After initial packing of the abdomen and stabilization of the patient, a retroperitoneal hematoma is found just above the renal veins. Proximal and distal control of the inferior vena cava is obtained and the blood pressure comes up to 100/60 mmHg. Which is the most appropriate management?

    (A) vascular repair of the injury
    (B) packing of the area with a definitive plan to return to the operating room in 48 hours
    (C) ligation of the inferior vena cava
    (D) use of intracava shunt to allow venous return while repairing the injury
    (E) use of Gore-Tex interposition graft to restore continuity

64. A 26-year-old woman in her sixth month of pregnancy is brought to the emergency department. She had been punched in the abdomen. She is found to have generalized abdominal pain, tenderness, abdominal distention, ileus, and absent fetal heart sounds. The patient's blood pressure is 80/60 mmHg; despite administration of 3 L of Ringer's lactate, her blood pressure only comes up to 90/60 mmHg. Which is the next step in management?

    (A) application of PASG
    (B) transfusion of two units of blood and reevaluate
    (C) exploratory laparotomy and vaginal hysterectomy
    (D) exploratory laparotomy with evacuation of the uterus and closure of the uterus disruption
    (E) CT scan of the abdomen

65. A 52-year-old secretary generally wears high heels and tight-fitting shoes. She saw her practitioner because of foot pain. His diagnosis of plantar fasciitis is characterized by which of the following?

    (A) It is an uncommon cause of persistent heel pain.
    (B) It causes pain on the lateral aspect of the calcaneum.
    (C) It results in part from poor selection of footwear.

(D) It does not reveal abnormality on x-ray.

(E) It occurs usually at rest.

66. A 43-year-old male clerk cuts his right hand on a broken glass door. In evaluating the hand, which should be kept in mind?

(A) The proximal wrist crease corresponds with the wrist joint.

(B) The distal wrist crease corresponds with the deep palmar arch.

(C) Hypothenar muscles are the short muscles of the thumb.

(D) The ulnar nerve supplies the medial three and one-half fingers on the palmar surface.

(E) The radial artery is the sole source of arterial supply to the hand.

67. A newborn boy was examined to exclude congenital dislocation of the hip (CDH). Which of the following tests is relative to the management of CDH?

(A) The diagnosis should be established between 2 and 4 years of age.

(B) Abduction of the flexed hip causes a click (Ortolani's sign) (Figure 1–5).

(C) Abduction of the hip is not limited.

(D) Apparent lengthening of the thigh with the hip and knee flexed may be seen.

(E) Open reduction usually is required.

68. A football player extends his right arm to make a tackle but experiences intense pain on tackle contact with subsequent inability to move the right arm. Examination reveals swelling and tenderness about the shoulder with loss of the normal deltoid contour. Which is the most likely diagnosis?

(A) brachial plexus injury

(B) anterior dislocation of the shoulder

(C) fracture of the proximal posterior portion of the humerus

(D) deltoid muscle rupture

(E) posterior dislocation of the shoulder

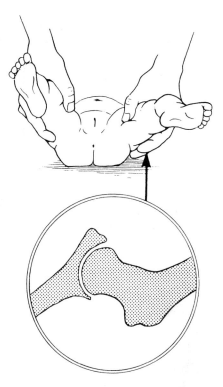

Figure 1–5. In Ortolani's sign, abduction and lifting with the fingers produces a corresponding jerk when the dislocated femoral head slides back into the acetabulum. (Reproduced, with permission, from Way, LW: Current Surgical Diagnosis & Treatment, 10th ed., Appleton & Lange, 1994.)

69. A 7-year-old boy falls off his bicycle, landing on the left elbow. He presents to the emergency room with massive tense swelling of the elbow with painful and restricted elbow motion. X-rays show a displaced fracture of the distal end of the humerus. Which is the most serious complication of this fracture?

(A) nonunion of fracture fragments

(B) nonunion of fracture fragments with deformity

(C) disruption of the growth plate at the distal end of the humerus

(D) forearm compartment syndrome (Volkmann's ischemia)

(E) ankylosis of the elbow joint

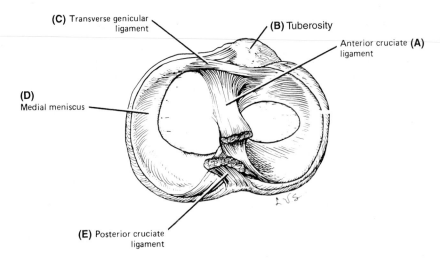

Figure 1–6. Superior aspect of the right tibia showing ligaments. (Reproduced, with permission, from Lindner, HH: Clinical Anatomy, Appleton & Lange, 1989.)

70. A 25-year-old man experiences pain in the right knee while skiing, causing his knee to twist and him to fall to the ground. His knee is swollen. He cannot bear full weight or fully extend or bend his leg. There is tenderness over the medial joint line (Figure 1–6). Emergency-room x-ray findings were normal, and the range of motion (ROM), although restricted, is stable to varus and valgus stress. Straight-leg raise is unrestricted. Which is the most likely type of injury?

   (A) anterior cruciate ligament
   (B) tuberosity
   (C) transverse genicular ligament
   (D) medial meniscus
   (E) posterior cruciate ligament

71. A 50-year-old man hears a "snap" and then feels pain in his right leg while lunging for a forearm drive playing tennis. He walks off the court with difficulty, but his leg is swollen and painful. Findings on x-rays of the leg and ankle in the emergency room are negative. Foot sensation is normal, but findings on the Thompson test (failure of plantar flexion to occur after squeezing the gastrocnemius) are positive. What is the diagnosis?

   (A) gastrocnemius muscle tear
   (B) acute thrombophlebitis

   (C) rupture of the Achilles tendon
   (D) acute compartment syndrome
   (E) fibula fracture

72. A 40-year-old housewife trips over the garden hose, landing on the patio with an outstretched hand. Swelling and pain in the wrist rapidly occur, but findings on emergency room x-rays are negative for fracture or dislocation. In addition to the swelling, there is restriction of wrist dorsiflexion and palmar flexion as well as some tenderness of the anatomic snuffbox at the base of the thumb. What is the best treatment?

   (A) Splint the wrist for 4 days until the swelling and wrist pain subside.
   (B) Apply a cast to the wrist and repeat the wrist x-ray in 10–14 days.
   (C) Apply a cast to the wrist for 8 weeks.
   (D) Apply an Ace wrap to the wrist and remove daily for range of motion and exercise in warm water.
   (E) Perform open exploration of the wrist.

73. A 55-year-old right-handed woman has left elbow pain laterally after cleaning up a flooded basement by wringing out water-soaked rags. X-ray findings are negative. There is tenderness and slight swelling over the lateral epicondyle of the humerus. Anatomically, this condition can be explained by which of the following?

(A) sprain of the lateral collateral elbow ligament

(B) rupture of the triceps muscle

(C) tendinitis of the wrist extensors

(D) synovitis of the left elbow joint

(E) rupture of pronator teres muscle

74. A 16-year-old cross-country runner experiences right midleg pain during workouts. Sometimes the pain prevents him from completing the prescribed mileage. There is midtibial tenderness but no deformity. ROM of the ankle and knee are full and painless. There is no calf tenderness or fullness, and the Achilles tendon is intact. X-ray findings for the tibia and fibula, including both the ankle and knee joints, are normal. What should the patient should be advised to do?

(A) Rest, take anti-inflammatory agents, and use crutches for 2 weeks.

(B) Wear a short leg cast for 3 weeks.

(C) Rest, take anti-inflammatory agents, use crutches, and undergo a bone scan.

(D) Continue running but increase stretching exercises before and after workout and apply analgesics to the painful area for 20 minutes after workout.

(E) Use steroids.

75. A 47-year-old man awakens with low back pain after a weekend of gardening. He recalls no specific incident of trauma and has never had back pain before. There is no radiation of the pain and no disturbance of normal bowel or bladder function. The ROM of the low back is painful and restricted in all planes, and there is paraspinal tenderness from L2 to L5 on the right. Scoliosis and kyphosis are absent. Findings on straight-leg-raising test are negative, reflexes are active and equal, and the patient can walk on his heels and toes. Findings on x-rays of the lumbar spine are normal. Which is the best treatment?

(A) bed rest for 48 hours, anti-inflammatory agents, heat to the low back, and non-narcotic analgesics

(B) bed rest for 7–10 days, heat to the lower back, anti-inflammatory agents, muscle relaxants, and analgesics

(C) hospitalization for pelvic traction, physical therapy, anti-inflammatory agents, intramuscularly analgesics, and muscle relaxants

(D) immediate magnetic resonance image (MRI) for the lumbar spine

(E) lumbar puncture

76. An 86-year-old woman experiences left hip pain after a fall at home. She cannot ambulate, her hip area is swollen and painful, and her left lower extremity is shortened and externally rotated. Before the fall, she was ambulatory and had no complaint of hip, pelvic, or knee pain. In addition to the fracture of the proximal portion of the left femur, the x-ray would show which of the following?

(A) arthritis of the left hip

(B) calcific bursitis of the left hip

(C) osteoporosis

(D) fracture of the pelvis

(E) dislocation of the head of the femur

77. A 70-year-old man has had a long-term "bow-legged" condition but recently his right knee has become warm, swollen, and tender. He reports no recent trauma and gets no relief with rest or Tylenol (paracetamol). He is otherwise in good health and takes no medication. X-rays show arthritis of the knee. Which would be the best treatment?

(A) bed rest, anti-inflammatory agents, analgesics, and a knee brace

(B) use of a cane for ambulating, restriction of knee-bending activities, and implementation of muscle-strengthening exercises

(C) intra-articular steroid injection, bed rest, and analgesics

(D) long leg cast and crutches for 3 weeks, analgesics, and anti-inflammatory agents

(E) urgent surgical correction

78. A 64-year-old woman is admitted to the emergency department with multiple injuries. She requires a central venous pressure line. To minimize the possibility of infection, the principal management of the catheter should be which of the following?

    (A) repeated attempts via the same cannula in the neck
    (B) after failure at one site, use of same cannula at another site
    (C) use of multiport catheters
    (D) avoidance of wound contamination by application of tincture of iodine for more than 4 seconds
    (E) selection of subclavian vein over femoral vein

79. A 40-year-old woman was involved in a car accident. She was unconscious for 5 minutes. X-ray revealed a depressed fracture in the frontal region. Which is true of skull fracture?

    (A) It always requires surgical exploration.
    (B) It is compound if multiple.
    (C) It requires burr holes if compound.
    (D) In the anterior cranial fossa, it may produce rhinorrhea.
    (E) It requires steroid administration.

80. A 32-year-old man underwent laparotomy for trauma because of multiorgan injuries. He was discharged after 2 weeks in the hospital only to be readmitted after 3 days because of abdominal pain and sepsis. The CT scan showed an accumulation of fluid in the subhepatic space. This space is likely to be directly involved following an injury to which of the following?

    (A) inferior pole of the right kidney
    (B) stomach
    (C) superior mesenteric artery
    (D) inferior mesenteric vein
    (E) right psoas muscle

81. Following a bullet wound penetrating the descending colon, necrotizing fasciitis of the anterior abdominal wall occurred postoperatively. Which is true for this condition?

    (A) It does not involve the superficial fascia.
    (B) It causes extensive localized abscess.
    (C) It is silent without pain in the majority of patients.
    (D) It is treated by wide excision and broad-spectrum antibiotics.
    (E) It is treated by immediate incision and drainage.

82. With regard to the injured pregnant patient, which of the following is true?

    (A) Hematocrit, blood volume, and blood pressure all decrease with advancing pregnancy.
    (B) CT scan is the diagnostic test of choice in pregnancy.
    (C) Amniotic fluid analysis has a very low sensitivity in detecting viability of the fetus.
    (D) The ideal position of transport of a pregnant patient is on her right side.
    (E) Pregnant patients who are injured are at high risk for the development of disseminated intravascular coagulapathy (DIC).

83. A 30-year old man sustained a pelvic fracture with a large pelvic hematoma. Rectal examination reveals a large laceration in the rectal wall and a nonpalpable prostate. His vital signs have stabilized with multiple transfusions. This patient requires which of the following?

    (A) resuscitation, blood transfusions, external fixature and exploratory laparotomy
    (B) resuscitation, angiography, embolization of the pelvic bleeders, exploratory laparotomy
    (C) resuscitation, broad-spectrum antibiotics, retrograde cystourethrogram, CT of abdomen and pelvis, suprapubic cystostomy and diverting colostomy
    (D) exploratory laparotomy, urinary diversion, sigmoid colostomy, presacral drainage and debridement of the rectal wall
    (E) ORIF of pelvic fracture by a posterior approach, colostomy, and suprapubic cystostomy

84. Which of the following is a contra-indication to nonoperative management of splenic injury?

(A) prior hematologic disorder
(B) HIV-positive patient
(C) hemodynamic instability
(D) multiple other solid organ injuries
(E) pediatric patient

85. Which is true of intraperitoneal colon injuries?

(A) They should never be repaired primarily.
(B) They may be treated by exteriorization of the repair.
(C) They should be treated with resection and colocolostomy.
(D) They require drainage after repair.
(E) Most can be treated by debridement and repair.

DIRECTIONS (Questions 86 through 101): Each set of matching questions in this section consists of a list of lettered options followed by several numbered items. For each numbered item, select the appropriate lettered option(s). Each lettered option may be selected once, more than once, or not at all. EACH ITEM WILL STATE THE NUMBER OF OPTIONS TO SELECT. CHOOSE EXACTLY THIS NUMBER. Select the most appropriate therapeutic option for each case.

Questions 86 through 88

(A) peritoneal lavage
(B) wound exploration
(C) sonogram
(D) paracentesis
(E) CT with intravenous and oral contrast
(F) IVP
(G) exploratory laparotomy
(H) CVP
(I) angiogram

86. A 16-year-old boy presents to the emergency department with a gunshot wound to the abdominal cavity. SELECT TWO.

87. A 60-year-old woman presents with a stab wound to the back just above the iliac crest. She is in stable condition. SELECT ONE.

88. A 26-year-old man presents with a tangential small-caliber gunshot wound of the anterior abdominal wall. SELECT ONE.

Questions 89 through 91

(A) splenorrhaphy with one suture
(B) partial splenectomy
(C) splenectomy
(D) splenorrhaphy with Dexon mesh
(E) packing
(F) subphrenic abscess
(G) pancreatitis
(H) left lower lobe pneumonia
(I) postsplenectomy sepsis
(J) gastric wall ulcer
(K) left colon perforation
(L) pneumococcal infection

89. A 48-year-old woman was brought to the emergency department after sustaining a stab wound to the left side of the abdomen. Exploration of the abdomen shows 1,000 mL of blood, clot, and feces. There is a bleeding laceration across the middle third of the spleen but not involving the pedicle, a 3-cm laceration of the left transverse colon, and through-and-through lacerations of the stomach and the left lobe of the liver. What should be the management of the splenic injury? SELECT ONE.

90. One week following splenectomy, a 12-year-old girl presents with nausea, vomiting, headache, and confusion. What is the most likely diagnosis? SELECT ONE.

91. Nine days following splenectomy, a 13-year-old patient presents with fever and leukocytosis. The chest x-ray shows free air under the diaphragm. What is the most likely diagnosis? SELECT ONE.

Question 92

    (A) flail chest

    (B) empyema

    (C) diaphragm rupture

    (D) cervical rib

    (E) sternal fracture

    (F) hemothorax

    (G) chylothorax

    (H) pectus excavation

    (I) paradoxical respiration

92. A 60-year-old man is in a car crash in which he is the driver. He did not have a seat belt or an airbag. He is found to have multiple rib fractures over his right chest. His pulse is weaker during inspiration. What are the most likely diagnoses? SELECT TWO.

Questions 93 and 94

    (A) medial meniscus

    (B) sacroiliac joint

    (C) neck of femur

    (D) lateral meniscus

    (E) intertrochanteric

    (F) pubic tuberosity

    (G) spine of ischium

    (H) ischial cruciate ligament

    (I) anterior cruciate ligament

    (J) posterior cruciate ligament

    (K) biceps femora

    (L) pectineal line

93. What injury to this tissue or structure causes lower leg extremities to be externally rotated? SELECT ONE.

94. Injuries to structures attached only to the tibia bone involve which of the following? SELECT TWO.

Questions 95 through 99

    (A) subclavian artery

    (B) subclavian vein

    (C) thoracic duct

    (D) congenital heart disease

    (E) inferior cervical ganglion

    (F) phrenic nerve

    (G) winging of the scapula

    (H) suprascapular nerve to supraspinatus muscle

    (I) trapezius muscle

    (J) blue naevus

    (K) sternomastoid muscle

    (L) subclavius muscle

    (M) ulnar nerve

    (N) wrist drop

    (O) biceps reflex

    (P) internal jugular vein

    (Q) vestibular vein

    (R) accessory spinal nerve

    (S) posterior rami

    (T) bed rest and elevation of the leg

    (U) heparinization

    (V) venous thrombectomy

    (W) femoral nerve

95. After sustaining multiple stab wounds to the right neck, a 26-year-old male jogger was unable to initiate abduction of the shoulder joint. On examination, there was a partly constricted right pupil (Horner syndrome). What did the injury involve? SELECT TWO.

96. On the 3rd day following admission to the hospital, it was noted that the patient's (see Question 95) right arm was swollen, but radial pulse was normal. He was dyspneic, and a chest x-ray revealed that the right diaphragm was elevated. What did the injury involve? SELECT TWO.

97. Inability to move the head to the left against resistance and shrug (upward) the right shoulder indicates what? SELECT THREE.

98. Phlegmasia cerulea dolens is diagnosed. SELECT THREE ITEMS relevant to this entity.

99. Examination reveals an absent knee reflex but present ankle reflex. What is the structure involved? SELECT ONE.

Questions 100 and 101

(A) observation and repeated blood transfusion only

(B) observation and, if necessary, laparotomy to control specific bleeding points

(C) hypogastric (internal iliac artery) ligation

(D) observation followed by femoral artery ligation

(E) infusion of fibrinogen to improve hemostasis

(F) urethral repair

(G) ureter

(H) trigone of bladder

(I) uterine artery

(J) superior gluteal artery

(K) obturator vein

100. After sustaining pelvic injury, a 28-year-old woman is noted on x-ray to have a pelvic fracture. She develops fever, and a CT scan of the pelvis reveals broad ligament hematoma. There is a further fall in blood pressure, but normal blood pressure is restored after blood transfusion. What is the next step in management? SELECT ONE.

101. Surgical intervention may result in ureteric injury, because of the close proximity of a vessel. SELECT ONE.

Answers and Explanations

1. **(B)** The priorities in patient care are to control hemorrhage in the abdomen and decompress the subdural hematoma. The optional initial surgical therapy of the supracondylar femur fracture is the insertion of a Steinman pin for traction (Figure 1–7). If traction fails to produce adequate alignment, open reduction can be performed at a later date.

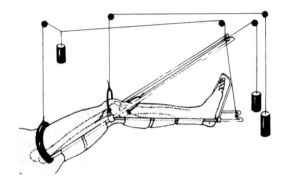

Figure 1–7. Method of suspension of lower extremity with biplanar skeletal traction for supracondylar fracture. (Reproduced, with permission, from Way, LW: Current Surgical Diagnosis & Treatment, 10th ed., Appleton & Lange, 1994.)

2. **(A)** In a patient presenting with a chest wound in shock, the priorities are airway, breathing, and circulation. Thus, aspiration of the right chest to rule out a tension pneumothorax should be performed first. Aspiration of the pericardium does not definitively rule out cardiac injury; a pericardial window provides both diagnosis and decompression. An echocardiogram is not indicated in an unstable patient.

3. **(C)** The most definitive test for aortic injury is the aortogram, even though only 20–30% of patients with widened mediastinum will demonstrate it. A transthoracic echocardiogram does not image the aorta wall; however, a trans-esophageal echocardiogram may have more value in experienced hands.

4. **(D)** The immediate treatment is the closure of the hole by any means available. Sucking chest wounds allow shift of the mediastinum to the opposite side. Thoracotomy is not usually required. Laparotomy is indicated for a gunshot wound below the fourth intercostal space, but it should follow respiratory stabilization. A chest tube will be required, following closure of the sucking wound, to prevent a tension pneumothorax.

5. **(D)** Either an esophagoscopy or a barium swallow—or both—can be used to rule out esophageal injury. The esophagogram should not be performed with Gastrografin because of its deleterious effects if aspirated into the lungs. Nasogastric tube aspiration showing blood is suggestive of an esophageal injury in this patient but is not specific. Peritoneal lavage is sensitive for an intra-abdominal injury, causing bleeding.

6. **(A)** In a patient with significant blunt mechanism of injury and head injury, the cervical spine should be protected against further injury. In an apneic patient with the potential for cervical spine injury, orotracheal intubation may be attempted with in-line stabilization of the neck. If this is unsuccessful, percutaneous cricothyroidotomy is the best definitive step.

7. **(D)** A patient without other sources of blood loss who presents to the emergency department with a stab wound to the abdomen and in shock should have an expeditious exploratory laparotomy. Hemorrhage control should take precedence over definitive management of a concomitant head injury. The other tests will waste precious time and are contraindicated in a patient in shock.

8. **(C)** The best means to establish the diagnosis is CT scan of the abdomen. It will demonstrate solid organ injury and the appropriate amount of fluid (blood) in the peritoneal cavity. It also serves as a baseline for a patient being treated conservatively for spleen and liver injuries.

9. **(B)** The initial operative step is packing of the liver to obtain control of the bleeding. A Pringle maneuver can then be performed. In this procedure, the proper hepatic artery is compressed between one finger inserted into the foramen omentalis (Winslow, epiloic) and another anterior to the free edge of the lesser (gastrohepatic omentum). Selective right hepatic artery is rarely useful, and ligation of the proper hepatic artery is contraindicated.

10. **(D)** The spleen is the most common solid organ injured by blunt trauma. Though gastric rupture could cause the clinical presentation described, it is very rare. Rib fracture in the midtorso alone generally does not cause the referred shoulder pain, because blood does not collect under the left diaphragm, as seen in splenic injuries.

11. **(D)** Most gunshot injuries to the right side of the colon should be closed primarily. Resection is required only where there is extensive devitalization of tissue or injury to the mesocolon causing devascularization of the bowel.

12. **(A)** Antibiotics should be given preoperatively to all patients with wounds penetrating the peritoneal cavity. Intraoperative and postoperative antibiotics fail to reduce postoperative abscesses and wound infections adequately.

13. **(D)** CT scan with oral and intravenous contrast is the most sensitive and specific study to diagnose injuries to the retroperitoneal duodenum. Findings on physical examination and peritoneal lavage are generally negative because of the retroperitoneal location of the posterior wall of the second portion of the duodenum. Rising amylase levels may increase suspicion of the injury but are not specific.

14. **(E)** The coiled-spring or stacked-coin appearance of the duodenum is diagnostic of a duodenal hematoma.

15. **(D)** Oral feeds and fluids are withheld, and hyperalimentation is administered. The upper GI study is repeated at 5- to 7-day intervals. Surgery can usually be avoided.

16. **(C)** Rupture of the duodenum would show in an extravasate Gastrografin study. Contusion of the head of the pancreas might show a widening of the duodenal C-loop.

17. **(C)** Distal pancreatectomy is the procedure of choice for distal pancreatic injuries. It is essential to avoid creation of an intestinal anastomosis (such as in pancreaticojejunostomy), which can leak. An intraoperative pancreatogram is indicated to rule out more proximal duct injuries. Debridement and drainage of the defect alone may result in a pancreatic fistula.

18. **(D)** A high-riding prostate on rectal examination indicates that the urethra has been torn and the prostate rides up with the bladder. The definitive study for suspected urethral injury is a urethrogram. Inability to void and a crushed pelvis also should raise the possibility of a urethral injury.

19. **(B)** Urine may extend in the subcutaneous layer to the anterior abdominal wall and scrotal skin. Fusion of Scarpa's fascia (part of superficial fascia) with fascia lata (deep fascia) explains why urine does not extend down the thigh (Figure 1–8).

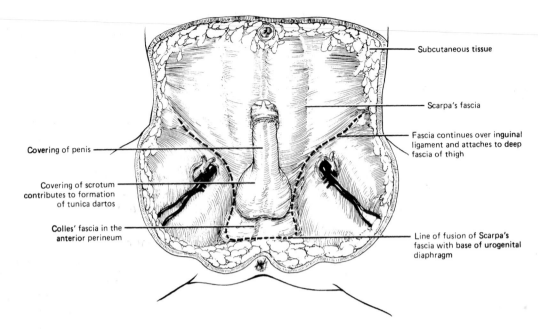

Figure 1–8. Scarpa's fascia showing continuation into the anterior male perineum. (Reproduced, with permission, from Way, LW: Current Surgical Diagnosis & Treatment, 10th ed., Appleton & Lange, 1994.)

20. **(A)** A small nonexpanding hematoma with no associated urine extravasation can be managed by observation with repeat CT scan or ultrasound. If the patient becomes hypotensive, exploration through a midline incision would be indicated.

21. **(C)** Early external fixation of the pelvis has been shown to reduce bleeding and mortality in patients in shock consequent to pelvic fractures. An unstable patient should not be sent for a CT scan. Selective angiography with embolization of the bleeding vessel may also be helpful in these patients. Laparotomy usually results in uncontrollable pelvic bleeding.

22. **(D)** Clearing the cervical spine usually consists of obtaining normal findings on AP, lateral, and odontoid views of the cervical spine. Flexion and extension views are rarely indicated and must be performed under careful supervision. Negative findings on physical examination alone are not reliable in a patient with an impaired sensorium.

23. **(C)** Midneck (zone II) stab wounds should be surgically explored if subcutaneous emphysema or expanding hematoma are found.

Zone II midneck lesions are those between the lower border of the mandible and hyoid cartilage. Further studies are indicated if the findings just listed are not present or the platysma has not been clearly violated.

24. **(C)** Because it is not possible to identify the specific vessels injured by physical examination, angiography with embolization is indicated. Insertion of a nasogastric tube in patients with midfacial trauma should be avoided because of the presence of a false passage to the brain.

25. **(B)** In a stable patient presenting with peripheral vessel occlusion following blunt trauma, angiography is indicated to plan the appropriate operative approach. An angiogram can also document preexisting arteriosclerosis, collateral circulation, and distal runoff. Doppler ultrasound is useful to localize the injury site but gives less information regarding collateral circulation. Immediate operation to control bleeding and restore flow is indicated if the patient's condition is unstable.

26. **(C)** Thoracentesis should be performed first to rule out a tension pneumothorax or hemothorax. However, if the patient does not re-

spond rapidly, early endotracheal intubation is necessary for patients with a flail segment of the chest wall. Intercostal nerve blocks and other means to control pain are important but should be performed after respiratory problems have been brought under control.

27. **(C)** In a patient with a massive midface injury, cricothyroidotomy or tracheostomy should be performed, depending on the urgency of the need for airway control (Figure 1–9). Cricothyroidotomy can usually be performed more quickly than can tracheostomy. Nasotracheal and endotracheal intubation may push blood and debris into the trachea.

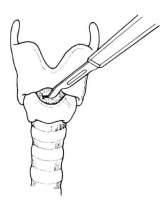

Figure 1–9. Incision for surgical cricothyroidectomy. Percutaneous cricothyroidotomy has largely replaced the open method. (Reproduced, with permission, from Lindner, HH: Clinical Anatomy, Appleton & Lange, 1989.)

28. **(A)** Loss of upward gaze is attributable to impairment of the superior rectus muscle and occasionally the inferior oblique muscle. Loss of upward gaze of the eye should not be confused with failure to elevate the upper eyelid (levator palpebrae superioris muscle), which contains both striated and nonstriated components.

29. **(B)** The bones injured describe a Le Fort II fracture, occasionally associated with a palatal split where the right and left maxillary are completely separated at the midline or the hard palate. Gently rocking the maxillary arch causes the maxilla and nasofrontal areas to move in concert. If there is a Le Fort III fracture, the entire face is detached from the cranial base.

30. **(C)** The physical findings are characteristics of a Le Fort III fracture. In this injury, the fracture passes through maxilla and nasal bones and above the zygomatic bone.

31. **(B)** Shift of the trachea strongly suggests a tension pneumothorax. Subcutaneous emphysema is also more common with a tension pneumothorax than with the other conditions listed. Simple pneumothorax and chest wall laceration are much less serious injuries than tension pneumothorax.

32. **(E)** A patient bleeding at a rate of more than 200 mL per hour should have an emergency thoracotomy. Autotransfusion of blood collected through chest tube should be considered for lesser degree of bleeding but is less reliable to succeed if bleeding does not decrease.

33. **(C)** Bleeding that is sufficient to require thoracotomy usually comes from vessels in the systemic circulation, particularly the internal thoracic (mammary) and intercostal arteries.

34. **(A)** Tamponade from blunt trauma to the heart is usually attributable to myocardial rupture or coronary artery laceration. The left coronary artery gives off the left anterior interventricular artery that passes between the left and right ventricle on the anterior surface of the heart. The right main coronary artery passes in the sulcus between the right atrium and the right ventricle on the anterior surface of the heart.

35. **(D)** Prednisone for 2 weeks in resistant cases is given and then tapered. The "shoulder–hand" syndrome is a reflex autonomic dystrophy occurring after an injury (usually shoulder) that causes immobilization of the ipsilateral extremity. Treatment is directed toward gradual physical therapy and nonsteroidal analgesic drugs. Stellate ganglion block may be helpful in resistant cases.

36. **(C)** CT scan with oral and intravenous contrast gives the best sensitivity and specificity in diagnosing blunt trauma to the pancreas. ERCP could be useful in studying the integrity of the pancreatic duct, but a CT scan is more accurate in revealing traumatic pancreatitis without

major ductal injury. An upper GI series may show widening of the duodenal C-loop. An isolated serum amylase elevation is not diagnostic of pancreatic injury. Repeated testing of amylase levels, if amylase levels increase with time, may be more diagnostic of traumatic pancreatitis than a single value.

37. **(C)** The patient should be brought to the OR prepared and draped, with the nasogastric tube and Foley catheter inserted, and then anesthetized immediately prior to laparotomy. Some surgeons initially control the aorta through a thoracotomy incision through the seventh intercostal space. Transfusion before control of bleeding causes more bleeding.

38. **(C)** Apply direct pressure with sterile gauze. Direct pressure is the best choice. Attempting to clamp vessels can cause further vascular or nerve injury. Tourniquet is used only if direct pressure fails. As soon as direct pressure is attempted, a second person should insert a large-bore peripheral intravenous line.

39. **(B)** A tense calf with comminuted fractures (fractures exposed to exterior) and pain on dorsiflexion necessitates a fasciotomy because of the very high probability of a compartment syndrome. Arterial injury is possible (but rare) in lower leg injuries if the pulses are palpable.

40. **(C)** Displace the uterus to the left. The first step in restoring cardiac return in a patient in the third trimester who has become hypovolemic is to displace the gravid uterus off the vena cava by pushing it to the left. The other choices (except for the use of the PASG) should be considered following displacement of the uterus.

41. **(D)** Fat embolus is usually associated with long bone or pelvic fractures and is associated with petechiae. Transfusion and antibiotic reactions causing hypotension would occur relatively quickly following administration.

42. **(B)** The most likely cause of the patient's persistent hypotension is the pelvic fracture; therefore, external fixation should be performed promptly. While the patient is undergoing external fixation in the OR, an exploratory laparotomy and colostomy should be performed for the rectal injury.

43. **(A)** In the patient who has no neurologic deficit preoperatively, every effort should be made to repair a carotid artery injury. Four-vessel angiography should be performed in stable patients with injuries in zones I and III. Careful judgment should be exercised in selecting patients with zone II injuries who are to have angiography (i.e., suspected injuries to bilateral carotid arteries or vertebral arteries) and in selecting those for observation. Carotid artery ligation might also be employed in patients who are unstable without a high incidence of neurologic deficit.

44. **(D)** Selective management of abdominal stab wounds, especially to the lower chest and upper abdomen, relies on physical examination and diagnostic peritoneal lavage (DPL) to identify the need for operative exploration. Small, isolated diaphragmatic lacerations may be asymptomatic and may not result in red blood cell counts required to cause a positive DPL These small diaphragmatic wounds are best detected by laparoscopy. Missed diaphragmatic injuries may cause late diaphragmatic hernias with potential morbidity and mortality.

45. **(D)** In a patient with respiratory distress and shock, adequate breathing is of higher priority than circulation. Insertion of an 18-gauge needle to rule out and/or treat a pneumothorax takes precedence over diagnostic tests.

46. **(E)** Tetanus toxoid plus human immunoglobulin and antibiotics with aerobic and anaerobic coverage. Patients who are taking steroids or who are immune suppressed should receive human immunoglobulin even though previously immunized. Tetanus booster and antibiotic therapy are also necessary.

47. **(D)** In general, most patients with significant head injury should be admitted for observation. Skull x-rays cannot be relied upon for the diagnosis of intracranial injury, because lesions

may still be present, even with normal skull x-ray. Elevated intracranial pressure may be present, even with the absence of papilledema. Bradycardia and hypertension (not hypotension) are the features of elevated intracranial pressure.

48. **(D)** Raccoons should be regarded as rabid animals unless the geographic area is known to be free of rabies. A 5-day course of vaccine and a single dose of HRIG should be administered. They should not be administered jointly into the gluteal area, because administration in this area results in lowering neutralizing antibody titers. Where feasible, up to half of the dose of HRIG should be infiltrated into the area around the wound.

49. **(D)** This patient's response is considered moderate to great in regard to envenomation and requires 3–5 vials of antivenin IV in 500 mL of normal saline. The tourniquet should not be removed until the antivenin therapy is instituted. Incision and suction will be of benefit only if accomplished within 30 minutes of sustaining the bite, and excision of the bite area is valuable only if performed within 1 hour.

50. **(E)** In considering management of neck wounds, three zones are described. Zone III refers to the area above and posterior to the angle of the mandible (see Figure 1–4). Angiographic definition of the site and extent of arterial injury is important because of the difficulty in exposure of internal carotid injuries near the base of the skull. Such injuries may require the use of extracranial–intracranial arterial bypass.

51. **(B)** Even those who advocate reconstruction of carotid arteries in patients with neurological deficit do not recommend attempted reconstruction in patients who are comatose. If the patient were not comatose, proximal and distal control with stenting and interposition graft would be the procedure of choice.

52. **(C)** Exsanguinating hemorrhage is the predominant risk, because bleeding may not be easily recognized, given that bleeding into the pleural cavity and mediastinum can occur. The abundant collateral blood supply gener-

ally protects against upper extremities or cerebrovascular compromise.

53. **(C)** Arteriography is used to assess possible renal artery injury in these circumstances. It is used if the kidney is not visualized with an IVP or CT a scan. Operative intervention without arteriography is not necessary in a stable patient. Peritoneal lavage is useful in determining the presence of intraperitoneal bleeding; if arteriography shows a need for surgery, peritoneal lavage will not be necessary.

54. **(D)** A patient with definitive negative findings on wound exploration can be discharged from the hospital for outpatient follow-up care. It is sometimes difficult to determine the depth of a stab wound to the back because of the thickness of the paraspinal muscles. Some authors have found that nearly 20% of patients with such injuries have negative findings on exploration. Such patients can be discharged. Deeper stab wounds to the back may injure peritoneal structures without penetration of the peritoneal cavity. Thus, peritoneal lavage is less useful than a CT scan with intravenous, oral, and (particularly) rectal contrast to rule out retroperitoneal colon injuries.

55. **(A)** Open the abdomen and use a large Richardson retractor to compress the abdominal aorta against the vertebrae just below the diaphragm. The advantages of occluding the subdiaphragmatic aorta (as opposed to the supradiaphragmatic aorta) are that it: (a) avoids opening another major cavity; and (b) results in less diminution of blood flow to the spinal cord and renal circulation. Further attempts to resuscitate the patient with whole blood will not be successful until bleeding sites are controlled; such measures may even increase bleeding by elevating blood pressure, which reopens vessels that have already stopped bleeding. Attempting to control individual bleeding sites with packing is difficult in a patient with multiple gunshot wounds who is exsanguinating.

56. **(D)** Contusion of the small bowel may be larger than apparent and may lead to necrosis and perforation. Contusions of 1 cm or less in diameter

may be turned in with mattress sutures. However, larger contusions should be resected. The advantage of a single-layer anastomosis is the speed of performance and the reduced likelihood of compromising the muscularis mucosa.

57. **(B)** The necrotic bowel is resected, the proximal end is constructed as an end colostomy, and the distal end is constructed as a mucous fistula. This is the best procedure, because it will avoid an anastomosis in a contaminated abdomen. Any procedure that involves either wound closure or anastomosis in an abdomen with extensive fecal contamination presents a significant risk of leakage and therefore should not be performed. Exteriorization should not be performed unless ischemic bowel is resected.

58. **(E)** Once a patient shows acidemia and hypothermia from significant blood loss, further operative manipulations will not likely result in control of persistent bleeding. It is best to pack the RUQ firmly and return to the OR in 36 hours. It is possible that the patient has a retrocaval hepatic vein injury, but attempting to insert an intracaval shunt in the presence of acidemia and hypothermia is not likely to be successful. Hepatic artery ligation has been used infrequently in recent years, because in most cases, hepatic bleeding is venous and therefore not altered by the ligation.

59. **(B)** A cholecystocholangiogram must be performed to ensure that the gallbladder is not leaking, and that there is free flow of dye in the duodenum if no abnormality is detected on the cholangiogram, the cholecystomy tube is removed. The patient should undergo follow-up gallbladder studies several months later, but routine removal of the gallbladder is not necessary.

60. **(A)** Although it may be technically possible to perform a primary anastomosis for a complete transection, these invariably lead to bile duct structure. It is important to remember that debridement of the duct following a gunshot wound increases the tension on the anastomosis. The best method for the early treatment of injuries to the common bile duct is a duct-to-small bowel anastomosis.

61. **(A)** Obstruction to the portal outflow causes acute splenic hypervolemia simultaneously with systemic hypovolemia. If not treated by overtransfusion of blood volume (in some cases, almost equal to the patient's normal blood volume), death may occur from hypovolemia. Vasopressors should never be used to correct blood pressure in the face of hypovolemia.

62. **(A)** Routinely performing distal pancreatectomy for all penetrating injuries to the body or tail of the pancreas significantly prolongs the operative time and contributes to additional hemorrhage and possible hypothermia. Approximately 25% of patients undergoing distal pancreatectomy develop an intra-abdominal abscess. Distal pancreatectomy is the procedure of choice if there is an obvious disruption of the pancreatic duct in the body or tail. Closed-suction drainage is preferred to suction drainage because of the lower incidence of abscess formation with closed-suction drainage. If there is an injury to the duodenum, a pancreaticogram can be performed through the injury site; however, a normal duodenum should not be opened to secure an intraoperative pancreaticogram.

63. **(A)** Although injuries in the inferior vena cava can be ligated if the repair is unduly time consuming for the patient with continued hypotension, every attempt must be made to repair a suprarenal vena cava injury. Packing of the injury should be performed only if acidemia and/or hypothermia develop, because packing of the vena cava is not likely to be effective for a very long period. If an interposition graft is necessary, vein graft should be obtained from the infrarenal cava or iliac veins. A synthetic graft is likely to thrombose. An intracaval shunt generally requires a thoracotomy to gain proximal control and is reserved for retrohepatic injuries to the vena cava.

64. **(D)** Exploratory laparotomy with evacuation of the uterus and closure of the uterus disrup-

tion is the procedure of choice despite continued hypotension. Blood administration should be instituted but is not as critical as gaining surgical hemostasis. A PASG may have a limited temporizing effect but should not be used as an alternative to exploratory laparotomy. Any patient with abdominal trauma who is hypotensive should not be sent for a CT scan.

65. **(C)** Plantar fasciitis may occur either with or without a calcaneal spur. Plantar fasciitis is more likely when footwear is inappropriate or there is excessive exercise (e.g., in athletes). There is pain either after exercise (in a patient who has had a period of rest) or at the end of prolonged activity. Tenderness is over the medial aspect of the plantar fascia close to the calcaneum. X-ray may reveal a tear in the periosteum or a calcaneal spur.

66. **(A)** The proximal wrist crease corresponds with the wrist joint, and the distal crease of the wrist corresponds with the proximal portion of the flexor retinaculum. The hypothenar muscles are on the ulnar side, and the thenar muscles are on the thumb side of the hand. The ulnar artery contributes predominantly to the superficial and the radial artery to the deep palmar arches in the hand.

67. **(B)** It is important to recognize congenital dislocation of the newborn soon after birth. Delay in initiating appropriate treatment may lead to permanent hip joint disease. There may be apparent shortening of the thigh, although with the hip and knee flexed.

68. **(B)** The mechanism of injury (abduction and external rotation) combined with the characteristic observable deformity of deltoid contour loss makes anterior dislocation the best choice. The common site of shoulder joint dislocation is inferior, because the rotator cuff muscles are absent there.

69. **(D)** Ischemia contracture may result in deformity and disability of the hand, which impairs function of the entire upper extremity, not only of the elbow area.

70. **(D)** Restriction of motion ("locking"), effusion ("swelling"), and medial joint-line tenderness are the hallmarks of meniscal tears. Stability-to-stress testing eliminates collateral ligament rupture, and the ability to elevate the straight leg eliminates patella dislocation and quadriceps tendon ruptures. In addition, patella dislocation would also be characterized by gross patella deformity laterally.

71. **(C)** Of all the conditions listed, only an Achilles tendon rupture will result in positive findings on the "squeeze" test (Thompson sign), whereby a squeezing of the gastrocnemius muscle fails to cause plantar flexion of the foot.

72. **(B)** Tenderness in the anatomic snuffbox (the interval between the extensor pollicis longus and the extensor pollicis brevis and abductor pollicis longus tendons) may signify a fracture of the carpal scaphoid (navicular) bone. Initial x-ray findings are often negative, but the fracture line often shows up in a repeat x-ray taken after 10–14 days.

73. **(C)** The act of wringing rags results in repeated and forceful wrist dorsiflexion, causing increased pressure on the wrist extensor muscles, which have their tendinous origins from the lateral humeral epicondyle. This results in an inflammatory condition at the bone tendon junction, lateral epicondylitis, or "tennis elbow." Although this condition is common in tennis players, it occurs more frequently in the general population.

74. **(C)** Although rest, anti-inflammatory agents, and crutches adequately treat the symptoms, the diagnosis of a stress fracture can be made only with a bone scan if the initial x-ray findings are negative for fracture.

75. **(A)** In the absence of bladder or bowel disturbance, or sciatic symptoms, a neurological defect caused by a herniated disk is unlikely. A short period of rest, along with heat, anti-inflammatory agents, and analgesics, is the best treatment for a soft-tissue inflammatory lesion of the lumbar region.

76. **(C)** Postmenopausal osteoporosis is the common denominator in all fractures involving elderly women. In this particular fracture, it is the twisting effect on an osteoporotic femur that causes the fracture rather than the impact of the fall itself.

77. **(B)** Acute synovial reactions of weight-bearing joints with underlying arthritis are a common occurrence. It is usually related to minor traumatic events. Complete immobilization may increase joint stiffness secondary to arthritis, but partial reduction of stressful motions (avoiding kneeling and squatting) and continued muscle activity would be beneficial. These will allow the synovial reaction to subside while decreasing the weakening and stiffness caused by the underlying arthritis.

78. **(E)** Where possible, a single-lumen cannula should be inserted into the vein to avoid repeated attempts. The tincture of iodine should remain in contact with the skin for 30 seconds before venipuncture. Unsterile adhesive must not be placed over the entry site.

79. **(D)** Skull fractures should be explored only if they are compound, if a depressed fracture is present, or if an intracranial lesion requires exploration. Compound fracture implies that the fracture site communicates with the exterior.

80. **(B)** Subhepatic space infection usually occurs after surgery or peritonitis in the supracolic compartment. It is an unlikely complication of biliary pancreatitis. Infections in the subhepatic space may extend to the infracolic compartment via the paracolic gutter (of Morrison).

81. **(D)** In addition to necrosis of the superficial and deep fascia, thrombosis of the microcirculation of the subcutaneous tissue occurs. Mortality rates have been reduced from 80% in the past to less than 12% in recent series. Polymicrobial infection is more commonly encountered, and gram-positive and gram-negative organisms are found in 70% of cases. Treatment is based on adequate debridement and use of appropriate broad-spectrum antibiotics.

82. **(E)** Hematocrit, blood volume, and BP all increase with pregnancy. Ultrasonography is the preferred method to evaluate the abdomen and can also determine fetal viability. Aspiration of amniotic fluid and determination of lecithin/sphingomyelin ratio is helpful in the determination of fetal prematurity. The pregnant patient should be placed on her left side so that the full-term uterus will not compress the inferior vena cava and interfere with venous return.

83. **(C)** This patient has a urethral injury and an open pelvic fracture. Continued resuscitation, broad spectrum antibiotics, and a CT scan of the abdomen and pelvis are important initial steps in management. A retrograde urethrogram will document the presence and type (complete or incomplete) of urethral injury. Suprapubic cystostomy and diverting colostomy are essential to prevent continued contamination of the pelvic hematoma. Angiography and embolization of bleeders are not necessary in all patients. Presacral drainage in a patient with pelvic hematoma can cause life-threatening hemorrhage.

84. **(C)** Hemodynamic instability is the most pressing indication for operative treatment in a patient with splenic injury. In all other situations listed a trial of nonoperative management may be continued.

85. **(E)** The modern treatment of civilian injuries of the colon emphasizes primary repair in the vast majority. The results are excellent in terms of suture line complications. Colocolostomy is reserved for a select few patients with the most optimal circumstances. Exteriorization after repair is no longer advised.

86. **(G, H)** All gunshot wounds clearly entering the abdominal cavity should be treated by emergency exploratory laparotomy. Over 80% of the time, injuries requiring repair will be found.

87. **(E)** A CT scan with intravenous and oral contrast can best rule out possible retroperitoneal injury caused by a stab wound.

88. **(B)** Wound exploration that convincingly documents failure of penetration through the posterior rectus fascia will most likely exclude abdominal injury from a tangential gunshot wound. A patient with negative findings on wound exploration can be discharged and followed as an outpatient. Peritoneal lavage would also rule out an intra-abdominal injury; however, it would require a subsequent period of hospital observation. A laparotomy would provide the most definitive evidence that an intra-abdominal injury did not occur, but a negative finding on laparotomy has a definitive associated complication rate.

89. **(C)** In a patient with significant bleeding, peritoneal contamination, and multiple injuries, splenectomy is indicated. Prompt packing of the liver injury and splenectomy are the first considerations at laparotomy.

90. **(I)** Postsplenectomy sepsis presents with sudden onset of nausea, vomiting, headache, confusion, and sometimes coma. Abdominal findings may be essentially normal following splenectomy. Inhibition of opsonization of leukocytes is evident with increased susceptibility to pneumococcal infection.

91. **(A)** Colon perforation is likely to show free air under the left hemidiaphragm. A subphrenic abscess presents with fever, leukocytosis, and a left pleural effusion. Gastric wall necrosis may likewise result in perforation with free air. There is air below the diaphragm following laparotomy, but it usually manifests symptoms clearly within the first week after operation.

92. **(A, I)** Flail chest should be excluded in multiple rib fractures where the individual rib is divided in two places. Paradoxical movement results in lung compression as the flail segment moves inward during inspiration.

93. **(C)** Both subcapital and petrochanteric fractures present with external rotation of the lower extremity. The lateral rotators are attached to the bone distal to the fracture line to cause this typical clinical sign. Trochanteric fractures have a better prognosis, because the blood supply to the proximal segment remains intact.

94. **(A, D)** The menisci are attached to the tibia, whereas, the cruciate ligaments extend between the tibia and femur. The medial meniscus is most commonly torn, because it is attached to the medial collateral ligament.

95. **(E, H)** The sympathetic chain passes from the thorax to the neck of the first rib. If the chain (and inferior cervical ganglion) is cut, sympathetic enervation leads to Horner syndrome (meiosis, ptosis, and unilateral anhydrosis). Injury to the suprascapular nerve will cause failure of the supraspinatus to initiate abduction.

96. **(B, F)** The scalenus anterior separates the deeply placed subclavian artery from the superficial subclavian artery. Occlusion of the vein may lead to swelling of the upper extremity. The phrenic nerve (C3–C5) passes downward anterior to scalenus anterior muscle; paralysis of the diaphragm is best demonstrated by failure of the right diaphragm to move downward on inspiration (tray image intensifies).

97. **(K, I, R)** The accessory spinal nerve (cranial nerve) innervates both sternomastoid and trapezius muscles. Paralysis of the right sternomastoid muscle will result in inability to rotate the head (against resistance) to the left. There will also be partial decrease in lateral flexion of the neck elevation of the right shoulder. The serratus anterior will assist trapezius in rotating (the scapula) in abduction.

98. **(T, U, V)** Phlegmasia cerulea (blue) dolens indicates that major venous obstruction has occurred. The standard treatment for postoperative thrombosis includes bed rest, anticoagulation, and leg elevation. Venous thrombectomy may be indicated when impending gangrene is noted. Vena cava filters are indicated in patients with established pulmonary emboli but may be considered prophylactically when ileofemoral thrombosis is massive. Thrombolysis of major venous thrombi requires systemic administration of urokinase and is, therefore, contraindicated in the postoperative period or period related to trauma.

99. **(W)** The femoral nerve supplies the quadriceps muscle (L3, L4), and thus the knee jerk will be absent if the nerve is cut. The gastrocnemius and soleus are supplied by the tibial nerve (S2, S2).

100. **(C)** Initial management of pelvic fractures is conservative, but further bleeding may require embolization or ligation of the internal iliac artery.

101. **(I)** The ureter crosses over the proximal portion of the external iliac artery just beyond the bifurcation of the common iliac vessels. In the female, it passes medially where it is inferior to the uterine artery.

CHAPTER 2

Shock and Homeostasis
Questions
Nanakram Agarwal

DIRECTIONS (Questions 1 through 95): Each of the numbered items or incomplete statements in this section is followed by answers or by completions of the statement. Select the ONE lettered answer or completion that is BEST in each case.

1. A 35-year-old man is admitted with systolic blood pressure of 60 mmHg and a heart rate of 150 bpm following a gunshot wound to the liver (Figure 2–1). What is the effect on the kidneys?

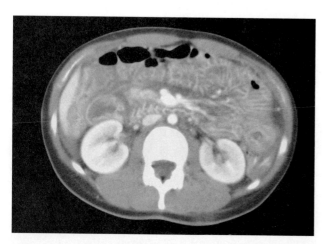

Figure 2–1. Axial image of CT scan of abdomen at level of both kidneys shows dense nephrogram, which is attributed to decrease in renal perfusion.

   (A) They tolerate satisfactorily ischemia of 3–4 hours' duration.
   (B) They undergo further ischemia if hypothermia is present.
   (C) They can become damaged, even though urine output exceeds 1,500 mL/d.
   (D) They are affected and cause an increased creatinine clearance.
   (E) They are prevented from further damage by a vasopressor.

2. Twenty-four hours after colon resection, urine output in a 70-year-old man is 10 mL/h. Blood chemistry analysis reveals sodium, 138 mEq/L; potassium, 6 mEq/L; chloride, 100 mEq/L; bicarbonate, 14 mEq/L. His metabolic abnormality is characterized by which of the following?

   (A) abdominal distension
   (B) peaked T waves
   (C) narrow QRS complex
   (D) cardiac arrest in systole
   (E) J wave or Osborne wave

3. A 24-year-old woman has acute renal failure following postpartum hemorrhage. Laboratory studies showed serum glucose, 150 mg/dL; sodium, 135 mEq/L; potassium, 6.5 mEq/L; chloride, 105 mEq/L; and bicarbonate, 15 mEq/L. Therapy should include which of the following?

   (A) decrease potassium chloride to 10 mEq/L
   (B) intravenous 0.9% sodium chloride
   (C) 100 mL of 50% glucose water with 10 U insulin
   (D) intravenous calcitonin
   (E) intravenous magnesium sulfate

4. A 60-year-old woman is oliguric after undergoing cholecystectomy. She weighs 65 kg, and her laboratory values are hemoglobin, 10.5 mg/dL; white blood cell (WBC) count, 12,000/mm^3; serum sodium, 138 mEq/L; serum potassium, 4 mEq/L; serum chloride, 100 mEq/L; serum bicarbonate, 28 mEq/L; serum creatinine, 1.0 mg/dL; and blood urea nitrogen (BUN), 20 mg/dL. The anion gap is which of the following?

(A) 10
(B) 18
(C) 30
(D) 38
(E) 42

5. A 55-year-old man with Crohn's disease had undergone resection of small bowel and anastomosis. Ten days later, he is found to have bilious drainage of 1 L/d from the drains. He is started on total parenteral nutrition (TPN). Four days later, his arterial blood gases (ABGs) are pH, 7.25; Po$_2$, 98 mmHg; and Pco$_2$, 40 mmHg. His anion gap is 10. The most likely cause is which of the following?

(A) diabetic ketoacidosis
(B) renal failure
(C) Hypovolemic shock
(D) Small-bowel fistula
(E) Uncompensated metabolic alkalosis

6. A 55-year-old man sustains numerous injuries involving the abdomen and lower extremities. During the intra- and postoperative periods, he is resuscitated with 10 L of Ringer's lactate and eight units of packed red blood cells. After initial improvement, he has severe dyspnea on the second postoperative day. The most useful initial diagnostic test is which of the following?

(A) electrocardiogram
(B) analysis of arterial blood gas
(C) insertion of a central venous line
(D) ventilation–perfusion scan
(E) CT scan of abdomen

7. A 20-year-old man involved in a car crash sustained severe injuries to the chest, abdomen, and lower extremities. He is intubated and requires increasing concentration of oxygen to maintain his Po$_2$. The pathologic changes do which of the following?

(A) They cause the alveolar capillary membrane to become more impermeable.
(B) They most frequently occur after severe injuries.
(C) They are associated with low compliance.
(D) They show a characteristic localized pattern on x-ray.
(E) They involve a decrease in dead-space ventilation.

8. A 24-year-old woman is scheduled for an elective cholecystectomy. The best method of identifying a potential bleeder is which of the following?

(A) platelet count
(B) a complete history and physical examination
(C) bleeding time
(D) Lee–White clotting time
(E) prothrombin time (PT)

9. A 24-year-old man who is admitted to the intensive care unit (ICU) following severe head injury develops seizures on the fourth day of hospitalization. His urine output is 500 mL over 24 hours, sodium is 115 mEq/L, and serum and urine osmolality are 250 and 800 mOsm, respectively. The metabolic abnormality is due to which of the following?

(A) administration of D$_5$W (5% dextrose in water) and 0.33 normal saline
(B) syndrome of inappropriate secretion of antidiuretic hormone (SIADH)
(C) decreased antidiuretic hormone (ADH) secretion
(D) nasogastric suction
(E) renal insufficiency

10. A 40-year-old man who weighs 65 kg is being observed in the ICU. Twenty-four hours postoperatively, he develops convulsions. His serum sodium is 118 mEq/L. Appropriate management includes which of the following?

(A) administration of normal saline (0.9%)

(B) administration of hypertonic saline (3%)

(C) emergency hemodialysis

(D) administration of vasopressin

(E) administration of Lasix, 40 mg IV

11. A 30-year-old man who weighs 60 kg has the following laboratory values: hemoglobin, 10 g/dL; serum sodium, 120 mEq/L; serum potassium, 4 mEq/L; serum chloride, 90 mEq/L; and serum CO_2 content, 30 mEq/L. What is his sodium deficit approximately?

(A) 20 mEq

(B) 200 mEq

(C) 400 mEq

(D) 720 mEq

(E) 120 mEq

12. A 65-year-old man has urine output of 10 mL/h following abdominal aortic aneurysmectomy. Acute tubular necrosis is suggested by the presence of which of the following?

(A) urine osmolality of more than 500 mOsm/kg

(B) urine sodium of more than 40 mEq/L

(C) fractional excretion of sodium of less than 1%

(D) BUN/serum creatinine ratio (SCR) of more than 20

(E) urine/plasma creatinine ratio (PCR) of more than 40

13. A 30-year-old man with a history of Crohn's disease of the small bowel is admitted with enterocutaneous fistula. The daily output from the fistula is 2 L. The approximate composition of the fluids in mEq/L is which of the following?

	Na	K	Cl	HCO$_3$
(A)	10	26	10	30
(B)	60	10	130	0
(C)	140	5	104	30
(D)	140	5	75	115
(E)	60	30	40	40

14. A 70-year-old woman has a small-bowel fistula with output of 1.5 L/d. Replacement of daily losses should be handled using the fluid solution that has the following composition in mEq/L.

	Na	K	Cl	HCO$_3$
(A)	130	4	109	28
(B)	154	0	154	40
(C)	77	0	77	0
(D)	167	0	0	167
(E)	513	0	513	0

Questions 15 and 16

A 70-year-old man has undergone anterior resection for carcinoma of the rectum. He is extubated in the operating room (OR). In the recovery room, he is found to be restless with a heart rate of 136 bpm and a blood pressure of 144/80 mmHg. ABG analysis on room air reveals pH, 7.24; Pco$_2$, 60 mm Hg; Po$_2$, 54; HCO$_3$, 25 mEq/L; and SaO$_2$, 90%.

15. The physiologic status can best be described as which of the following?

(A) respiratory alkalosis

(B) respiratory acidosis

(C) metabolic acidosis

(D) metabolic alkalosis

(E) combined respiratory and metabolic acidosis

16. Appropriate management for this patient should be which of the following?

(A) to administer 40% oxygen by mask

(B) morphine, 2 mg IV

(C) Ringer's lactate, 250 mL over 1 hour

(D) intubation and ventilatory support

(E) deep breathing and coughing

17. A 60-year-old woman with mild hypertension is admitted for elective hysterectomy. On pre-operative evaluation, she is found to have os-teoarthritis; over the previous 6 months, she had noted watery diarrhea that was becoming progressively worse. The serum potassium is 3.0 mEq/L. Which is the most likely cause of hypokalemia?

    (A) myoglobinemia
    (B) villous adenoma of colon
    (C) high-output renal failure
    (D) massive blood transfusion
    (E) spironolactone (Aldactone)

Questions 18 and 19

A 64-year-old man underwent major abdominal sur-gery to remove a ruptured aortic aneurysm. Four days after the operation, an attempt was made to wean him off the ventilator. ABG analysis reveals pH, 7.54; P_{CO_2}, 30 mmHg; P_{O_2}, 110 mmHg; HCO_3, 30 mEq/L; and SaO_2, 99%.

18. Blood gas analysis reveals which of the following?

    (A) respiratory acidosis
    (B) metabolic alkalosis
    (C) respiratory alkalosis
    (D) compensated respiratory acidosis
    (E) combined respiratory and metabolic alkalosis

19. What will be the most likely complication due to the metabolic changes experienced by the patient?

    (A) hypokalemia
    (B) shift of oxyhemoglobin dissociation to the right
    (C) hyperkalemia
    (D) hypercalcemia
    (E) hyperchloremia

20. A 42-year-old man with small-bowel fistula has been receiving total parenteral nutrition (TPN) with standard hypertonic glucose–amino acid solution for 3 weeks. The patient is noticed to have scaly, hyperpigmented lesions over the acral surfaces of elbows and knees, similar to enterohepatic acrodermatitis. What is the most likely cause of the condition?

    (A) copper deficiency
    (B) essential fatty acid deficiency
    (C) excess glucose calories
    (D) hypomagnesemia
    (E) zinc deficiency

Questions 21 through 23

A 27-year-old man is involved in a car crash while traveling in excess of 70 mph. He sustains an intra-abdominal injury and a fracture of the femur. The blood pressure is 60/40 mmHg, and the hematocrit is 16%.

21. Which physiologic changes will ensue?

    (A) peripheral vasodilation
    (B) inhibition of sympathetic tone
    (C) temperature rise to 103°F
    (D) eosinophilia
    (E) lactic acidosis

22. There is likely to be a proportionately greater increase in blood flow to which of the follow-ing?

    (A) kidneys
    (B) liver
    (C) heart
    (D) skin
    (E) thyroid gland

23. Initial resuscitation is best done by adminis-tration of which of the following?

    (A) D_5W
    (B) D_5W and 0.45% normal saline
    (C) Ringer's lactate solution
    (D) 5% plasma protein solution
    (E) 5% hydroxyethyl starch solution

24. A 30-year-old man is brought to the emer-gency department following a high-speed car accident. He was the driver, and the wind-shield of the car was broken. On examination, he is alert, awake, oriented, and in no respira-

tory distress. He is unable to move any of his four extremities; however, his extremities are warm and pink. His vital signs on admission are: heart rate 54 bpm and blood pressure 70/40 mmHg. What is the diagnosis?

(A) hemorrhagic shock
(B) cardiogenic shock
(C) neurogenic shock
(D) septic shock
(E) irreversible shock

Questions 25 through 28

A 48-year old man with severe vomiting as a result of gastric outlet obstruction is admitted to the hospital. There is marked dehydration, with urine output 20 mL/h, and the hematocrit is 48%.

25. Clinical confirmation of pyloric obstruction is most readily established by which of the following?

(A) observation of peristalsis from left to right
(B) observation of peristalsis from right to left
(C) percussion of the upper abdomen
(D) succussion splash
(E) auscultation of the upper left abdomen

26. What is the predominant metabolic abnormality?

(A) aspiration pneumonia with respiratory alkalosis
(B) hypochloremic alkalosis
(C) salt-losing enteropathy
(D) intrinsic renal disease
(E) metabolic acidosis

27. Initial treatment for this patient should include which of the following?

(A) Administration of 10% dextrose ($D_{10}W$) in one-third saline solution intravenously
(B) antiemetic
(C) Hemodialysis to correct azotemia
(D) saline fluid replacement with appropriate potassium administration
(E) Ringer's lactate solution

28. Severe hypochloremic metabolic alkalosis fails to respond to standard therapy. His metabolic abnormality can be corrected by infusing which of the following?

(A) normal saline
(B) Ringer's Lactate Solution
(C) hypertonic Saline
(D) 0.1 N hydrochloric acid
(E) 1.0 N hydrochloric acid

29. In the absence of malignancy, further treatment after appropriate resuscitation should include which of the following?

(A) jejunostomy feeding
(B) vagotomy and drainage
(C) steroids
(D) no foods given orally for 6 weeks
(E) pyloromyotomy alone

Questions 30 through 32

During cholecystectomy in a 67-year-old woman, there is severe bleeding from accidental injury to the hepatic artery. The patient requires transfusion of 2,000 mL of blood. After the operation, 24-hour urine output varies between 1,250 and 2,700 mL/d. She was adequately hydrated, but BUN levels continue to rise 10–12 mg daily over a 5-day period.

30. What is the main finding?

(A) progressive bleeding
(B) high-output renal failure
(C) postcholecystectomy syndrome
(D) glomerulonephritis
(E) obstructive jaundice

31. Metabolic changes likely to occur include which of the following?

(A) hyperkalemia
(B) hyponatremia
(C) hypophosphatemia
(D) metabolic alkalosis
(E) hypomagnesemia

32. Management includes which of the following?

    (A) restriction of fluids to 750 mL/d
    (B) 8 L of fluid daily to remove urea
    (C) replacement of fluid loss plus insensible loss
    (D) 80 mEq potassium chloride (KCl)/12 h
    (E) ammonium chloride intravenously

Questions 33 and 34

A 14-year-old boy with a known bleeding tendency since infancy has severe epistaxis. Examination reveals an equinus contracture of the right leg and a large hemarthrosis.

33. What is the most likely diagnosis?

    (A) diethylstilbestrol (DES) was taken by the mother during pregnancy
    (B) aplastic anemia
    (C) Henoch–Schönlein purpura
    (D) hemophilia
    (E) Wilson's disease with cirrhosis

34. Treatment should include which of the following?

    (A) penicillamine
    (B) transfusion of factor VIII to 30% of normal
    (C) transfusion of factor VIII to 10% of normal
    (D) platelet transfusion
    (E) exploration of joint

35. A 10-year-old boy with history of prolonged bleeding after minor injury is scheduled for tonsillectomy. The bleeding time, PT, and fibrinogen are normal. What would be the most helpful investigation?

    (A) fibrinolysis (euglobulin clot lysis time)
    (B) platelet count
    (C) thrombin time
    (D) partial thromboplastin time (PTT)
    (E) factor VII assay

Questions 36 to 38

A 22-year-old man is brought into the emergency department in profound shock after a fall from the fourth floor of a building. After resuscitation, small-bowel resection and hepatic segmentectomy are performed at laparotomy. He receives 15 U of blood, 4 U of fresh-frozen plasma, and 8 L of Ringer's lactate. On closure, diffuse oozing of blood is noted.

36. What is the most likely cause?

    (A) hepatic failure
    (B) hypersplenism
    (C) platelet deficiency
    (D) factor IX (Christmas factor) deficiency
    (E) congenital hypoprothrombinemia

37. Which test is most likely to be helpful in management of this patient?

    (A) platelet count
    (B) bone marrow biopsy
    (C) liver–spleen scan
    (D) factor VIII assay
    (E) smear for Howell–Jolly bodies

38. Bleeding persists despite all appropriate blood coagulant replacement, and laparotomy reveals multiple sites of bleeding from the liver and the rest of the abdomen. Treatment should include which of the following?

    (A) hepatic artery ligation
    (B) packing with laparotomy towels
    (C) immediate closure
    (D) a large dose of heparin
    (E) Solu-Medrol, 1 g 1V

39. A 50-year-old suffering from chronic alcoholism is admitted to the hospital. He has muscle tremors and hyperactive tendon reflexes. Serum magnesium is 1.8 mEq/L (normal 1.5 to 2.5 mEq/L). Concerning magnesium, which of the following statements is true?

    (A) It is mainly extracellular.

(B) Excess may cause a positive Chvostek's sign (carpopedal spasm).

(C) Deficiency is treated with parenteral bicarbonate.

(D) Symptoms are due to deficiency of magnesium.

(E) It may become elevated in acute pancreatitis.

Questions 40 and 41

A 30-year-old man with multiple injuries has severe renal insufficiency. On the third day of hospitalization, he is lethargic with generalized weakness and decreased deep tendon reflexes. An electrocardiogram (ECG) reveals a widened QRS complex with elevated T waves.

40. What is the most likely cause of the patient's condition?

(A) hypokalemia

(B) hyponatremia

(C) hypermagnesemia

(D) hypocalcemia

(E) hypophosphatemia

41. What should be the immediate management of the patient?

(A) administration of potassium chloride

(B) administration of calcium chloride

(C) restriction of fluid intake

(D) use of Kayexylate enemas

(E) administration of hypertonic saline

42. A 45-year-old male with a known history of alcoholism is admitted with acute pancreatitis. His serum calcium is 7 mg/dL. Management is based upon which of the following?

(A) One-fourth of calcium in serum is ionized.

(B) Alkalosis increases the ionized calcium component.

(C) Hypocalcemia may cause polyuria and polydypsia.

(D) Determination of serum albumin is necessary.

(E) Treatment should involve intravenous administration of calcium chloride.

43. A 36-year-old diabetic woman develops metabolic changes following salpingo-oophorectomy. Serum osmolality of the blood can be calculated from serum values of which of the following?

(A) sodium, potassium, chloride, and bicarbonate

(B) sodium, potassium, urea, and hemoglobin

(C) sodium, potassium, glucose, and urea

(D) sodium, albumin, urea, and glucose

(E) sodium, potassium, albumin, and glucose

44. In a 12-year-old boy who sustained severe head injury caused by a fall from the third floor of a building, the syndrome of diabetes insipidus is characterized by which of the following?

(A) low serum sodium

(B) high urinary specific gravity or osmolality

(C) high serum osmolality

(D) low urine output

(E) expanded extracellular fluid volume

45. In a 40-year-old woman receiving TPN for small-bowel fistula, what finding can be attributed to hypophosphatemia?

(A) increased cardiac output

(B) diarrhea

(C) increased energy production

(D) rhabdomyolysis

(E) increased WBC function

Questions 46 and 47

A 60-year-old woman who underwent a mastectomy for breast cancer 2 years earlier presents to the emergency department with headache, backache, and frequent vomiting. She is extremely thirsty and stuporous.

46. Which test is most likely to identify the cause?

(A) computed tomography (CT) scan of the head

(B) x-ray of spine

(C) serum sodium determination

(D) serum calcium determination

(E) serum glucose determination

47. What should be the initial management of the patient?

   (A) restrict fluid intake
   (B) normal saline infusion
   (C) D₅W infusion
   (D) thiazide
   (E) hemodialysis

48. A 40-year-old man is found to have severe metabolic acidosis with a high anion gap. What is the most likely cause?

   (A) diarrhea
   (B) methanol ingestion
   (C) proximal renal tubular acidosis
   (D) distal renal tubular acidosis
   (E) ureterosigmoidostomy

49. An 18-month-old boy slipped and hurt his right knee while walking. He presents with a tender, swollen, warm knee with significant hemarthrosis. His PT is 12 (normal, 13 seconds), PTT is over 100 (normal 25 seconds), platelet count is 300,000/mm³, and bleeding time is normal. Management should consist of which of the following?

   (A) fresh-frozen plasma
   (B) aspiration of knee
   (C) factor VIII concentrate
   (D) passive exercise
   (E) all of the above

50. A 30-year-old woman with a history of an uneventful tonsillectomy at age 4 is scheduled for exploratory laparotomy. Preoperative assessment that identifies the risk of intraoperative bleeding is which of the following?

   (A) bleeding time
   (B) platelet count
   (C) PT and PTT
   (D) complete blood cell count
   (E) none of the above

51. A 43-year-old woman with von Willebrand's disease is scheduled for cholecystectomy. It can be stated that preoperative evaluation will reveal which of the following?

   (A) normal bleeding time, PT, and PTT
   (B) platelet aggregate with restocetin
   (C) increased bleeding time and PTT, and normal PT
   (D) increased bleeding time and PT, and normal PTT
   (E) increased bleeding time, and normal PT and PTT

52. Following admission to the emergency department, a 26-year-old woman with severe menorrhagia states that both her father and sister have a bleeding disorder. The hemostatic disorder transmitted by autosomal-dominant mode is which of the following?

   (A) factor X deficiency
   (B) von Willebrand's disease
   (C) factor VIII deficiency (true hemophilia)
   (D) factor IX deficiency (Christmas disease)
   (E) factor V deficiency (parahemophilia)

53. A 75-year-old man is found to have prolonged bleeding from intravenous puncture sites. Platelet aggregation is inhibited by which of the following?

   (A) adenosine diphosphate (ADP)
   (B) calcium
   (C) magnesium
   (D) aspirin
   (E) serotonin

54. A 45-year-old woman with deep-vein thrombosis is taking warfarin (coumadin), 5 mg/d. Seven days after initiation of therapy, she has warfarin-induced skin necrosis. Which following statement regarding this condition is true?

   (A) It commonly occurs after warfarin therapy.
   (B) It usually involves the upper extremities.
   (C) It improves with an increase in the dose of Coumadin.
   (D) It improves with a decrease in the dose of Coumadin.
   (E) It requires cessation of Coumadin and infusion of heparin.

55. A 50-year-old man with atrial fibrillation is taking warfarin (coumadin). The effect of Coumadin is decreased by which of the following?

(A) the presence of vitamin K deficiency
(B) phenylbutazone
(C) quinidine
(D) barbiturates
(E) thyrotoxicosis

56. After undergoing a transurethral resection of the prostate, a 65-year-old man experiences excessive bleeding attributed to fibrinolysis. It is appropriate to administer which of the following?

(A) heparin
(B) warfarin (Coumadin)
(C) volume expanders and cryoprecipitate
(D) ε-amino caproic acid
(E) fresh-frozen plasma and vitamin K

Questions 57 and 58

A 64-year-old woman undergoing radical hysterectomy under general anesthesia is transfused with 2 U of packed red blood cells (RBCs).

57. A hemolytic transfusion reaction during anesthesia will be characterized by which of the following?

(A) shaking chills and muscle spasms
(B) fever and oliguria
(C) hyperpyrexia and hypotension
(D) tachycardia and cyanosis
(E) bleeding and hypotension

58. The specific test to identify the cause of transfusion reaction for the patient is which of the following?

(A) PT
(B) PTT
(C) platelet count
(D) bleeding time
(E) free plasma hemoglobin

59. A 41-year-old woman has an episode of mild right upper quadrant (RUQ) pain associated with jaundice that resolves completely with antibiotics. Workup reveals numerous large stones in the gallbladder. The patient has polycythemia vera, a hematocrit of 58%, and a platelet count of 1.8 million. What is the preferred course of treatment for this patient?

(A) She should be referred to the medical clinic for follow-up care and be observed.
(B) She should undergo phlebotomy and then be scheduled for cholecystectomy.
(C) She should be treated with chlorambucil for 6 weeks and then undergo cholecystectomy.
(D) She should receive miniheparin and urgent cholecystectomy.
(E) She should undergo cholecystectomy.

60. A 56-year-old man underwent prostatectomy. He bled excessively and urgently required blood over and above that which had been requested before surgery. In deciding on an appropriate blood transfusion protocol, what should be kept in mind?

(A) Group AB is the universal donor.
(B) Serum from the recipient stored for 1 week is suitable for testing.
(C) Hypothermia is indicated if cryoglobulin is found.
(D) Cross-matching should be done before dextran administration.
(E) All of the above should be remembered.

61. A 60-year-old man with carcinoma of the esophagus is admitted with severe malnutrition. Nutritional support is to be initiated. What should his daily caloric intake be?

(A) 1 kcal/kg body weight/day
(B) 5 kcal/kg body weight/day
(C) 15 kcal/kg body weight/day
(D) 30 kcal/kg body weight/day
(E) 100 kcal/kg body weight/day

62. TPN is initiated in a 44-year-old woman with Crohn's disease. In parenteral alimentation, carbohydrates should be provided in an optimal ratio of which of the following?

    (A) 1 kcal/g nitrogen
    (B) 5 kcal/g nitrogen
    (C) 10 kcal/g nitrogen
    (D) 100 kcal/g nitrogen
    (E) 1,000 kcal/g nitrogen

63. After undergoing subtotal gastrectomy for carcinoma of the stomach, a 64-year-old woman is receiving peripheral parenteral nutrition. To increase calories by the peripheral route, what should be prescribed?

    (A) D_5W in normal saline
    (B) multivitamin infusion
    (C) $D_{25}W$ (25% dextrose in water)
    (D) soybean oil
    (E) lactulose

64. A 35-year-old man with duodenal stump leak after partial gastrectomy is receiving central parenteral nutrition containing the standard $D_{25}W$, 4.25% amino acid solution. Which is true of essential fatty acid deficiency seen after hyperalimentation?

    (A) It occurs if soybean oil is given only once weekly.
    (B) It is usually noted at the end of the first week.
    (C) It causes dry scaly skin with loss of hair.
    (D) It is accompanied by hypercholesterolemia.
    (E) It is treated with insulin.

65. In metabolic alkalosis, there is which of the following?

    (A) gain in fixed acid
    (B) loss of base
    (C) hyperkalemia
    (D) rise in base excess
    (E) hyperchloremia

66. Following urinary tract infection associated with extraction of a bladder stone, a 64-year-old woman developed gram-negative septicemia. Which statement is true for gram-negative bacterial septicemia?

    (A) *Pseudomonas* is the most common organism isolated.
    (B) Many of the adverse changes can be accounted for by endotoxin release.
    (C) The cardiac index is low.
    (D) Central venous pressure (CVP) is high.
    (E) Endotoxin is mainly a long-chain peptide.

67. In septic shock, which of the following is true?

    (A) The mortality rate is between 10% and 20%.
    (B) Gram-negative organisms are involved exclusively.
    (C) The majority of patients are elderly.
    (D) The most common source of infection is the alimentary tract.
    (E) Two or more organisms are responsible in most cases.

68. A 68-year-old man has a history of myocardial infarction. He undergoes uneventful left hemicolectomy for carcinoma of the colon. In the recovery room, he is hypotensive and given a fluid bolus of 500 mL Ringer's lactate over 30 minutes. He is intubated, and his neck veins are distended. His heart rate is 130 bpm, his blood pressure is 80/60 mmHg, and his urine output is 20 mL over the last hour. What should be the next step in his management?

    (A) administration of Ringer's lactate, 500 mL over 1 hour
    (B) administration of dopamine
    (C) insertion of a Swan–Ganz catheter
    (D) administration of lasix
    (E) extubation of the patient

69. A 75-year-old woman in the ICU after undergoing cholecystectomy for acute cholecystitis is hypotensive and tachycardic. Pulmonary capillary wedge pressure (PCWP) is elevated to 18 mmHg, and cardiac output is 3 L/min. She is in shock best described as which of the following?

(A) hypovolemic shock

(B) septic shock

(C) cardiogenic shock

(D) anaphylactic shock

(E) neurogenic shock

70. A 40-year-old woman with deep-vein thrombosis is being treated with intravenous heparin, 1,000 U/h. On the seventh day of treatment, her laboratory values are hemoglobin, 14 g/dL; WBC count, 7,600/mm³; platelet count, 30,000/mm³; PT, 13 seconds (control, 12.5 seconds); and PTT, 50 seconds (control, 26 seconds). What management would be appropriate?

(A) Continue with heparin at the same dosage.

(B) Increase heparin.

(C) Decrease heparin.

(D) Discontinue heparin.

(E) Continue heparin and start warfarin (Coumadin).

71. A 55-year-old man involved in an automobile accident is unresponsive and is intubated at the scene. On arrival in the emergency department, he responds to painful stimulation. His systolic blood pressure is 60 mmHg, his heart rate is 140 bpm, his neck veins are distended, and his breath sounds are absent on the left side. Immediate management should involve which of the following?

(A) insertion of a central venous line on the right side

(B) insertion of an 18-gauge needle in the left second intercostal space

(C) pericardiocentesis

(D) peritoneal lavage

(E) CT scan of head

72. A 25-year-old man sustained laceration of the liver and rupture of the spleen in an automobile accident. He was hypotensive for more than 1 hour and received 10 L of crystalloids and 10 U of blood. On the second postoperative day, he is intubated, his heart rate is 120 bpm, his blood pressure is 110/60 mmHg, his urine output is 40 mL/h, and his CVP is 13 cm H₂O. His ABGs on 70% oxygen reveal a pH of 7.42, a

PO_2 of 58 mmHg, and a PCO_2 of 35 mmHg. What is the most appropriate management?

(A) Increase the fraction of inspired oxygen (FIO_2)

(B) Increase the tidal volume (V_T).

(C) Administer Lasix, 20 mg IV.

(D) Institute positive end-expiratory pressure (PEEP).

(E) Decrease FIO_2.

73. A 40-year-old paraplegic is taken to the OR for cholecystectomy for acute cholecystitis. She is given succinylcholine before intubation. Immediately after induction of anesthesia, she develops cardiac arrest. What is the most likely cause?

(A) esophageal intubation

(B) hyperkalemia

(C) perforation of gallbladder

(D) hypovolemic shock

(E) myocardial infarction

74. A 70-year-old woman has low cardiac output with increased PCWP and increased systemic vascular resistance. What should be the drug of choice?

(A) dopamine

(B) norepinephrine

(C) dobutamine

(D) epinephrine

(E) phenylephrine

75. A 60-year-old man had undergone exploratory laparotomy for perforated gastric ulcer with severe peritoneal contamination. Six hours after surgery, he is tachycardic, hypertensive, and has shallow respirations. Intubation and institution of ventilatory support is indicated in the presence of which of the following?

(A) respiratory rate of 23 breaths per minute

(B) $PaCO_2$ of 45 mmHg

(C) PaO_2 of 55 mmHg on room air

(D) heart rate of 140 bpm

(E) blood pressure of 150/100 mmHg

76. A 60-year-old man is being weaned from a ventilator in the ICU. The likelihood that weaning is going to fail is suggested by the presence of which of the following?

    (A) a respiratory rate of 24 breaths per minute
    (B) a PaO_2 of 80 mmHg on FIO_2 of 40%
    (C) a vital capacity (VC) of 5 mL/kg body weight
    (D) A minute ventilation of 8 L/min
    (E) A maximum negative inspiratory pressure of -30 cm H_2O

77. Successful weaning from a ventilator is suggested by the presence of which of the following?

    (A) an alveolar arterial gradient of more than 350 mmHg
    (B) a PaO_2/FIO_2 ratio of less than 200
    (C) a $PaCO_2$ over 55 mmHg
    (D) a tidal volume (VT) of over 5 mL/kg
    (E) all of the above

78. A 55-year-old man with oat-cell carcinoma of the lung is suspected to have SIADH. This is characterized by which of the following?

    (A) decreased total body water (TBW)
    (B) low serum sodium
    (C) increased urine output
    (D) urine sodium of less than 10 mEq/L
    (E) low urinary specific gravity

79. Following surgery for a perforated appendix with generalized peritonitis and multiple intra-abdominal abscess, a 25-year-old man is admitted to the ICU. On the third postoperative day, he continues to be febrile and has a nasogastric tube. What is the metabolic characteristic seen in him?

    (A) a decrease in energy expenditure
    (B) fat as his primary fuel
    (C) respiratory quotient of 0.6–0.7
    (D) proteolysis
    (E) decreased hepatic synthesis of protein

80. Increase in energy expenditure by 100% over normal, or two times greater than normal, is seen in a patient with which of the following?

    (A) pyloric obstruction from chronic duodenal ulcer
    (B) fractured femur
    (C) perforated diverticulitis of colon
    (D) severe thermal burns of more than 30% total body surface area (BSA)
    (E) right inguinal herniorrhaphy for incarcerated inguinal hernia

81. A 30-year-old man with a gunshot wound to the abdomen has severe injuries involving the liver, duodenum, pancreas, and colon. Why is parenteral nutrition support preferred over enteral nutrition support?

    (A) It is less expressive.
    (B) It preserves gut mucosal mass and mucosal immunity.
    (C) It prevents gut permeability and translocation.
    (D) It is easy to start and administer nutrient requirement rapidly.
    (E) It attenuates hypermetabolic response to surgery.

82. A 24-year-old man with multiple injuries is receiving standard total parenteral nutrition. The following is true regarding glutamine.

    (A) It is a major fuel for the brain.
    (B) It is an essential amino acid.
    (C) It is a major fuel for the gut.
    (D) It is synthesized de novo in the kidney.
    (E) It is a component of TPN solutions.

83. A 50-year-old man with small-bowel fistula has been receiving TPN for the previous 3 weeks through a single-lumen central venous catheter. He is scheduled for exploratory laparotomy and closure of fistula. On the morning of the day of surgery, TPN is discontinued and intravenous infusion with balanced salt solution (Ringer's lactate) is started. An hour later, the patient is found to be anxious, sweating, and tachycardic. What is the most likely cause?

    (A) anxiety
    (B) hypoglycemia
    (C) hypovolemia

(D) unexplained hemorrhage

(E) hyperglycemia

84. A 40-year-old woman with inflammatory bowel disease has been receiving TPN for over 3 weeks. Workup reveals pelvic abscess. She undergoes exploratory laparotomy, resection of small bowel with anastomosis, and drainage of pelvic abscess. During surgery, TPN is maintained at the original rate of 125 mL/h. In the recovery room, the patient is found to have a urine output of 200 mL/h. CVP is 1, and laboratory results are Na, 149; K, 3.5; Cl, 110; HCO_3, 18; BUN, 40; and creatinine, 1.0 mg/dL. Which of the following statements is true regarding this condition?

(A) The patient's urine output is secondary to fluid overload during surgery.

(B) The patient is in high-output renal failure.

(C) Hyperosmolar–nonketotic coma will develop if the condition is not aggressively treated.

(D) Diuresis is a normal response to stress of surgery.

(E) Potassium supplementation is not indicated.

85. A 42-year-old man who weighs 60 kg is receiving 3 L of standard hypertonic 25%/glucose–amino acid solution. He has no history of smoking or bronchial asthma. In the ICU, he is alert, afebrile, and hemodynamically stable, but he remains intubated and attempts to wean him off the ventilator have been unsuccessful. What is the most likely cause?

(A) copper deficiency

(B) excess fat calories

(C) excess glucose calories

(D) excess amino acids

(E) inadequate glucose calories

86. What ensues immediately following pancreaticoduodenectomy (Whipple's operation) for carcinoma of the head of the pancreas in a 50-year-old man?

(A) Serum catecholamine levels are decreased.

(B) Serum cortisol levels are normal.

(C) Serum glucagon level is increased.

(D) Serum insulin level is increased.

(E) Catabolism is decreased.

87. A 50-year-old woman with adult respiratory distress syndrome (ARDS) is intubated. The oxyhemoglobin curve is shifted to the right with increased oxygen delivery by which of the following?

(A) metabolic acidosis

(B) older age

(C) decreased 2,3-diphosphoglycerate (DPG)

(D) decreased thyroid hormone level

(E) hypothermia

88. A 60-year-old man with no significant past medical history is scheduled for elective cholecystectomy. He has been taking aspirin daily. Preoperative recommendations should include which of the following?

(A) determination of PT

(B) estimation of platelet count

(C) discontinuation of aspirin 2 days before surgery

(D) discontinuation of aspirin at least 1 week before surgery

(E) none of the above

89. A 70-year-old man was administered 20,000 U of heparin before femoral artery embolectomy. Following surgery, he is noted to have generalized bleeding from the wound margins. Immediate management should consist of administration of which of the following?

(A) fresh-frozen plasma

(B) cryoprecipitate

(C) platelet transfusion

(D) intravenous protamine sulfate

(E) intravenous sodium bicarbonate

90. A 70-year-old female has serum potassium 2.3 mEq/L. Her potassium deficit is approximately which of the following?

(A) 50 mEq
(B) 100 mEq
(C) 200 mEq
(D) 300 mEq
(E) 500 mEq

91. A 34-year-old male has serum sodium of 114 mEq/L. Correction of hyponatremia can be done by raising serum sodium by which amount?

(A) 1 mEq/L/h
(B) 3 mEq/L/h
(C) 5 mEq/L/h
(D) 7 mEq/L/h
(E) 10 mEq/L/h

Questions 92 and 93

A 47 year-old woman with chronic renal failure has been maintained on chronic dialysis for several years. She had undergone kidney transplantation but because of rejection, she was placed back on dialysis. She had repeated bouts of pain in the right upper quadrant and was intolerant to fatty meals. Ultrasound showed cholelithiasis.

92. Following elective cholecystectomy, severe bleeding occurred. This was most likely attributed to which of the following?

(A) elevated PT
(B) elevated PTT
(C) low platelet count
(D) decreased platelet aggregation
(E) sepsis

93. The most appropriate management of this patient is the administration of which of the following?

(A) heparin
(B) protamine sulfate
(C) fresh frozen plasma
(D) desmopressin
(E) factor VIII concentrate

94. A 70-year-old man, who weighs 70 kg, is admitted with acute cholecystitis. His calculated daily fluid requirement for maintenance is approximately which of the following?

(A) 1.0 L
(B) 2.0 L
(C) 2.5 L
(D) 3.0 L
(E) 4.0 L

95. A 90-year-old woman with a fractured neck of femur is receiving low molecular weight heparin (LMWH). Which following statement regarding LMWH is true?

(A) It has molecular weight below 4,000 daltons.
(B) Its anticoagulant effect is by binding to Antithrombin III.
(C) It should be administered two to three times a day.
(D) It has lower bioavailability than standard heparin.
(E) It has a greater rate of heparin-associated thrombocytopenia.

DIRECTIONS (Questions 96 through 102): Each set of matching questions in this section consists of a list of lettered options followed by several numbered items. For each numbered item, select the appropriate lettered option(s). Each lettered option may be selected once, more than once, or not at all. EACH ITEM WILL STATE THE NUMBER OF OPTIONS TO SELECT. CHOOSE EXACTLY THIS NUMBER.

Questions 96 through 98

(A) copper deficiency
(B) chromium deficiency
(C) zinc deficiency
(D) manganese deficiency
(E) vitamin A deficiency
(F) vitamin D deficiency
(G) vitamin E deficiency
(H) vitamin K deficiency
(I) vitamin C deficiency

96. A 45-year-old man receiving TPN has signs of retarded wound healing. SELECT ONLY THREE.

97. A 40-year-old woman with no previous history of diabetes is receiving TPN. After 4 weeks, she is hyperglycemic, and it is difficult to control her glucose despite insulin therapy. SELECT ONLY TWO.

98. A 42-year-old man with small-bowel fistula has been receiving TPN with standard hypertonic glucose–amino acid solution for the previous 3 weeks. The patient is noticed to have scaly, hyperpigmented lesions over the acral surfaces of elbows and knees, similar to enterohepatic acrodermatitis. What is the most likely cause of this condition? SELECT ONLY ONE.

Questions 99 through 101

  (A) factor II (prothrombin)
  (B) factor V
  (C) factor VII
  (D) factor VIII
  (E) factor IX
  (F) factor X
  (G) factor XII
  (H) calcium
   (I) fibrin split products

99. A 72-year-old man requires blood transfusion. He was initially given stored plasma. He is most likely to show a deficiency of what? SELECT TWO.

100. What is the coagulation factor involved exclusively in the extrinsic coagulation system? SELECT ONE.

101. A 48-year-old man with severe liver cirrhosis is admitted to the hospital with a hematemesis. What coagulation factors are not synthesized in the liver? SELECT TWO.

Question 102

A 20-year-old man has undergone appendectomy for perforated appendicitis with generalized peritonitis. Seven days postoperatively, his temperature continues to spike to 103°F despite antibiotic therapy with ampicillin, gentamicin, and metronidazole. A CT scan reveals a large pelvic abscess. Soon afterward, he has bleeding from the mouth and nose with increasing oozing from the surgical wound and all intravenous puncture sites.

  (A) anaphylactoid reaction to intravenous dye
  (B) disseminated intravascular coagulation (DIC)
  (C) antibiotic-induced coagulopathy
  (D) liver failure
  (E) congenital bleeding disorder
  (F) allergy to penicillin
  (G) intracerebral bleed
  (H) intravenous heparin
   (I) drainage of pelvic abscess
  (J) cortisone
  (K) platelet transfusion

102. What is the most likely diagnosis? SELECT ONLY ONE.

Answers and Explanations

1. **(C)** High-output renal failure should be suspected if the BUN continues to rise with urine output greater than 1,000–1,500 mL/d. It is associated with mild to moderate renal insufficiency; in comparison, severe renal injury results in oliguric renal failure. The kidneys do not tolerate ischemia for more than 30–90 minutes. Hypothermia is protective. There is a decrease in creatinine clearance. Vasopressors aggravate the deleterious effects of shock.

2. **(B)** Hyperkalemia can manifest by gastrointestinal (GI) or cardiovascular signs. GI symptoms include nausea, vomiting, intestinal colic, and diarrhea. Abdominal distension as a result of paralytic ileus is due to hypokalemia. An ECG is useful to monitor potassium levels. Hyperkalemia is characterized by peaked T waves. ECG changes also include ST segment depression, widened QRS complex, and heart block. Cardiac arrest occurs in diastole with increasing levels of potassium. Osborne (J) wave is seen in hypothermia.

3. **(C)** In hyperkalemia, all oral and intravenous potassium must be withheld. Sodium chloride worsens the metabolic acidosis. Sodium bicarbonate intravenously is given to divert potassium intracellularly by causing alkalosis. Calcium gluconate (1 g [10 mL of 10% solution]) is given to counteract the effect of potassium on the myocardium. The hypertonic glucose solution stimulates the synthesis of glycogen, which causes cellular uptake of potassium. Small amounts of insulin (1 U/5 g of glucose) is helpful. The usual recommended dose is 100 mL of 50% glucose with 10 U of insulin. Calcitonin is used for treating hyper-calcemia. Serum magnesium is also elevated in renal failure.

4. **(A)** Anion gap is calculated by subtracting sum of serum chloride and bicarbonate from serum sodium value. The normal value is 10–15 mEq/L. In this patient, the anion gap is:

$$Na - (Cl + HCO_3)$$
$$138 - (100 + 28) = 138 - 128 = 10$$

5. **(D)** This patient has metabolic acidosis with normal anion gap. The normal value of anion gap is 10–15. Loss of bicarbonate (e.g., small-bowel fistula, pancreatic fistula, or diarrhea) and gain of chloride (e.g., administration of ammonium chloride or HCl and decreased excretion as in distal renal tubular acidosis) result in metabolic acidosis with normal anion gap. In contrast, in acidosis due to increased production of an organic acid (e.g., ketoacids in diabetes, sulfur and phosphoric acid in renal failure, and lactic acid in shock), the anion gap is increased.

6. **(B)** The patient has ARDS. Measurement of ABGs provides initial evaluation of pulmonary function in terms of oxygenation and ventilation. ECG is valuable for diagnosing myocardial ischemia or cardiac arrhythmias. Ventilation perfusion scanning is used for diagnosing pulmonary embolism. A central venous line provides information regarding the volume status of the patient, which may be low to normal in ARDS.

7. **(C)** Increased airway resistance (stiff lung) may be noted early in shock lung. The alveolar

capillary membrane becomes more permeable. There is a leak of a high-protein fluid from the capillary to the interstitial tissues and then into the alveoli. This is commonly called ARDS. Sepsis syndrome is the most frequent cause of ARDS (39%), followed by aspiration, multiple transfusion, massive soft-tissue injury, multiple trauma, near drowning, fat embolism, DIC, and pancreatitis. ARDS is associated with ventilation–perfusion imbalance. In some areas of lung, there is ventilation with no perfusion; whereas, in other areas, nonventilated alveoli are being perfused. The net result is decrease in functional residual capacity, shunting, and increased dead space ventilation. Chest x-ray reveals diffuse alveolar infiltration, and findings are normal in the initial stage.

8. **(B)** A history of bleeding should alert the clinician to evaluate the underlying cause. The bleeding time is influenced by those factors affecting platelet and capillary integrity. Prolongation of the PT may be attributed to decreased absorption of fat-soluble vitamin K, liver impairment, or decrease in the blood components because of consumption.

9. **(B)** Possible causes of this syndrome include head injury, central nervous system (CNS) disorders, neoplastic diseases, pulmonary diseases, drugs, and idiopathic. It results in impaired water excretion characterized by oliguria, hyponatremia, significantly decreased serum osmolality, and increased urinary osmolality.

10. **(B)** Hyponatremia occurs because of overhydration and/or inadequate sodium replacement. When serum sodium is less than 130 mEq/L, acute symptomatic hyponatremia is manifested by CNS symptoms due to increased intracranial pressure. Muscle twitching and increased tendon reflexes seen in moderate hyponatremia progress to convulsions, loss of reflexes, and hypertension with severe hyponatremia. Oliguric renal failure may become irreversible if not immediately treated. Mild asymptomatic hyponatremia is treated with fluid restrictions. In the presence of CNS symptoms, the patient should be given hypertonic saline.

11. **(D)** Sodium deficit is estimated by multiplying the decrease in serum sodium times the total body water, which is 60% of body weight:

$$(\text{normal serum sodium} - \text{observed serum sodium})$$
$$\times\ 0.6\ \text{total} \times \text{total body weight}$$
$$= (140 - 120) \times 0.6 \times 60 = 720\ \text{mEq}$$

Half of this amount should be administered over 12–18 hours.

12. **(B)** Oliguria may be prerenal or renal. The following table characterizes findings in prerenal failure versus those observed in intrinsic renal failure:

	Prerenal Failures	Intrinsic Renal Failures
Urine osmolality (mOsm/kg)	>500	<350
Urine sodium (mEq/L)	>20	>40
Fractional excretion of sodium	<1%	>2%
BUN/SCR	>20	<10
Urine/PCR	>40	<20

13. **(C)** The composition of various GI secretions is different. They are as follows: **A**, saliva; **B**, gastric; **C**, ileal; **D**, pancreatic; and **E**, colonic. The composition of intestinal fluid is the closest to that of plasma.

14. **(A)** The composition of small-intestinal fluid is sodium, 140 mEq/L; potassium, 5 mEq/L; chloride, 104 mEq/L; and bicarbonate, 30 mEq/L. Daily losses are best replaced by administration of balanced salt solution (Ringer's lactate) whose composition is depicted in **A**. **B** represents normal saline (0.9%), **C** is half normal saline (0.45%), **D** is M/6 sodium lactate, and **E** is 3% sodium chloride.

15. **(B)** A decrease in pH below 7.4 indicates acidosis. P_{CO_2} is increased over 40 mmHg, suggesting respiratory acidosis. To differentiate "pure" from "combined" acidosis, pH is calculated based on changes in CO_2. A change of 10 mmHg from 40 mmHg changes pH by 0.08 from 7.4. In this case, there is a 20 mmHg increase in P_{CO_2}, which would decrease pH by

$2 \times 0.08 = 0.16$ from 7.4 or 7.24. The measured pH is 7.24. Therefore, the patient has pure respiratory acidosis.

16. **(D)** Respiratory acidosis in the immediate postoperative period is due to inadequate ventilation. Adequate ventilation needs to be restored by prompt intubation and ventilatory support. Use of morphine will further depress the respiration.

17. **(B)** Villous adenoma of colon can result in watery diarrhea and hypokalemia. Massive tissue injury producing myoglobinemia is associated with significant release of intracellular potassium. Massive blood transfusion results in release of large amounts of potassium. The ability to excrete potassium is impaired in high-output renal failure. Spironolactone is a potassium-sparing diuretic.

18. **(E)** A change in P_{CO_2} of 10 mmHg from the normal value of 40 mmHg produces a 0.08 change in pH (from 7.4). A P_{CO_2} of 30 mmHg, representing a decrease of 10 mmHg, can account for an increase in pH by 0.08 (i.e., 7.4–7.48). The patient's measured pH is 7.54. The additional increase in pH is due to metabolic alkalosis.

19. **(A)** Alkalosis is associated with hypokalemia. Hypokalemia can be sudden and severe. It is related to: (a) intracellular shift of potassium in exchange for hydrogen and (b) excessive urinary potassium loss. The oxyhemoglobin dissociation curve is shifted to left, and a decrease in levels of ionized calcium can result in tetany and convulsions.

20. **(E)** Zinc is one of the metalloenzymes involved in lipid, carbohydrate, protein, and nucleic acid metabolism. Skin lesions similar to enterohepatic acrodermatitis are the most common sign seen in zinc deficiency. Other manifestations include hypogonadism, diminished wound healing, and immunodeficiencies. Copper deficiency is characterized by microcytic hypochromic anemia.

21. **(E)** The fall in pressure will signal changes via baroreceptors located in the arch of the aorta and carotid sinus and will cause sympathetic stimulation with tachycardia, peripheral vasoconstriction, and hypothermia. Eosinopenia rather than eosinophilia is more likely to be present. There is a switch from aerobic to anaerobic metabolism. Lactic acid accumulation indicates an adverse prognosis in shock. There is a progressive deterioration in prognosis as the blood lactate level increases from 1 to above 3 mm/L.

22. **(C)** The fall in cardiac output results in a relatively larger proportion of blood to be distributed to the heart. The changes are mediated mainly by sympathetic stimulation. There is increased arteriolar and precapillary sphincter tone in the skin and in the renal and splanchnic circulation. In the heart, coronary artery vasodilation occurs, which is brought about partly by local release of vasodilator substances (due to hypoxemia and acidosis).

23. **(C)** Initial resuscitation of a trauma patient is best done by administering Ringer's lactate, because it is isotonic, and it is similar to plasma in electrolyte composition. There is no conclusive evidence that colloid solutions (albumin, plasma protein solution, or hydroxyethyl starch solution) improve the rate of resuscitation or eventual outcome. D_5W and D_5W and 0.45% normal saline are hypotonic.

24. **(C)** Neurogenic shock is secondary to high spinal cord injury as evidenced by inability to move all four extremities. Neurogenic shock is clinically manifested by warm skin, bradycardia, and hypotension. In septic shock, while the skin is warm, the patient usually has tachycardia. In all other types of shock, the skin is cold. Treatment consists of volume replacement with balanced salt solution (lactated Ringer's solution). On rare occasions, some patients may need vasoconstrictors (e.g., phenylephrine hydrochloride).

25. **(D)** Succussion splash is elicited by placing one hand behind and the other in front of the left abdomen and rib cage and rocking the patient gently between the two hands. In pyloric obstruction, one can feel the fluid hitting the

fingers (succussion). Peristalsis is likely to be observed in infants with congenital pyloric stenosis.

26. **(B)** Duodenal ulcer and gastric carcinoma are the most likely causes of pyloric obstruction in adults. Metabolic alkalosis results from loss of fixed acids from the stomach. The bicarbonate content of the blood accompanies the elevation in pH. In severe metabolic alkalosis, paradoxical loss of acid (hydrogen) in the urine occurs in an attempt to conserve potassium. Hypokalemia worsens the metabolic consequences of metabolic alkalosis.

27. **(D)** Potassium should not be given initially until moderate hydration has been achieved, and urine flow is adequate. Normal saline is required initially to correct the hypochloremia.

28. **(D)** Initial management of hypochloremic metabolic alkalosis includes administration of isotonic sodium chloride solution with replacement of potassium chloride. In patients refractory to standard therapy use of O.1 N and 0.2 N hydrochloric acid has been shown to be safe and effective therapy. Ammonium chloride solution has also been used, but this can lead to ammonia toxicity, especially in patients with hepatic insufficiency.

29. **(B)** The actual surgical treatment for obstruction caused by peptic ulcer is controversial. Appropriate gastric surgery with drainage usually is required if pyloric stenosis is severe. Drainage procedures include pyloroplasty, gastrojejunostomy, or antrectomy. An alternative to vagotomy and drainage would be vagotomy, antrectomy with gastrojejunostomy, or a Billroth II subtotal gastrectomy with gastrojejunal anastomosis. It is important to be certain that a gastric carcinoma is not the cause of the pyloric outlet obstruction.

30. **(B)** The presence of an adequate urine output does not preclude a diagnosis of high-output renal failure. The mechanism is based in part on prior ischemia to the nephron structure of the kidneys. There may be an initial period of oliguria. Urea, potassium, and acids are still partly excreted in the urine, and lac-

tate or bicarbonate is given to avoid development of acidosis.

31. **(A)** Potassium should not be given, and potassium levels must be monitored carefully to avoid hyperkalemia. Phosphorous and magnesium levels may be increased, and hypernatremia is likely to occur when fluid is restricted and a solute-poor urine is excreted. Autopsy in patients dying early shows that the distal nephron is affected more than the proximal nephron. Although mortality figures are high, if the patient survives the postoperative period, satisfactory renal function can be anticipated.

32. **(C)** Marked fluid restriction may result in hypernatremia. If the condition is treated appropriately, urea nitrogen usually falls after 1 or 2 weeks. In elderly and cardiac patients, pulmonary edema occurs more readily, and diuretics may be contraindicated because azotemia may be made more severe. Ammonium chloride would make the acidosis worse. Potassium has to be monitored carefully, because severe hyperkalemia is readily induced.

33. **(D)** Hemophilia (factor VIII deficiency) usually occurs during infancy. It is sex-linked recessive and affects males almost exclusively. DES administered during the mother's pregnancy has not been incriminated in coagulation disorders but is associated with vaginal carcinoma in adolescent girls. Henoch–Schönlein purpura usually occurs about 3 weeks after a streptococcal infection and includes joint pain, purpura, and nephritis. Wilson's disease is associated with a disturbance in copper metabolism.

34. **(B)** Spontaneous bleeding occurs when factor VIII is reduced below 2–3%. Once serious bleeding occurs, a higher factor VIII activity—probably approaching 30%—is required for adequate hemostasis. The half-life of factor VIII is 8–12 hours. In minor lesions, 10 U/kg body weight of factor VIII is administered. For severe lesions, the dosage is 40–50 U/kg body weight of factor VIII. After major surgical procedures, factor VIII must be given daily for 7–10 days. Penicillamine is used to inhibit excess copper deposition (e.g., in Wilson's disease).

35. **(D)** The clinical picture is suggestive of hemophilia. The normal bleeding time excludes capillary fragility or platelet deficiency. If fibrinolysis was evident, the fibrinogen level would be reduced. In the presence of a normal PT, a prolonged PTT indicates a deficiency of factor VIII, IX, XI, or XII. The PT evaluates the extrinsic coagulation pathway. The normal PT excludes factor VII deficiency. The thrombin time evaluates fibrinogen to fibrin conversion with an external source of thrombin and will be normal as fibrinogen levels are normal.

36. **(C)** Thrombocytopenia is the major hemostatic disorder in massive blood transfusion. Platelet transfusion usually is indicated when more than 6–8 U of blood is transfused rapidly. There is the risk of causing hepatitis. Stored blood is deficient in factors V and VIII; as such, PT and PTT may be slightly prolonged after massive blood transfusion. Fresh-frozen plasma is the source of factors V and VII, which would be deficient in banked blood. Unless there is previous liver cirrhosis, the procedures enumerated are unlikely to lead to liver failure. Hypersplenism occurs in patients with enlarged spleens.

37. **(A)** Platelet deficiency is likely to be evident, but tests to exclude other causes of bleeding are indicated. The possibility of defibrinogenation, intravascular coagulopathy, or fibrinolysis must be excluded by appropriate coagulation studies. Bleeding from a vein or artery, incompatible blood transfusion, DIC, acidosis, and hypothermia are other considerations to explain any unusual bleeding after a major surgical procedure.

38. **(B)** In desperate cases where bleeding persists despite all other measures, packing the abdomen with laparotomy packs may offer temporary control. The patient is taken to the OR 24–48 hours later for removal of packing after stabilization of hemodynamic status and correction of coagulopathy.

39. **(D)** Symptoms are due to magnesium deficiency. Magnesium is mainly intracellular. Magnesium deficiency occurs in the presence of starvation, malabsorption syndrome, acute pancreatitis, and chronic alcoholism. Symptoms are characterized by neuromuscular and CNS hyperactivity, such as muscle tremors, hyperactive tendon reflexes, and tetany with a positive Chvostek sign. The syndrome of magnesium deficiency can exist in the presence of normal serum magnesium levels. Magnesium deficiency is treated with parenteral magnesium sulfate or magnesium chloride.

40. **(C)** Symptomatic hypermagnesemia is seen after early thermal injury, massive trauma, surgical stress, and in the presence of severe renal insufficiency. ECG changes resemble those seen with hyperkalemia. Hypokalemia and hypophosphatemia can cause symptoms of generalized weakness, but potassium and phosphorus are increased in renal failure. Hypokalemia is characterized by flattening of T waves and U waves. Hypocalcemia is characterized by hyperactive tendon reflexes. Hyponatremia is characterized by nervous irritation as restlessness and convulsions with no specific ECG changes.

41. **(B)** Administer calcium chloride. Management of hypermagnesemia involves correction of extracellular volume deficit and acidosis and withholding exogenous magnesium. Calcium chloride should be administered to reverse the ECG changes temporarily. Peritoneal dialysis or hemodialysis is necessary for persistent symptoms or toxicity.

42. **(D)** Determination of serum albumin or protein level is necessary for proper determination of serum calcium level. For every 1 g decrease of serum albumin, the serum calcium level is corrected by 0.8. Intravenous administration of calcium chloride is indicated in the presence of symptoms. Approximately 45% of serum calcium is ionized and responsible for neuromuscular stability. Half of the calcium in the blood is bound to protein, and an additional 5% is attached to substances other than protein. Alkalosis decreases the ionized component. Hypercalcemia causes polydipsia and polyuria.

43. **(C)** Serum osmolality is calculated from serum values of sodium, potassium, glucose, and BUN by using the formula 2 (Na + K) + BUN/ 2.8 + glucose/18.

44. **(C)** Injury to the pituitary stalk in major skull fractures involving the base of the skull can result in decreased secretion of vasopressin. There is increased urine output that is diluted (osmolality < 270 mOsm/kg). The extracellular fluid volume is contracted, resulting in high serum osmolality (> 300 mOsm/kg) and increased serum sodium.

45. **(D)** Hypophosphatemia results in decreased synthesis of phosphorylated intermediate metabolites such as adenosine triphosphate (ATP), 2, 3-DPG, and cyclic adenosine monophosphate (cAMP). Deficiency can result in erythrocyte membrane instability, WBC dysfunction, platelet dysfunction, congestive heart failure, arrhythmias, weakening of respiration muscles, hemolysis, and rhabdomyolysis.

46. **(D)** The symptoms are suggestive of hypercalcemia. Major causes of hypercalcemia are cancer with bony metastasis and hyperparathyroidism. Symptoms involve the GI, renal, musculoskeletal, and central nervous systems.

47. **(B)** Patients with hypercalcemia have decreased extracellular fluid volume due to vomiting and polyuria. Vigorous resuscitation with salt solution will lower the serum calcium by dilution and increased renal excretion. Furosemide and not thiazides increase renal excretion of calcium. Additional therapy includes administration of oral or intravenous inorganic phosphates, corticosteroid, mithramycin, and calcitonin.

48. **(B)** Methanol ingestion results in increased production of lactic acid causing an increased anion gap. The other conditions listed are associated with normal anion gap. Diarrhea, proximal renal tubular acidosis, and ureterosigmoidostomy result in loss of bicarbonate, while distal renal tubular acidosis is associated with decreased acid excretion.

49. **(C)** The boy has hemophilia. Management consists of infusion of factor VIII concentrate. Bed rest and local cold packs are helpful. Aspiration of the knee to remove blood and passive exercise are not recommended for fear of recurrent bleeding. In contrast, active exercise is beneficial, because movement beyond the point when bleeding can recur is limited owing to pain. Fresh-frozen plasma has a low level of factor VIII (0.6 U/mL) and is not useful, because the required volume is excessive.

50. **(E)** Obtaining a detailed history is the most important preoperative information that predicts the risk of unexpected intraoperative bleeding complication. It is even more reliable than laboratory tests.

51. **(C)** von Willebrand's disease is characterized by decreased level of factor VIIIc (procoagulant). It has autosomal-dominant inheritance. These patients have prolonged bleeding times and PTT, with normal PTs. In contrast to platelets of normal patients that aggregate when restocetin is added, in von Willebrand's disease, platelets fail to aggregate in presence of restocetin.

52. **(B)** von Willebrand's disease is the most common hemostatic disorder transmitted by autosomal-dominant mode. Other disorders transmitted by this mode are hereditary hemorrhagic telangiectasia and factor XI deficiency. Diseases transmitted by an autosomal-recessive mode are factor X, factor V, factor VII, and factor I deficiencies. Factor VIII (true hemophilia) and factor IX (Christmas disease) deficiencies are sex-liked recessive.

53. **(D)** ADP, serotonin, and thromboxane A_2 are important mediators of platelet aggregation. In the presence of calcium, magnesium, and platelet factor 4, they cause release of platelet content and their granules resulting in the formation of a "platelet plug." This process is inhibited by aspirin.

54.   **(E)** Requires cessation of Coumadin and infusion of heparin. Warfarin (Coumadin)-induced skin necrosis is a rare complication with high morbidity and mortality. It usually occurs 3–10 days after initiation of therapy, affects women more commonly than men, and most often involves the skin of thighs, buttocks, abdomen, and breast. The exact mechanism is unknown but may be related to depression of protein C levels in some patients. Management involves immediate cessation of Coumadin and administration of heparin intravenously.

55.   **(D)** Patients receiving barbiturates, oral contraceptive agents, and corticosteroids often require larger amounts of Coumadin to maintain adequate anticoagulation. In patients with vitamin K deficiency or impaired liver function and in those with thyrotoxicosis, there is increased effect of Coumadin. Also, the cholesterol-lowering agent clofibrate, D-thyroxine, and certain antibiotics given concomitantly with Coumadin enhance its anticoagulant effect. It is important to adjust the dose of Coumadin when initiating anticoagulation therapy in such patients.

56.   **(D)** Fibrinolysis may be primary or acquired. Primary fibrinolysis is seen after fibrinolytic therapy with streptokinase or urokinase; surgical procedures on the prostate gland (which is rich in urokinase) and severe liver failure. Secondary fibrinolysis is most commonly seen in DIC. If the PT, PTT, and platelet count are normal, DIC is unlikely to be present. ε-Amino caproic acid inhibits plasminogen activation to plasmin and can be used if there is excessive fibrinolysis. It must not be given in DIC, because serious intravascular clotting may occur.

57.   **(E)** In the anesthetized patient, the classic signs of transfusion reaction are masked. The sudden unexplained onset of bleeding and hypotension should include transfusion reaction in the differential diagnosis. In the conscious patient, chills, fever, pain in the lumbar region, a tight sensation over the chest, flushing of the face, and dark-colored urine may be evident.

58.   **(E)** Acute hemolytic transfusion reaction due to transfusion of incompatible blood in a patient under general anesthesia usually presents as generalized bleeding due to DIC. PT, PTT, and bleeding time will be abnormally high, and platelets may be decreased because of DIC. The most specific tests to determine hemolysis are free plasma hemoglobin and hemoglobinuria. The laboratory criteria are hemoglobinuria with a concentration of free hemoglobin over 5 mg/dL, a serum hepatoglobin level below 50 mg/dL, and serological criteria to show antigen incompatibility of the donor and recipient blood.

59.   **(C)** Patients with polycythemia vera do poorly in general surgery if they have not had appropriate treatment to reduce the RBC and platelet count. With chlorambucil treatment, elective cholecystectomy should be performed to avoid the possible need to perform the operation on an emergency basis when the patient is not fully prepared.

60.   **(D)** Cross-matching should be done before dextran administration. Group O is the universal donor, and if there is insufficient time to do appropriate cross matching of blood, this type of blood should be used. Serum of the recipient should be less than 24 hours old, because antigenicity may be altered in blood stored for a longer time. Before hypothermia is undertaken, the patient's (recipient's) blood should be tested for cold agglutinin titer. Cryoglobulin may be present in patients with lymphoma or leukemia. Blood must be given at room temperature to such patients.

61.   **(D)** In general, total caloric needs for the majority of patients ranges between 25 and 35 kcal/kg/d. An alternative formula for calculating daily caloric requirements is the Harris–Benedict equation, which is based on sex, age, weight, and height. The caloric requirements of humans also varies by amount of activity, degree of stress of surgery, trauma, sepsis, or burns.

62. **(D)** The baseline protein requirements are calculated as 1 g/kg/d. Following stress, there is an increased protein requirement, and protein intake should be 1.5 g/kg/d after surgery, 2.0 g/kg/d after polytrauma, and 2.5 g/kg/d after sepsis. Glucose and amino acids must be infused simultaneously to obtain maximal nitrogen used, and the ideal ratio is 100 nonprotein kilocalories per gram of nitrogen. In starvation, the nonprotein calorie-to-nitrogen ratio of 150 kcal/g is adequate.

63. **(D)** Lipid emulsions derived from soybean or safflower oils are widely used. One of the real advantages of lipid emulsion is that a large amount of calories can be provided through a peripheral vein. The 10% solution provides 4.62 kJ/mL and the 20% solution, 9.24 kJ/mL. Dextrose concentration in peripheral route is 10%. Concentrations greater than 10% require administration into a central vein to prevent phlebitis owing to hypertonicity of the solutions. Lactulose is used to treat hepatic encephalopathy.

64. **(C)** Essential fatty acid deficiency usually occurs if hyperalimentation is extended for more than 1 month and when soybean oil is not administered at least twice a week. There is a decrease in linolenic, linoleic, and arachidonic acids and an increase in oleic and palmitoleic acid. In addition to the skin changes, there may be poor wound healing, increased susceptibility to infection, lethargy, and thrombocytopenia. It is characterized by a triene:tetraene ratio greater than 0.40.

65. **(D)** In metabolic alkalosis, there may be a loss of fixed acids or excess of base. It is associated with hypokalemia because of renal conservation of H^+ ions and urinary potassium loss. Loss of hydrochloric acid as seen in vomiting in patients with pyloric obstruction results in hypochloremic hypokalemic metabolic alkalosis.

66. **(B)** Many of the adverse changes can be accounted for by endotoxin release. *Escherichia coli* is the most common organism involved in gram-negative septicemia, followed by *Klebsiella, Aerobacter, Proteus,* and *Pseudomonas.* The cardiac index is high, peripheral resistance is decreased, and CVP is low to normal. The most common conditions leading to gram-negative sepsis are those of the urinary tract, followed by respiratory and biliary tract and abdominal visceral infections. Endotoxins are lipopolysaccharide complexes. The lipid A portion is probably responsible for the toxicity.

67. **(C)** Most patients are elderly. The underlying conditions leading to septic shock occur more commonly in elderly patients. The mortality is higher in this patient population. The overall mortality rate exceeds 40–50%. Gram-positive organisms, parasites, or fungi also may be responsible. The genitourinary and respiratory tracts are more common sources for initiating sepsis. Two or more organisms are found in 10–20% of cases.

68. **(C)** The patient's clinical picture is suggestive of cardiogenic shock. However, he may still be hypovolemic, because distension of neck veins does not accurately reflect the filling pressures of the heart. A Swan–Ganz catheter should be inserted for appropriate assessment of hemodynamic status and institution of appropriate therapy. Fluid therapy will worsen cardiogenic shock, and Lasix will make the patient hypovolemic. Dopamine will increase blood pressure but is deleterious to the heart. The patient should not be extubated until he is stable.

69. **(C)** Low cardiac output in the presence of elevated filling pressures is characteristic of cardiogenic shock. PCWP is decreased in all the other types of shock.

70. **(D)** Thrombocytopenia is a common complication of heparin therapy. The most common form, type I (seen in up to 30% of patients), is a milder form that occurs after 2–3 days of heparin therapy. The platelet count remains over 50,000/mm³ and has no clinical significance. Type II, seen in 1–2%, usually occurs 7–10 days after heparin treatment. It is immune mediated and can be caused by heparin therapy in any form, in any dose, including heparin flushes and heparin-bonded intravenous catheters. Treatment consists of immediate cessation of heparin administration in any form.

71. (B) The patient has tension pneumothorax, as evidenced by distended neck veins and absent breath sounds. Increased intrathoracic pressure interferes with venous return to the heart, resulting in shock. Immediate management should be insertion of a large-bore needle in the left second intercostal space, followed by insertion of a chest tube. In a trauma patient, venous access should be achieved by inserting two large-bore (16-gauge) angiocatheters in the cubital veins. Insertion of a central venous line on the right side should not be done, because it carries the risk of producing pneumothorax in the opposite side.

72. (D) Institute positive end-expiratory pressure (PEEP). This patient has developed ARDS, which is associated with a significant decrease in functional residual capacity (FCR) of the lungs from collapse of alveoli and increased shunt from perfusion of unventilated alveoli. The most appropriate way to improve his oxygenation is by instituting PEEP.

73. (B) Administration of a depolarizing anesthetic agent such as succinylcholine in quadriplegics, in paraplegics, or after burns and severe trauma can result in life-threatening hyperkalemia from release of intracellular potassium.

74. (C) Dobutamine is the drug of choice for improving cardiac function. It is a β_1-receptor agonist and increases myocardial contractibility and also reduces afterload by β_2 effect. Dopamine at low doses (1–3 µg/kg/min) stimulates dopaminergic receptors and increases renal blood flow. At moderate doses (3–10 µg/kg/min), it stimulates β-receptors, resulting in a positive inotropic and chronotropic effect. Systolic and mean blood pressure are increased; whereas, diastolic blood pressure is usually unchanged. At higher doses (10–20 µg/kg/min), stimulation of α-receptors occurs and it significantly increases SVRI. Norepinephrine, epinephrine, and phenylephrine are powerful vasoconstrictors.

75. (C) The criteria for need for ventilatory support are apnea, respiratory rate greater than 30 breaths per minute, PaO_2 less than 60 mmHg on room air, and $PaCO_2$ greater than 55 mmHg (except in patients with chronic obstructive pulmonary disease [COPD]).

76. (C) vital capacity (VC) 5 mL/kg body weight. See Answer 77.

77. (D) Successful weaning from the ventilator is suggested by the presence of:

a. PaO_2 of 70 mmHg or more with an FIO_2 of 0.35 or less
b. An alveolar arterial gradient of less than 350 mmHg
c. A PaO_2/FIO_2 ratio of greater than 200
d. A $PaCO_2$ of over 30 mmHg and less than 55 mmHg
e. A vital capacity of more than 10–15 mL/kg
f. A maximum negative inspiratory force of more than –25 cm H_2O
g. A minute ventilation of less than 10 L/min
h. A tidal volume of over 5 mL/kg
i. A respiratory rate of less than 30 breaths per minute

78. (B) Patients with SIADH have low urinary output with hyponatremia. Urine-specific gravity or osmolality is increased, urinary excretion of sodium is increased (> 20 mEq/L) and TBW is increased as manifested by low serum osmolality. SIADH is seen after various CNS disorders, in neoplastic disease, in pulmonary diseases, and with some drugs and may be idiopathic.

79. (D) The metabolic response to stress is different to that seen following starvation, as illustrated in Table 2–1.

Table 2–1.

	Starvation	Stress
Resting energy expenditure	Decreased	Increased
Respiratory quotient	(0.6–0.7)	(0.8–0.9)
Mediator activation	NA	+++
Primary fuels	Fat	Mixed
Proteolysis	+	+++
Branched-chain oxidation	+	+++
Hepatic protein synthesis	+	+++
Ureagenesis	+	+++
Urinary nitrogen loss	+	+++
Glucogenesis	+	+++
Ketone body production	++++	+

80. **(D)** Resting energy expenditure is decreased following starvation (e.g., in the patient with pyloric obstruction) and increased after the stress of surgery, trauma, or sepsis. The increase in energy expenditure correlates with the severity of insult being 1.2 times greater after minor operation (e.g., right inguinal herniorrhaphy), 1.35 times greater after skeletal trauma (e.g., fractured femur), 1.60 times greater after major sepsis (e.g., perforated diverticulitis), and 2 times greater after severe thermal burns.

81. **(D)** It is easy to start and administer nutrient requirement rapidly. Parenteral nutrition should be administered when enteral access cannot be obtained, when enteral nutrition support fails to meet nutritional requirements, or when feeding into the GI tract is contraindicated. Current evidence suggests that in addition to safety, convenience, and cost, enteral feeding is well tolerated, preserves gut mucosal mass and normal gut flora, prevents increased gut permeability to bacteria and other toxins, maintains mucosal immunity, and attenuates the hypermetabolic response to surgery. As compared to parenteral nutrition, enteral nutrition is also associated with significantly reduced septic complications. Therefore, enteral feeding is preferred over TPN when feasible.

82. **(C)** It is a major fuel for the gut. It is readily synthesized de novo in skeletal muscle, lung, and liver. Glutamine is a nonessential amino acid. It is not a component of presently available TPN solutions because of its lack of stability. Glutamine is a major fuel for the small intestinal mucosa and other replicating cells such as lymphocytes, macrophages, fibroblasts, and endothelial cells. Glucose is the primary source of fuel for the brain.

83. **(B)** Patients on TPN with hypertonic glucose solutions have elevated islet-cell production of insulin. Sudden cessation of TPN can lead to rebound hypoglycemia, because pancreatic islet-cell insulin secretion is not immediately downregulated. Symptoms are attributable to high catecholamine release secondary to hypoglycemia. In general, the TPN rate should be reduced to 50 mL/h during surgery. This prevents both hypoglycemia and the hyperglycemia seen with higher infusion rates. Weaning from TPN should be done gradually over 24–48 hours. In instances where TPN is discontinued suddenly, a solution of $D_{10}W$ should be administered in the interim.

84. **(C)** Hyperosmolar–nonketotic coma is a serious complication seen when an excessive amount of glucose is given, especially in the presence of sepsis, steroids, or inadequate insulin. Furthermore, the combination of surgery and sepsis results in an increased insulin-resistant state. The increased urine output is secondary to osmolar load from blood glucose. Low CVP, hypernatremia, and BUN-creatinine ratio over 20 suggest hypovolemia and not fluid overload. Normal creatinine level and BUN-creatinine ratio over 20 rules out high-output renal failure. The stress of surgery is characterized by water retention and not diuresis. Management consists of aggressive hydration, discontinuation of TPN, and insulin drip. Insulin drives the potassium intracellularly and potassium must be replaced.

85. **(C)** Glucose infusion should not exceed 4–5mg/kg/min, equivalent to 365–432 g for this patient. The patient is receiving 750 g of glucose. Glucose has a respiratory quotient of 1. Excess glucose results in increased production of CO_2, making it difficult to wean the patient off ventilator. Treatment consists of reducing glucose load and providing fat calories (up to 40% of total calories). Fat has a respiratory quotient of 0.7, resulting in decreased production of CO_2.

86. **(C)** Serum glucagon level is increased. There is hypermetabolism, hypercatabolism, and skeletal muscle proteolysis, resulting in a negative nitrogen balance. The nervous and endocrine systems are mainly involved in regulating the metabolic response to stress of surgery or injury. This response is characterized by substantial increase in the secretion of adrenocorticotropic hormone, cortisol, catecholamine, glucagon, growth hormone, arginine vasopressin (AVP), and angiotensin II. It is also characterized by a reduced secretion of insulin.

87. **(A)** The oxyhemoglobin dissociation curve is a convenient method to study the affinity of hemoglobin for oxygen. It is S-shaped, which provides an efficient method of uptake and release of oxygen. It holds on to the oxygen at high concentrations, and as the blood enters the lower pressures encountered in the capillaries, it releases the oxygen. Hemoglobin is 75% saturated at a Po_2 of 40 mmHg and 50% saturated at a Po_2 of 27 mmHg. At the peripheral tissues, a right or left shift does have a real impact on the affinity of hemoglobin for oxygen. If the S-curve is shifted to the right, there is a decreased affinity of hemoglobin for oxygen (more oxygen is released). A right shift occurs with increase in 2,3-DPG, acidosis, increase in temperature, and increase in hormones (cortisol, thyroid, or aldosterone). A left shift occurs with a decrease in temperature, alkalosis, low DPG, carboxyhemoglobinemia, and old age.

88. **(D)** Discontinuation of aspirin at least 1 week before surgery. Aspirin inactivates platelet cyclo-oxygenase and thus inhibits platelet aggregation. The effect of aspirin is irreversible and lasts for the entire life span of the platelets. Therefore, aspirin should be discontinued for at least 1 week before surgery.

89. **(D)** Intravenous protamine sulfate. The cause of bleeding is circulating heparin. The anticoagulative effect of heparin can be immediately neutralized by intravenous protamine sulfate. One milligram of protamine sulfate usually neutralizes 100 U of heparin. Fresh-frozen plasma is given to counteract the effect of warfarin (Coumadin). Cryoprecipitate is useful in treating patients with hemophilia. Intravenous sodium bicarbonate is indicated after mismatched blood transfusion to alkalinize the urine. Platelet transfusions are necessary to correct dilutional thrombocytopenia seen after massive blood transfusion.

90. **(E)** Decrease is serum potassium from 4.0 and 3.0 mEq/L is associated with a loss of 100 to 200 Eq of total body potassium. Further decrease from 3.0 to 2.0 mEq/L indicates a deficit of 400 to 800 mEq. This patient's total deficit is approximately 380 to 760 mEq/L. $(100 + 400 \times 0.7 \text{ to } 200 + 800 \times 0.7)$.

91. **(A)** Rapid correction of hyponatremia greater than 1–2 mEq/L/h can lead to central ponitine myelionlysis. Serum sodium level should not be raised greater than 25 mEq/L within 48 hours of starting therapy.

92. **(D)** Abnormal hemostasis, common in chronic renal failure, is characterized by prolongation of bleeding time, decreased activity of platelet factor 3, abnormal platelet aggregation and adhesiveness. This can be reversed with desmopressin or cryoprecipitate.

93. **(D)** The coagulation changes can be reversed with desmopressin or cryoprecipitate.

94. **(C)** Daily maintenance fluid requirements are calculated on the basis of 100 mL/kg for the first 10 kg of body weight; 50 mL/kg for the second 10 kg of body weight and 20 mL/kg for each additional kg of body weight (i.e., $100 \times 10 + 50 \times 10 + 20 \times 50 = 2,500$ mL). Hourly fluid requirement can be calculated using the 4, 2, 1 rule as flows: 4 mL/kg, for the first 10 kg, 2 mL/kg for second 10 kg; and 1 mL/kg for each additional kg of body weight (i.e., $4 \times 10 + 2 \times 10 + 1 \times 50 = 110$ mL/h).

95. **(B)** Low molecular weight heparins (LMWH) are fragments of unfractionated standard heparin with mean molecular weights between 4,000 and 64,000 daltons. They bind to and accelerate the activity of antithrombin III. LMWH has greater bioavailability, more effective anticoagulant effect, lower incidence of heparin-associated thrombocytopenia, and can be administered once daily.

96. **(C, E, I)** Zinc deficiency, vitamin A deficiency, and vitamin C deficiency. Zinc is a metalloenzyme involved in protein and nucleic acid metabolism. Deficiency results in diminished wound strength and healing rates. Vitamin A deficiency results in delayed wound healing, specifically epithelization. Vitamin C deficiency results in defective sulfonated mucopolysaccharides and chondroitin sulfate with retarded wound healing.

97. **(B, D)** Chromium is an insulin cofactor. Deficiency state results in hyperglycemia. Manganese is a cofactor of enzyme of energy and protein metabolism and also fat synthesis. Besides causing glucose intolerance, manganese deficiency also causes hypocholesterolemia.

98. **(C)** Zinc is one of the metalloenzymes involved in lipid, carbohydrate, protein, and nucleic acid metabolism. Skin lesions similar to enterohepatic acrodermatitis are the most common signs seen in zinc deficiency. Other manifestations include hypogonadism, diminished wound healing, and immunodeficiencies. Copper deficiency is characterized by microcytic hypochromic anemia.

99. **(B, D)** Factor V and factor VIII are deficient in stored plasma. In contrast, fresh-frozen plasma contains all the coagulation factors. The major disadvantage of plasma administration, however, is the risk of hepatitis.

100. **(C)** There are two coagulation pathways: extrinsic and intrinsic. In the extrinsic system, tissue thromboplastin (a lipoprotein) interacts with factor VII. The intrinsic pathway requires factors XII, XI, IX, and VIII. Factor XII is the initial step in the coagulation cascade. Factor XII, activated by contact with a nonendothelial substance, will activate factor XI (plasma thromboplastin antecedent). However, factor XI can be activated even when factor XII is deficient. Calcium is required for nearly all of the enzyme reactions in both the intrinsic and extrinsic systems. The amount of ionized calcium required for these reactions is extremely small, and clinical hypocalcemia itself is not a cause of abnormal bleeding. Fibrin split products are not part of the normal pathway in either the intrinsic or extrinsic system. The excessive breakdown of fibrinogen results in measurable amounts of the breakdown products of fibrinogen in the blood. Their presence may signal DIC if the PT and platelet count are deranged. In pure fibrinolysis, fibrinogen breakdown product levels also may be increased.

101. **(D, H)** All the coagulation factors except thromboplastin, calcium, and factor VIII are synthesized in the liver. Factors II, VII, IX, and X are vitamin K dependent.

102. **(B)** Disseminated intravascular coagulation (DIC) is characterized by diffuse intravascular coagulation, thrombosis, and fibrinolysis. It results in thrombocytopenia, hypofibrinogenemia, prolongation of PT and PTT, and increased concentration of fibrin degradation products in plasma. Sepsis is a major factor that can trigger DIC.

CHAPTER 3

Stomach, Duodenum, and Esophagus
Questions

Max Goldberg, Simon Wapnick, and John Savino

1. A newborn boy weighs 7 lb and is noted to have distension of the abdomen, which is attributed to a midgut anomaly. What is the abnormality?

   (A) pyloric obstruction
   (B) jejunal atresia
   (C) choledochocoele
   (D) esophageal atresia
   (E) splenic cyst

Questions 2 and 3

A 4-week-old boy presents with projectile vomiting containing no bile. Immediately after vomiting, the child cries excessively for further feeds. After feeding, examination reveals peristaltic waves passing from left to right across the upper abdomen. A mass is palpable in the right upper quadrant (RUQ) during feeding.

2. Select the most likely diagnosis.

   (A) intracranial hemorrhage
   (B) duodenal atresia
   (C) volvulus neonatorium (high intestinal obstruction)
   (D) hypertrophic pyloric stenosis of infants
   (E) esophageal atresia

3. What is the most appropriate treatment for this condition?

   (A) cimetidine and alkalis
   (B) emergency laparotomy and bowel resection
   (C) gastric resection, vagotomy, and pyloroplasty
   (D) antiemetic and atropine for 4 months
   (E) pyloromyotomy

4. A 2-day-old boy has been vomiting since birth and rapidly losing weight. An abdominal x-ray shows a "double bubble" (stomach and duodenum). The vomitus contains bile. What is the most likely diagnosis?

   (A) congenital hypertrophic pyloric stenosis
   (B) duodenal atresia
   (C) intussusception
   (D) esophageal atresia
   (E) Hirschsprung's disease

5. A 45-year-old man complains of classic symptoms of duodenal ulcer. Diagnosis is best confirmed by which of the following?

   (A) basal acid studies and an augmented histamine test
   (B) serum gastrin levels
   (C) barium meal examination
   (D) upper endoscopy
   (E) upper endoscopy, biopsy, and culture for *Helicobacter pylori*

6. A 64-year-old woman with arthritis who has taken nonsteroidal anti-inflammatory drugs (NSAIDs) for several years develops severe abdominal pain. She is informed that she has an ulcer adjacent to the pyloric sphincter. Which is true of the pyloric sphincter in humans?

(A) It cannot be palpated at laparotomy in most cases.
(B) It is not covered completely by omentum.
(C) It is a distinct anatomic entity at operation.
(D) It is a true physiological sphincter.
(E) It is a site where cancer is rare.

7. Which of the following is the best indication for elective surgical therapy in duodenal ulcer disease?

(A) episode of melena in a 30-year-old man
(B) repeated episodes of pain
(C) pyloric outlet obstruction due to stenosis of the duodenal lumen
(D) frequent recurrence of ulcer disease
(E) referral of pain to the back, suggestive of pancreatic penetration

8. A 44-year-old dentist was admitted to the hospital with a 1-day history of hematemesis caused by a recurrent duodenal ulcer. He had shown considerable improvement following operative treatment by truncal vagotomy and pyloroplasty 10 years previously. Which is true of truncal vagotomy?

(A) It can be performed exclusively via the thorax.
(B) It can be performed in the neck.
(C) If complete, it will result in increased acid secretion.
(D) It requires a gastric drainage procedure.
(E) It has been abandoned as a method to treat ulcer disease.

9. A 42-year-old business executive with chronic duodenal ulcer disease was recommended by his attending physician to undergo surgery. Of the various options available, he requested that a parietal (highly selective [superselective]) vagotomy be performed because he learned that,

as compared to gastrectomy, this operation has which outcomes?

(A) It results in a lower incidence of ulcer recurrence.
(B) It benefits patients with antral ulcers the most.
(C) It reduces acid secretion to a greater extent.
(D) It reduces many postoperative complications.
(E) It includes removal of the antrum.

Questions 10 through 13

A 63-year-old woman is admitted to the hospital with severe abdominal pain of 3 hours duration. Examination reveals generalized board-like rigidity, guarding, and rebound tenderness. Her blood pressure is 100/50 mmHg, respiratory rate 30, and pulse 110. She has mild cardiac failure.

10. Before scheduling the operation, the main priority in management is to provide which of the following?

(A) 6 L of intravenous fluids given over 1 hour
(B) antibiotics only
(C) 2 L of hypertonic saline over 2 hours
(D) Swan–Ganz catheter to monitor fluid administration
(E) pH measurements

11. What is the next test requested?

(A) plain supine abdominal x-rays
(B) upright radiograph of the chest
(C) gastrografin swallow
(D) computed Tomogram (CT) of the abdomen
(E) sonography

12. At laparotomy, a large amount of copious fluid is detected in the peritoneal cavity. There is an anterior perforation of a duodenal ulcer. What is the next step in management?

(A) lavage of peritoneal cavity alone
(B) lavage and suture closure of the ulcer

(C) total gastrectomy

(D) lavage, vagotomy, and gastro-enterostomy

(E) laser of ulcer

13. On further questioning, 3 months after recovery from an operation to treat peptic ulcer disease, it is noted that she has had difficulty, in eating a larger meal. A ^{99m}Tc-labeled chicken liver scintigraphy test confirms marked delay in gastric emptying. Delay in gastric emptying may be due to which of the following?

(A) Zollinger–Ellison syndrome

(B) steatorrhea

(C) massive small bowel resection

(D) previous vagotomy

(E) hiatus hernia

14. A 64-year-old director of a supermarket developed diarrhea involving more than 20 bowel movements daily following an elective operation for duodenal ulcer disease. Medication was ineffective. The exact details of the operation could not be ascertained. What is the most likely operation that was performed?

(A) Billroth I gastrectomy and gastro-duodenostomy

(B) gastric surgery combined with cholecystectomy

(C) truncal vagotomy

(D) superselective vagotomy

(E) selective vagotomy

15. A 40-year-old man has had recurrent symptoms suggestive of peptic ulcer disease for 4 years. Gastroscopy reveals an ulcer located in the greater curvature of the stomach and mucosal biopsy reveals H. pylori with a positive rapid urease test (RUT). What is true about H. pylori?

(A) It can be confirmed by serologic tests in the blood.

(B) It is protective against gastric carcinoma.

(C) It is associated with chronic gastritis.

(D) It causes gastric ulcer but not duodenal ulcer.

(E) It can be detected by urea breath test in <60% of cases.

16. A 63-year-old man had a gastrointestinal (GI) study for abdominal pain. The only abnormal finding was in the antrum, where the mucosa prolapsed into the duodenum. There were no abnormal findings on gastroscopy. What should he do?

(A) sleep with his head elevated

(B) be placed on an H_2 antagonist

(C) undergo surgical resection of the antrum

(D) be observed and treated for the pain accordingly

(E) have laser treatment of the antral mucosa

17. A 58-year-old man was admitted to the hospital for severe bilious vomiting following gastric surgery. This occurs in which circumstance?

(A) following ingestion of gaseous fluids

(B) spontaneously

(C) following ingestion of fat foods

(D) following ingestion of bulky meals

(E) in the evening

18. A 63-year-old man underwent gastric resection for severe peptic ulcer disease. He had complete relief of symptoms but developed the "dumping syndrome." This patient is most likely to complain of which of the following?

(A) gastric intussusception

(B) repeated vomiting

(C) severe diarrhea

(D) severe vasomotor symptoms after eating

(E) intestinal obstruction

19. A 64-year-old man was evaluated for moderate protein deficiency; he underwent gastrectomy 20 years earlier. Now he is most likely to show which of the following?

(A) porphyria

(B) hemosiderosis

(C) aplastic anemia

(D) hemolytic anemia

(E) iron-deficiency anemia

20. A 68-year-old woman has been shown to have a benign ulcer located on the greater curvature of the stomach, 5 cm proximal to the antrum. After 3 months of standard medical therapy, she continues to have guaiac-positive stools, anemia, and abdominal pain with failure of the gastric ulcer to heal. Biopsies of the gastric ulcer have not identified malignancy. The next step in management is which of the following?

(A) treatment of the anemia and repeat all studies in 6 weeks

(B) endoscopy and bipolar electrocautery or laser photocoagulation of the gastric ulcer

(C) admission of the patient for total parenteral nutrition (TPN), treatment of anemia, and endoscopic therapy

(D) surgical therapy, including partial gastric resection

(E) surgical therapy, including total gastrectomy

21. A 64-year-old man has had intermittent abdominal pain as a result of duodenal ulcer disease for the past 6 years. Symptoms recurred 6 weeks before admission. He is most likely to be which group?

(A) A and secretor (blood group antigen in body fluids)

(B) B and Lewis antigen

(C) AB

(D) O and nonsecretor

(E) O and secretor

22. Over the past 6 months, a 60-year-old woman with long-standing duodenal ulcer disease has been complaining of anorexia, nausea, weight loss, and repeated vomiting. She recognizes undigested food in the vomitus. Examination and workup reveal dehydration, hypokalemia, and hypochloremic alkalosis. What is the most likely diagnosis?

(A) carcinoma of the fundus

(B) penetrating ulcer

(C) pyloric obstruction due to cicatricial stenosis of the lumen of the duodenum

(D) Zollinger–Ellison syndrome

(E) anorexia nervosa

23. A 50-year-old woman presents with flagrant duodenal ulcer disease and high basal secretory outputs. Secretin stimulated serum gastrin levels in excess of 1,000 pg/mL. She has a long history of ulcer disease that has not responded to intense medical therapy. What is the most likely diagnosis?

(A) hyperparathyroidism

(B) pernicious anemia

(C) renal failure

(D) Zollinger–Ellison syndrome

(E) multiple endocrine adenopathy

24. Investigations of a 43-year-old woman with pluriglandular syndrome were scheduled to determine if a gastrinoma (Zollinger–Ellison syndrome) was present. The serum gastrin level was slightly elevated. Further assessment to establish a diagnosis of Zollinger–Ellison syndrome can be made by repeating the serum gastrin level after stimulation with which of the following?

(A) phosphate

(B) potassium

(C) calcium

(D) chloride

(E) magnesium

25. A 44-year-old man underwent partial resection of the stomach. Following the operation, there was a reduction in serum gastrin levels (Figure 3–1). The site of resection of the stomach that removed the normal source of gastrin is which of the following?

(A) gastroduodenal junction

(B) lower esophagus

(C) pyloric antrum

(D) body of the stomach

(E) fundus of the stomach

26. A 50-year-old man presents with vague gastric complaints. Findings on physical examination are negative. The serum albumin level is markedly reduced—1.8 g/100 mL. Barium x-ray shows massive gastric folds within the proximal stomach. This is confirmed at endoscopy. Which is the correct diagnosis?

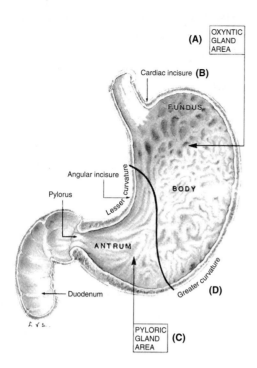

Figure 3–1. Site of gastrin release. (Reproduced, with permission, from Way, LW: Current Surgical Diagnosis & Treatment, 10th ed., Appleton & Lange, 1994.)

(A) hypertrophic pyloric stenosis

(B) gallstone ileus

(C) Mallory–Weiss tear

(D) hypertrophic gastritis (Ménétrier's disease)

(E) Crohn's disease

27. Following admission to the intensive care unit, a 64 year-old female is diagnosed on endoscopy to have acute erosive gastritis "stress" ulcer. Which statement is true of acute erosive gastritis?

(A) Bleeding resulting from acute erosive gastritis has increased dramatically in recent years.

(B) It is treated initially by H_2 receptor antagonists alone.

(C) Treatment by sucralfate offers protection even in an acid environment.

(D) On gastrocopy, it shows lesions noted initially in the antrum.

(E) Gastrectomy procedures are contra-indicated.

28. A 70-year-old woman is diagnosed, by barium examination, as having a 2-cm ulcer on the greater curvature of the stomach. Gastric analysis to maximal acid stimulation shows achlorhydria. What is the next step in management?

(A) antacid, H_2 blockers, and repeat x-ray in 6–8 weeks

(B) proton pump inhibitor (omeprazole [Prilosec]) and repeat x-ray in 6–8 weeks

(C) prostaglandin E (misoprostol [Cytotec]) and repeat x-ray in 6–8 weeks

(D) immediate elective surgery

(E) gastroscopy with multiple biopsies (at least 8 or 9) of the ulcer

29. The most appropriate treatment for a persistent gastric lesser curvature ulcer in a patient whose condition has failed to respond to intensive medical treatment over a 3-month period is which of the following?

(A) treatment with H_2 blockers

(B) vagotomy alone without additional surgery

(C) endoscopy and laser treatment of the ulcer

(D) distal gastrectomy (Billroth I—gastroduodenal anastomosis)

(E) elevating the head of the bed when asleep

30. A 63-year-old woman complains of abdominal discomfort, anorexia, and a 10-lb weight loss over a 3-month period. Endoscopy reveals a polypoid lesion in the gastric antrum. She is informed that she has "early gastric cancer." Why?

(A) because it involves only the mucous membrane and does not invade the muscularis or the muscular wall of the stomach

(B) because this is demonstrable on barium x-ray

(C) because this has a 5-year survival rate of 5%

(D) because surgery always cures it

(E) because this does not require tumor-free margins when resected

31. Which statement is true of gastric cancer?

    (A) It is increasing in frequency in the United States.
    (B) Its incidence is greater than in the colon.
    (C) It infrequently causes severe epigastric pain on presentation.
    (D) It results in a palpable epigastric mass in about one-half of cases.
    (E) If bulky and polypoid, it usually occurs in the antrum.

32. A 62-year-old man presents with guaiac-positive stools. He is otherwise asymptomatic. Workup reveals an ulcerating carcinoma, 2 cm in diameter, situated on the antral lesser curvature. Tumor markers are negative. A CT scan is negative for metastatic disease. Liver function tests are normal. What is the correct treatment for this patient?

    (A) chemotherapy
    (B) radiotherapy
    (C) combination of chemotherapy and radiotherapy
    (D) total gastrectomy
    (E) distal subtotal gastrectomy with wide dissection of the lymphatic drainage area

33. A 55-year-old man complains of abdominal discomfort, tiredness, and anorexia. He has lost 20 lbs over the last 4 months. The contrast barium study showed an ulcer at the incisura. Endoscopy and biopsy confirm the diagnosis of carcinoma of the stomach. Where is the incisura located?

    (A) cardia
    (B) fundus
    (C) greater curvature
    (D) lesser curvature
    (E) gastrocolic ligament

34. A 36-year-old man presents with weight loss and a large palpable tumor in the upper abdomen. Endoscopy reveals an intact gastric mucosa without signs of carcinoma and multiple biopsies show normal gastric mucosa. Barium x-ray demonstrates a mass in the stomach. At surgery, a 3-kg mass is removed by partial gastrectomy. It is necessary to remove the left side of the transverse colon. What is the most likely diagnosis?

    (A) gastric cancer
    (B) leiomyosarcoma
    (C) choledochoduodenal fistula
    (D) eosinophilic gastroenteritis
    (E) linitis plastica

35. A 74-year-old man presents with an isolated non-Hodgkin's lymphoma of the stomach. What is the usual therapy?

    (A) chemotherapy alone
    (B) immunotherapy
    (C) radiation and chemotherapy
    (D) surgery, radiation, and chemotherapy
    (E) surgery alone

36. A 63-year-old woman is admitted to the hospital with upper GI bleeding that subsides spontaneously within a short time after admission. Barium examination shows gastric ulceration that is described by the radiologist as a "doughnut sign." What is the most likely diagnosis?

    (A) lipoma
    (B) gastric ulcer
    (C) ectopic pancreas
    (D) leiomyoma
    (E) carcinoma

37. A 50-year-old woman is found, on gastroscopy and biopsies, to have multiple hyperplastic polyps in the stomach. How are these best treated?

    (A) total gastrectomy
    (B) partial gastrectomy
    (C) staged endoscopic removal after brushing for cytological examination
    (D) ablation by laser
    (E) no treatment other than repeated endoscopic and multiple-brush biopsies

38. During a routine surveillance gastroscopy, a 35-year-old woman who was successfully treated for multiple familial polyposis of the colon is found to have several polyps in the

gastric antrum. Biopsies show adenomatous polyps. What is the best therapy?

(A) observation and repeated gastroscopy at frequent intervals

(B) antrectomy

(C) endoscopic polypectomies with repeat endoscopies to monitor subsequent polyp development

(D) endoscopic laser ablation of the polyps

(E) total gastrectomy to remove all existing and potential future polyps

39. A 64-year-old woman presents with severe upper abdominal pain and retching of 1 day's duration. Attempts to pass a nasogastric tube are unsuccessful. Plain x-rays show an air–fluid level in the left side of the chest in the posterior mediastinum, behind the heart. Strangulated paraesophageal hernia and gastric volvulus is diagnosed. What is the next step in management?

(A) insertion of weighted bougie to untwist the volvulus

(B) elevation of the head of the bed

(C) placing patient in Trendelenburg position with the head of the bed lowered

(D) laparotomy and vagotomy

(E) surgery, reduction of the gastric volvulus, and repair of the hernia

40. A 78-year-old woman undergoes an uncomplicated minor surgical procedure, under local anesthesia. At the completion of the operation, she suddenly develops pallor, sweating, bradycardia, hypotension, abdominal pain, and gastric distension. What is the next step in management?

(A) rapid infusion of 3 L of Ringer's lactate

(B) digoxin

(C) insertion of a nasogastric tube

(D) morphine

(E) neostigmine

41. Which of the following predisposes towards gastric carcinoma?

(A) hypersecretory chronic gastritis (Type B)

(B) autoimmune chronic gastritis (Type A)

(C) Menetrier's disease

(D) duodenal ulcer

(E) hiatus hernia

42. A 60-year-old woman remains partly stuporous for 3 weeks following a motor vehicle accident. She had two episodes of aspiration pneumonia associated with an indwelling nasogastric tube. It is anticipated that she will not be able to eat for at least a further 3 months. She should have which of the following?

(A) gastrostomy performed by endoscopic technique

(B) the nasogastric tube changed once

(C) the nasogastric tube changed daily

(D) a feeding jejunostomy

(E) gastrostomy performed under general anesthesia using a Foley catheter

43. A 48-year-old man undergoes surgery for chronic duodenal ulcer. At operation, he undergoes truncal vagotomy and which of the following?

(A) gastroenterostomy

(B) removal of the duodenum

(C) closure of the esophageal hiatus

(D) routine appendectomy

(E) no further operation

44. A 75-year-old patient, in good physical health, suffers from persistent bleeding from a duodenal ulcer. Medical management and endoscopic measures fail to stop the bleeding. What is the next step in management?

(A) a further trial of transfusion of 8 U of blood

(B) administration of norepinephrine

(C) oversew of the bleeding point

(D) oversew of the bleeding point and vagotomy and pyloroplasty

(E) hepatic arterial ligation

45. Following removal of the antrum, what will happen to the serum gastrin level?

    (A) It will increase slightly.
    (B) It will remain the same.
    (C) It will fall.
    (D) It will become zero.
    (E) It will increase markedly.

46. A 60-year-old woman undergoes vagotomy and pyloroplasty for duodenal ulcer disease. Gallstones are noted at the time of the original operation. Eight days following surgery, she develops abdominal pain and right upper quadrant tenderness. To determine if the gallbladder is the cause of the symptoms, she should undergo which of the following?

    (A) supine x-ray
    (B) hepatobiliary scan (HIDA or DESIDA)
    (C) ultrasound
    (D) erect x-ray
    (E) intravenous cholangiography

47. The most common site of GI sarcomas is which of the following?

    (A) esophagus
    (B) stomach
    (C) jejunum
    (D) ileum
    (E) colon

48. A 38-year-old woman is admitted to the hospital with hematemesis. At gastroscopy, she is noted to have a small antral mass. Biopsy reveals sarcoma. What does she require?

    (A) fulguration of the tumor
    (B) distal gastrectomy
    (C) laser therapy and postoperative radiotherapy
    (D) chemotherapy alone
    (E) total gastrectomy

49. A 67-year-old woman complains of paresthesia in the limbs, and examination shows loss of vibration, position sense, and light touch in the lower limbs. She is found to have pernicious anemia. Endoscopy reveals an ulcer in the body of the stomach. What does she most likely have?

    (A) excess of vitamin B_{12}
    (B) deficiency of vitamin K
    (C) cancer of the stomach
    (D) gastric sarcoma
    (E) esophageal varices

Questions 50 and 51

A 79-year retired opera singer presents with dysphagia, which has become progressively worse during the past 5 years. He states that he is sometimes aware of a lump on the left side of his neck and gurgling sounds during swallowing. He sometimes regurgitates food during eating.

50. What is the likely diagnosis?

    (A) carcinoma of the esophagus
    (B) foreign body in the esophagus
    (C) Plummer–Vinson (Kelly–Patterson) syndrome
    (D) pharyngoesophageal diverticulum
    (E) scleroderma

51. The next step in management following a barium swallow test would most likely include which of the following?

    (A) H_2-blockers
    (B) anticholinergic drugs
    (C) elemental diet
    (D) bougienage
    (E) Surgery—cricopharyngeal myotomy and diverticulectomy

52. An epiphrenic diverticulum may be associated with which of the following?

    (A) duodenal ulcer
    (B) gastric ulcer
    (C) cancer of the tongue
    (D) cancer of the lung
    (E) hiatal hernia

53. A 64-year-old man develops increasing dysphagia over many months. A barium-swallow

study is performed. What is the most likely cause of his clinical presentation?

(A) carcinoma of the esophagus

(B) achalasia

(C) sliding hiatal hernia

(D) paraesophageal hernia

(E) esophageal diverticulum

54. A 63-year-old woman from Norway, visiting the United States, presents with dysphagia. On endoscopy, an esophageal web is identified, and the diagnosis of Plummer–Vinson syndrome is established. What would be the next step in the management?

(A) esophagostomy

(B) dilation of the web and iron therapy

(C) esophagectomy

(D) gastric bypass of the esophagus

(E) cortisone

55. A 53-year-old moderately obese woman presents with heartburn aggravated mainly by eating and lying down in the horizontal position. Her symptoms are suggestive of gastroesophageal reflux disease (GERD). Which of the following statements is true?

(A) It is best diagnosed by an anteroposterior (AP) and lateral film of the chest.

(B) It may be alleviated by certain drugs, especially theophylline, diazepam, and calcium-channel blockers.

(C) It may be relieved by smoking.

(D) If associated with dysphagia, it suggests a stricture or motility disorder.

(E) It should immediately be treated surgically.

56. A 64-year-old man has had symptoms of reflux esophagitis for 20 years. The barium study below (Figure 3–2) shows a sliding hiatal hernia. Which is true in sliding esophageal hernia?

(A) A hernia sac is absent.

(B) The cardia is displaced into the posterior mediastinum.

(C) Reflux esophagitis always occurs.

(D) A stricture does not develop.

(E) Surgery should always be avoided.

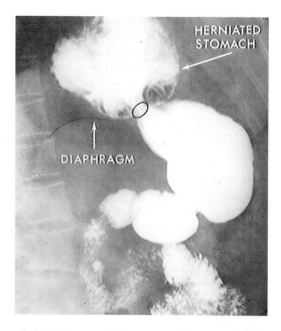

Figure 3–2. Large sliding hiatal hernia. Diaphragmatic hiatis is encircled. (Reproduced, with permission, from Way, LW: Current Surgical Diagnosis & Treatment, 10th ed., Appleton & Lange, 1994.)

57. A 45-year-old man presents with a long history of heartburn, especially at night. He uses three pillows and has medicated himself with a variety of antacids over the past 15 years. Recently, he has been complaining of dysphagia, which he localizes to the lower precordial area. Which is the most likely diagnosis?

(A) adenocarcinoma of the esophagus

(B) angina pectoris

(C) benign peptic stricture of the esophagus

(D) achalasia of the esophagus

(E) lower esophageal ring (Schatzki's ring)

58. A 45-year-old man presents with dysphagia, which has become more severe in the past few months. He noted that his complaints of heartburn, which had troubled him for 20 years, had also been alleviated recently during the similar time period that the dysphagia had worsened. Diagnosis based upon GI series, endoscopy, and biopsy indicates that the most likely cause is benign esophageal stricture. He has not been on any medications other than antiacid secretory drugs. *H. pylori* are absent from gastric mucosal examination. The results of esophageal manometry are normal. What is true in benign esophageal stricture?

(A) Dilation therapy should be avoided.

(B) Surgical therapy consists of an antireflux operation with pre- and postoperative dilation of the stricture.

(C) Emergency esophagectomy is required.

(D) The stricture is due to liver cirrhosis.

(E) Most peptic strictures are located in the upper esophagus.

59. A 54-year-old man presents with dysphagia, heartburn, belching, and epigastric pain. Barium swallow shows a sliding hiatal hernia and a stricture situated higher than usual in the midesophagus. Barium swallow and endoscopy findings are reported as Barrett's esophagus (ectopic gastric epithelium lining the esophagus). Marked esophagitis with linear ulcerations are noted at esophagoscopy. Biopsy shows columnar epithelium at the affected area and normal squamous epithelium above, confirming the diagnosis. What statement is true regarding this condition?

(A) Adenocarcinoma is less common in Barret's esophagus.

(B) Most patients do not have associated gastroesophageal reflux.

(C) The presence of ectopic gastric lining protects against aspiration during sleep, and prevents recurrent pneumonitis.

(D) The present treatment is aimed at preventing esophagitis.

(E) When strictures form, they are always malignant.

60. A 75-year-old woman presents with a para-esophageal hiatal "rolling" hernia. Diagnosis is made by radiologic studies, as shown in Figure 3–3. What can this patient be told about paraesophageal hernias?

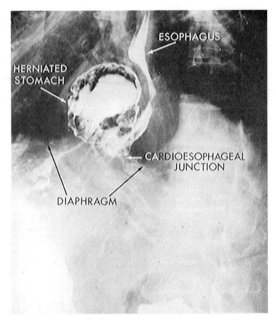

Figure 3–3. Paraesophageal hernia. (Reproduced, with permission, from Way, LW: Current Surgical Diagnosis & Treatment, 10th ed., Appleton & Lange, 1994.)

(A) They constitute about 50% of all esophageal hiatal hernias and are more common in women over the age of 60.

(B) They cause the gastroesophageal junction to become displaced from its normal position below to above the diaphragm.

(C) They prevent herniation of stomach and intestine above the diaphragm.

(D) They may result in rotation and strangulation of the stomach, gastric ulcer, and bleeding.

(E) They are treated medically with attention to diet, position during sleep, antacids and omeprazole [H^+/K^+ adenosine triphosphatase (ATP-ase) pump inhibitor].

61. A 52-year-old gastroenterologist suffers from intermittent dysphagia attributed to the presence of a lower esophageal stricture (Schatzki's ring). The doctor's condition is characterized by which of the following?

   (A) a full-thickness scar in the upper esophagus
   (B) symptoms of mild to moderate dysphagia
   (C) a low incidence in men
   (D) the absence of a sliding hiatal hernia in most cases
   (E) the need for antireflux surgery at an early stage

62. A 54-year-old female clerk complains of having had dysphagia for 15 years. The clinical diagnosis of achalasia is established on barium swallow. What is true in this condition?

   (A) The most common symptom is dysphagia.
   (B) In the early stages, dysphagia is more pronounced for solids than for liquids.
   (C) The incidence of sarcoma is increased.
   (D) Recurrent pulmonary infections are rare.
   (E) Endoscopic dilation should be avoided.

63. A 69-year-old man is admitted to the emergency department with acute upper GI hemorrhage following a bout of repeated vomiting. Fiberoptic gastroscopy reveals three linear mucosal tears at the gastroesophageal junction. What is the diagnosis?

   (A) reflux esophagitis with ulceration
   (B) Barrett's esophagus
   (C) carcinoma of the esophagus
   (D) Mallory–Weiss lesion
   (E) scleroderma

Questions 64 and 65

A 50-year-old man presents with excruciating pain. The pain follows an episode of violent vomiting that occurred after a heavy meal. Subcutaneous emphysema was noted in the neck. Plain x-rays showed air in the mediatinum and neck and a fluid level in the left pleural cavity.

64. What is the most likely diagnosis?

   (A) perforated duodenal ulcer
   (B) spontaneous rupture of the esophagus
   (C) spontaneous pneumothorax
   (D) inferior-wall myocardial infarction
   (E) dissecting aortic aneurysm

65. What should be the next step in management?

   (A) administration of intravenous antibiotics and TPN
   (B) administration of intravenous antibiotics and TPN plus insertion of a chest tube and nasogastric tube
   (C) insertion of a nasogastric tube with intravenous antibiotics and administration of TPN
   (D) emergency surgery either by laparotomy or thoracotomy
   (E) resuscitation; administration of antibiotics, fluids, and electrolytes; and, if necessary, blood transfusion to improve the patient's general condition, followed by elective operation when the general status of the patient improves

66. In evaluating findings of the CT scan of the superior mediastinum at the lower border of T4 level, which structure is remote from the esophagus?

   (A) trachea
   (B) recurrent laryngeal nerves
   (C) aorta
   (D) azygos vein
   (E) brachiocephalic vein

67. A full-term newborn boy regurgitates initial feedings. X-rays confirm the presence of atresia of the upper third of the esophagus. The mother is anxious and inquires about her baby's condition. What should she be informed about congenital atresia of the esophagus?

(A) It frequently is associated with an esophagorespiratory tract fistula.

(B) It is one of the rarest anomalies of the esophagus.

(C) It may be associated with a fistula that communicates mostly between the esophagus and the skin surface.

(D) It is usually associated with cystic fibrosis.

(E) It is mostly nontreatable.

68. A 69-year-old male is informed that the cause of his dysphagia is a benign lesion. The barium-swallow study is shown in Figure 3–4. What should he be informed about benign tumors and cysts of the esophagus?

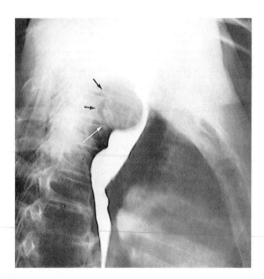

Figure 3–4. Note smooth rounded density causing extrinsic compression of esophageal lumen. (Reproduced, with permission, from Way, LW: Current Surgical Diagnosis & Treatment, 10th ed., Appleton & Lange, 1994.)

(A) They occur more commonly than malignant tumors.

(B) They are symptomatic at an early stage.

(C) Diagnosis is best confirmed on chest x-ray.

(D) Leiomyoma is by far the most common benign tumor encountered in the esophagus.

(E) Malignant transformation of a benign leiomyoma into a malignant leiomyosarcoma is common.

69. In severe reflux esophagitis, lower esophageal sphincter (LES) is decreased. Physiologically, this may be increased by which of the following?

(A) pregnancy

(B) acetylcholine

(C) gastrin

(D) secretin

(E) glucagon

70. A 28-year-old executive director complains of mild chest pain and dysphagia of several months duration. Manometric studies indicate diffuse esophageal spasm DES. What is true regarding DES?

(A) It usually occurs in individuals who have an emotional overlay.

(B) It is similar to the nutcracker esophagus.

(C) Manometry confirms low-amplitude contractions.

(D) The lower esophageal sphincter fails to relax.

(E) It usually requires esophagectomy.

71. A 46-year-old man had a long history of heartburn (GERD). His x-ray showed an irregular, ulcerated area in the lower third of the esophagus. There are marked mucosal disruption and overhanging edges. What is the most likely diagnosis?

(A) sliding hiatal hernia with GERD

(B) paraesophageal hernia

(C) benign esophageal stricture

(D) squamous carcinoma of the esophagus

(E) adenocarcinoma arising in a Barret's esophagus

72. A 46-year-old man presents with dysphagia of recent onset. His esophagram shows a lesion in the lower third of the esophagus, which, on biopsy, proves to be an adenocarcinoma. His general medical condition is excellent, and his metastatic workup findings are negative. What should he undergo?

(A) chemotherapy

(B) radiotherapy

(C) insertion of a wide esophageal tube to improve swallowing

(D) surgical resection of the esophagus

(E) a combination of chemotherapy and radiotherapy

73. An 8-lb newborn boy has severe respiratory distress with gasping immediately after birth. An x-ray of the chest reveals a left solid area with the heart displaced to the right. Diagnosis of congenital diaphragmatic (pericardioperitoneal [Bochdalek]) hernia is established. What should the treatment be?

(A) nasal oxygen

(B) controlled endotracheal ventilation

(C) nasogastric feeding

(D) expansion of the lung by positive pressure above 50 cm H_2O

74. A 25-year-old man is admitted to the emergency department in respiratory distress following an automobile accident. Among other findings, chest x-rays show abdominal viscera in the left hemithorax. What is the most likely diagnosis?

(A) traumatic rupture of the diaphragm

(B) sliding esophageal hernia

(C) short esophagus with intrathoracic stomach

(D) rupture of the esophagus

(E) Bochdalek hernia

75. In preparing for surgery for resection of a cancer of the esophagus, what does the surgeon note about this organ?

(A) It receives its arterial supply from the pulmonary trunk.

(B) It partly drains into the left gastric (coronary) vein.

(C) It drains into the suprarenal glands.

(D) It commences at the level of the fourth thoracic vertebra.

(E) It is innervated by the phrenic nerve.

76. A 44-year-old woman has lost 12 lb over 3 months. She complains of abdominal distension and fullness. At laparotomy, she has extensive thickening around the loops of small and large intestine. Frozen section confirms the diagnosis of pseudomyxoma peritonei. What is true in this condition?

(A) It is a malignant lesion.

(B) It spreads by the bloodstream.

(C) It may arise from an ovarian mucinous carcinoma.

(D) It may arise from a pleomorphic adenoma.

(E) It is treated by irradiation and wide small-bowel resection.

77. A 32-year-old man undergoes laparotomy for trauma due to multiorgan injuries. He is discharged after 2 weeks in the hospital only to be readmitted 3 days later because of abdominal pain and sepsis. The CT scan shows an accumulation of fluid in the subhepatic space (Figure 3–5). This space is likely to be directly involved following an injury to which of the following?

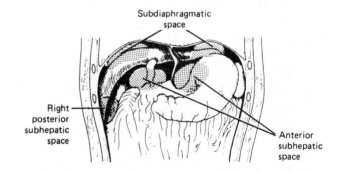

Figure 3–5. Subhepatic space; anterior view. (Reproduced, with permission, from Way, LW: Current Surgical Diagnosis & Treatment, 10th ed., Appleton & Lange, 1994.)

(A) inferior pole of the right kidney

(B) stomach

(C) uncinate process of the pancreas

(D) aortic bifurcation

(E) right psoas muscle

Questions 78 and 79

A 38-year-old male came home and found his wife with a stranger in the bedroom. In a rage, he fatally stabbed her. He attempted suicide by ingesting drain cleaner fluid. The police admitted him to the emergency room of the local hospital.

78. What should be done in his management?

    (A) Copious neutralizing (acid) solutions should be given.
    (B) Emetics should be administered.
    (C) One can anticipate that stricture formation is inevitable.
    (D) Oral fluid and solid feeds can usually be commenced several days after the injury.
    (E) Esophagoscopy should be performed to visualize the distal end of the lesion.

79. On the day following admission to hospital, he is noted to have severe chest pain, and on palpation, subcutaneous crepitus is detected in the neck. His pulse is 120 per minute, and a chest x-ray shows widening of the mediastinum with pleural effusion. What is found in evaluating his condition?

    (A) He most likely has a rupture of the arch of the aorta.
    (B) Alkali solutions usually cause coagulation necrosis.
    (C) Esophageal perforation has occurred.
    (D) He has no esophageal lesions, because the oropharynx has minimal changes.

80. Following emergency operation for severe hypotension caused by hepatic and splenic trauma, the surgeon inserts a finger in the foramen of Winslow (epiploic, omental) in an attempt to reduce bleeding. What is true of the hepatic artery?

    (A) It is called common hepatic at this level.
    (B) It is on the left of the common bile duct and anterior to the portal vein.
    (C) It is posterior to the portal vein.
    (D) It is posterior to the inferior vena cava.
    (E) It forms the superior margin of the foramen epiploic.

Questions 81 and 82

A 44-year-old patient develops a mass on the anterior abdominal wall. He notes that the swelling has gradually increased in size over the past 3 months. On examination, the lesion was palpated as a 5- × 8-cm mass in the left iliac fossa and hypogastrium.

81. Which test will help establish whether the tumor arises from the abdominal wall or the abdominal cavity?

    (A) needle biopsy
    (B) ability to elicit a cough impulse
    (C) transillumination
    (D) examination of the mass with the patient in the prone position
    (E) examination of the mass with the patient instructed to attempt sitting up

82. The histology of the tumor is reported as sarcoma. What is the most likely diagnosis?

    (A) synovial sarcoma
    (B) malignant fibrous histiosarcoma
    (C) liposarcoma
    (D) leiomyosarcoma
    (E) rhabdomyosarcoma

DIRECTIONS (Questions 83 through 100): Each set of matching questions in this section consists of a list of lettered options followed by several numbered items. For each numbered item, select the appropriate lettered option(s). Each lettered option may be selected once, more than once, or not at all. EACH ITEM WILL STATE THE NUMBER OF OPTIONS TO SELECT. CHOOSE EXACTLY THIS NUMBER.

Question 83

    (A) It decreases basal (baseline) acid.
    (B) It causes basal acid to remain constant.
    (C) It causes basal acid to rise substantially within 1 hour.
    (D) It causes rise in basal acid after a latent period of 6 hours.
    (E) It causes fall and then rise in basal acid.
    (F) It passes into the portal system to the stomach and intestinal mucosa.

(G) It will promote healing of peptic ulcer.

(H) It involves a potent enzyme.

83. What does the release of gastrin do? SELECT ONLY TWO.

Questions 84 through 86

(A) blood group B

(B) gastric remnant following distal gastrectomy

(C) corrosive gastritis

(D) lipoma of the stomach

(E) pernicious anemia

(F) ampullary cancer

(G) lymphosarcoma

(H) ectopic pancreas

(I) gastric volvulus

(J) acute gastric dilation

(K) adenomatous gastric polyps

84. What is considered as predisposing to gastric cancer? SELECT ONLY THREE.

85. What causes vasovagal attack following anesthesia? SELECT ONLY ONE.

86. During laparotomy, an incidental nonepithelial benign tumor in the stomach is found. SELECT ONLY TWO.

Questions 87 and 88

(A) hypertrophic pyloric stenosis

(B) hemangioma

(C) neurofibromatosis

(D) adenomatous gastric polyps

(E) chordoma

(F) teratoma

(G) leiomyosarcoma

(H) epulis

(I) lymphosarcoma

(J) linitis plastica

(K) hypoalbuminemia

(L) ampullary carcinoma

87. A 46-year-old man has remained free of recurrent disease following total colectomy 24 years ago for familial adenomatous polyposis. He now presents with undulating obstructive jaundice of 1 month's duration and guaiac-positive stools. He does not have calculus disease. What is the diagnosis? SELECT ONLY ONE.

88. Long-term survival of malignant alimentary tract tumor with involvement of surrounding organs is found. What is the diagnosis? SELECT ONLY ONE.

Question 89

(A) blood group AB

(B) Lewis antigen

(C) excess of pepsinogen

(D) excess gastrin

(E) excess of gastrin volume

(F) RH compatibility

(G) blood group A

(H) blood group antigen in tissue fluids

(I) Blood group O

89. What does secretor status imply? SELECT ONLY ONE.

Questions 90 through 92

(A) acid secretion

(B) reduced rate of back diffusion of hydrogen ions

(C) H_2 blockers

(D) mucus and alkaline secretion

(E) submucosal edema

(F) serum B_{12} levels

(G) gastric mucosal blood flow

(H) acute erosive gastritis

(I) antacids

(J) gastric lavage

(K) obstructive jaundice

(L) Mallory–Weiss tear of the cardioesophageal junction

90. A critically ill 50-year-old man, suffering from multiple trauma as a result of a traffic accident, begins to bleed massively from the stomach 2 days after hospital admission. What is the probable cause? SELECT ONLY ONE.

91. What does the pathogenesis of erosive gastritis involve? SELECT ONLY THREE.

92. What is the initial treatment of bleeding from erosive gastritis? SELECT ONLY THREE.

Question 93

   (A) gastric ulcer
   (B) hiatal hernia
   (C) duodenal ulcer
   (D) Mallory–Weiss tear
   (E) gastric carcinoma
   (F) esophagitis
   (G) achalasia
   (H) esophageal atresia

93. What is the most likely cause of bleeding in a patient presenting to the hospital with hematemesis? SELECT ONLY TWO.

Questions 94 and 95

A 33-year-old man is admitted for diagnosis and treatment of a gastrojejunal ulcer. At age 25, he was treated surgically by omental patch for perforated duodenal ulcer. At 30, he was treated by truncal vagotomy and antrectomy for a chronic duodenal ulcer. He now has a stomal (gastrojejunal) ulcer that is refractory to medical therapy.

   (A) serum gastrin level
   (B) acid secretion
   (C) H₂-blockers
   (D) intrinsic factor
   (E) cortisone
   (F) adrenaline
   (G) *H. pylori*
   (H) prostaglandin E (misoprostol [cytotec])

94. Which is the item that, although effective in protecting the gastric mucosa, has not proved useful in management of erosive gastritis, because of its diarrheal side effect. SELECT ONLY ONE.

95. Which facts are relevant? SELECT ONLY TWO.

Questions 96 through 98

   (A) acid secretion
   (B) submucosal islet cells
   (C) serum gastrin levels
   (D) H₂ blockers
   (E) prostaglandin E (misoprostol [Cytotec])
   (F) proton pump inhibitors (omeprazole [Prilosec])
   (G) acute erosive gastritis
   (H) chronic duodenal ulcer
   (I) *H. pylori*
   (J) serum glucose
   (K) endoscopy, bipolar electrocautery, or laser
   (L) photocoagulation
   (M) urgent gastric surgery
   (N) triple therapy with antibiotics (e.g., biaxin or tetracycline, metronidazole, and bismuth subsalicylate)
   (O) elective gastric surgery

96. A 73-year-old woman is admitted with mild upper GI hemorrhage, which stops spontaneously. She did not require transfusion. She has ingested large amounts of aspirin in the past 4 months to relieve the pain caused by severe rheumatoid arthritis. Endoscopy confirms the presence of a duodenal ulcer. Cultures were taken. What are the next steps in the management of duodenal ulcer with a positive culture for *H. pylori*? SELECT ONLY TWO.

97. What are the most important causes of duodenal ulcer other than *H. pylori*? SELECT ONLY TWO.

98. Bleeding from the ulcer commences and cannot be controlled by attempts at both local endoscopic therapy and vigorous, conservative therapy. What is the next step in therapy? SELECT ONE.

Question 99

    (A) It is safe to leave cancer at cut edges.

    (B) There is a favorable response to radio-therapy.

    (C) The 5-year survival rate is about 12%.

    (D) There is an increased rate in patients with duodenal ulcer.

    (E) There is an increased rate in patients with gastric ulcer.

    (F) Drainage lymph nodes should not be extensively removed.

    (G) It is associated with hyperchlorhydria.

    (H) It is caused by diverticulitis.

99. Which statement is true regarding gastric cancer? SELECT TWO

Question 100

    (A) central hyperalimentation

    (B) intralipids 3 L daily

    (C) percutaneous endoscopic gastrostomy

    (D) nasogastric feeding

    (E) glucose 10%, 4 L IV daily

    (F) peripheral hyperalimentation

    (G) gastrojejunostomy

    (H) cervical esophagostomy

    (I) rectal feeding

100. What treatment should a nursing-home patient who is alert but has weight loss caused by permanent neurologic disease that interferes with swallowing receive? SELECT ONLY ONE.

Answers and Explanations

1. **(B)** There are three major divisions of the alimentary tract during fetal development. The foregut is supplied by the celiac vessels (cardia to ampulla of Vater), the midgut by superior mesenteric vessels (ampulla of Vater to distal transverse colon), and the hindgut by the inferior mesenteric vessels (distal transverse colon to lower anus). The duodenum beyond the ampulla of Vater arises from the midgut.

2. **(D)** The clinical diagnosis rests on the findings of vomiting, visible peristalsis, and the presence of a lump in the right upper abdomen. Male infants are most commonly affected between the 3rd and 6th weeks of life. The vomitus does not contain bile.

3. **(E)** Infants born with hypertrophic pyloric stenosis rarely have symptoms immediately after birth and are more likely to have projectile vomiting between the 4th and 6th weeks of life. Examination may reveal a hard, small mass (due to pyloric hypertrophy) in the right upper abdomen close to the midline. Pyloromyotomy (not pyloroplasty) is the operation of choice. Milder cases have been treated by spasmolytic drugs if surgery is not undertaken.

4. **(B)** There is stenosis of the duodenum, usually in the region of the ampulla of Vater. Frequently, there are other congenital defects. Vomiting occurs from birth and contains bile, in contradistinction to congenital pyloric stenosis, which occurs at a later stage. The classic x-ray finding is the "double bubble." Treatment is by duodenojejunostomy. Annular pancreas and an abnormal (Ladd) band associated with malrotation may also present with a "dou-

ble bubble" on x-ray. In a newborn infant the "double bubble" sign may be an entirely normal feature within the first 12 hours after birth.

5. **(E)** Upper endoscopy is the most accurate diagnostic method. The presence of *H. pylori* is an indication to prescribe appropriate therapy that may include Biaxin, metranidazole, bismut subsalicylate, and drugs to reduce acid secretion. *H. pylori* can also be detected by the rapid urea test (RUT) of the mucosal biopsy and the urea breath test.

6. **(C)** It is palpable at laparotomy but is not a true physiological sphincter, because it does not show reciprocal contraction when the rest of the stomach relaxes or relaxation when the stomach undergoes contraction.

7. **(C)** Following appropriate correction of fluid and electrolyte balance and nutrition, treatment is nearly always surgical. Intractable pain is less commonly considered an indication for surgery. Noncompliance with medical therapy is often the cause of failure to show improvement.

8. **(D)** If vagotomy alone is performed, gastric stasis occurs in more than 40% of cases. Although truncal vagotomy can be performed via the supradiaphragmatic approach, it would be necessary to add a drainage procedure (e.g., pyloroplasty) by an abdominal incision. In the neck, accidental severance of the vagus would result in recurrent laryngeal nerve palsy.

9. **(D)** In highly selective vagotomy (Figure 3–6), the nerve supply to the muscle of the pyloric

Truncal   Selective   Parietal cell (highly selective)

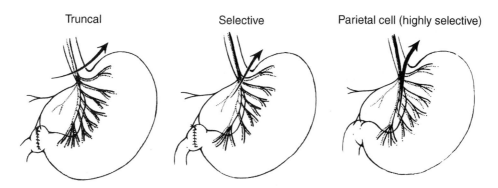

Figure 3–6. Various types of vagotomy currently popular for treating duodenal ulcer disease. (Reproduced, with permission, from Way, LW: Current Surgical Diagnosis & Treatment, 10th ed., Appleton & Lange, 1994.)

antrum is left intact. The branches of the vagus nerves that supply the parietal cell mass are all meticulously divided, leaving the main anterior and posterior nerves of Latarjet intact. The main vagal trunks are left intact, thus also sparing the nerve supply to the liver and gallbladder and to the pancreas and intestine. To improve completeness of the procedure, great care is taken to divide the proximal (criminal) nerve of Grassi. Because the antral nerves are left intact, drainage procedures are not required.

10. (D) It is important to rehydrate patients with perforated peptic ulcer rapidly before operation. Elderly patients who have had the perforation for more than several hours may require considerable fluids to achieve this goal. A Swan–Ganz catheter is essential in ill, elderly, or cardiac patients to gauge the exact amount of fluid that can be administered safely.

11. (B) Upright radiograph of the chest will demonstrate free air below the diaphragm in about 70–75% of patients presenting with perforation of a duodenal ulcer.

12. (B) Although surgery generally is recommended, treatment by conservative measures can be considered if the diagnosis is established early after perforation, if the patient has not eaten recently, and the clinical course shows rapid clinical improvement. Boardlike rigidity of the abdomen is a characteristic presenting sign of perforated duodenal ulcer. It occurs as a result of chemical peritonitis. After 8–12 hours, the initial signs are less prominent,

and the diagnosis may be more difficult to establish because of the onset of paralytic ileus.

13. (D) Following truncal and selective vagotomy, gastric emptying is delayed. If a vagotomy procedure is performed, it is necessary to perform a drainage operation (such as pyloroplasty). Disturbance in gastric motility with delay in gastric emptying may occur following mechanical gastric obstruction, diabetes, myxedema, hypokalemia, and the administration of anticholinergic or opiate drugs. Rapid gastric emptying may be seen in the Zollinger–Ellison syndrome, retained gastric antrum syndrome, steatorrhea, and massive small bowel resection where there is impaired ability to reduce gastric acid secretion. Failure of the switch off mechanism in inhibiting acid secretion also results in increased motility and emptying of the stomach.

14. (C) Although a milder type of diarrhea is not uncommon after gastrectomy, fulminant diarrhea may be a real problem after vagotomy. The exact mechanism is not known. It occurs in about 1–2% of patients following truncal vagotomy and is less likely to be found after selective or superselective vagotomy.

15. (C) *Helicobacter pylori* (previously called *Campylobacter pylori*) is also associated with duodenal ulcer, gastric ulcer, and gastric cancer. Gastric cancer (in sites beyond the cardia) is increased threefold in patients who grow *H. pylori* as compared to control patients who are negative for infection.

16. **(D)** Prolapse of gastric mucosa into the duodenum may cause difficulty in distinguishing it from a polyp in the antrum. It may be detected in a patient who is asymptomatic; therefore, surgical correction should be reserved for those patients who have clear gastric holdup with vomiting.

17. **(B)** Bilious vomiting is usually spontaneous and should be differentiated from vomiting that occurs after food. The most likely cause of this complication is reflux of bile into the stomach. Bile gastritis with intestinalization of the gastric mucosa is a likely cause.

18. **(D)** The dumping syndrome is a symptom complex occurring after gastric surgery and is characterized by tiredness, abdominal distension, pain, and vasomotor symptoms caused by the rapid entry of food into the small intestine. Tachycardia, sweating, and a feeling of faintness after eating are other symptoms that patients with this syndrome may experience.

19. **(E)** There is a varying degree of impairment in carbohydrate, fat, protein, and mineral absorption after gastrectomy. These changes are most severe after a Billroth II (subtotal gastrectomy plus gastrojejunostomy) (see Figure 3–7). However, in most patients, these changes are mild and can be corrected.

Subtotal gastrectomy
(Billroth II)

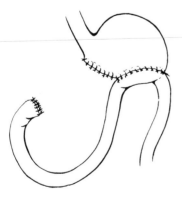

Figure 3–7. Subtotal gastrectomy; Billroth II. (Reproduced, with permission, from Way, LW: Current Surgical Diagnosis & Treatment, 10th ed., Appleton & Lange, 1994.)

20. **(D)** In general, vagotomy with a gastric drainage procedure is less satisfactory in the treatment of primary gastric ulcer. The standard treatment for a gastric ulcer is a partial distal gastrectomy with gastroduodenal anastomosis (Billroth I gastrectomy). The indications for corrective surgery in peptic ulcer therapy has decreased as alternative medical antiulcer treatment (including eradication of *H. pylori*) has become more effective.

21. **(D)** Blood group O is more common than others in patients with duodenal ulcer. In patients who have bled from a duodenal ulcer, this difference is even more striking. Secretors have an excess of blood group antigen that is absent in nonsecretors. The secretor antigen on the red blood cell appears in body fluids also. Nonsecretors are more prone to develop duodenal ulcers than secretors.

22. **(C)** Chronic duodenal ulcer, with recurrent episodes of healing and repair may lead to pyloric obstruction due to scarring and stenosis of the duodenum. Painless vomiting of undigested food may occur once or twice a day. Surgical intervention should be carried out after correction of fluid and electrolyte balance and nutrition.

23. **(D)** This syndrome is characterized by flagrant duodenal ulcer disease, high basal acid secretory output, and a pancreatic tumor. Stimulated serum gastrin levels may be in excess of 1,000 pg/mL or as high as 10,000 pg/mL. Zollinger–Ellison syndrome is due to a true tumor in adults, but hyperplasia may be evident in children. Growth of the tumor is usually slow and survival is often prolonged.

24. **(C)** In Zollinger–Ellison syndrome, gastrin levels may be only mildly elevated but can be increased by provocation with intravenous calcium or secretin. Most patients with gastrinoma have serum gastrin levels that exceed 500 pg/mL. When the range is lower than 200–500 pg/mL, a stimulation test is performed to confirm the diagnosis. A rise of 200 pg/mL after 15 minutes or a doubling of the fasting level is diagnostic.

25. **(C)** Gastrin is found in the pyloric antrum, duodenum, and small intestine. It is not present in the fundus of the stomach. When the distal stomach is removed, gastrin levels are particularly lowered.

26. **(D)** Hypertrophic gastritis (Ménétrier's disease) is characterized by massive loss of plasma protein through the affected gastric mucosa. Most cases can be managed medically by maintenance of adequate nutrition. An increased incidence of gastric cancer has been reported in some series.

27. **(C)** Sucralfate offers protection, even in an acid environment. The use of antacids to prevent or treat erosive gastritis is superior to that of H_2 receptor antagonists alone. There is an advantage in adding H_2 antagonists with antacids. Sucralfate is cytoprotective and destroys some of the oropharyngeal enteric colonized bacteria; it may reduce complications of pneumonia. The initial lesion of acute erosive gastritis is in the fundus of the stomach and if bleeding persists surgical intervention may be required.

28. **(E)** The distinction between a benign and malignant ulcer can still be difficult, and a 5% false-negative rate exists. The presence of achlorhydria rules out peptic ulceration. If the ulcer persists, further follow-up measures with x-rays, endoscopy, biopsy, and possible operation are indicated. Gastric ulcers are conveniently divided into:

    Type I—confined to stomach (excluding prepyloric region)
    Type II—is associate with duodenal ulcer disease
    Type III—prepyloric ulcer
    Type II and III gastric ulcers have acid secretory characteristics (and hence treatment protocols) similar to those of duodenal ulcer disease.

29. **(D)** An appropriate operation for antral ulcer is the Billroth I partial gastrectomy with gastroduodenal anastomosis. There is a high success rate after surgery, as judged by patient satisfaction. Vagotomy is not nearly as effective in preventing recurrences. It is important to realize that the management of gastric and duodenal ulcer are not identical.

30. **(A)** Gastric cancer is defined as "early" if the mucous membrane alone is involved. Early gastric cancer may be overlooked on a barium upper GI series. The treatment is by gastric resection with care taken to ensure that the resected margins and anastomosis are tumor free.

31. **(C)** Gastric cancer seems to be decreasing in incidence, and colon cancer is now encountered more commonly. Most patients present with vague abdominal discomfort and dyspeptic symptoms. Severe pain is unusual in early cases. If there is a bulky polypoid lesion, it is often encountered in the proximal stomach.

32. **(E)** Distal subtotal gastrectomy with wide dissection of the lymphatic drainage area remains the hallmark of appropriate surgical treatment for possible cure of gastric cancer.

33. **(D)** The incisura is the distal portion of the lesser curvature as seen on barium x-ray studies. The fundus is that part of the stomach that is above a horizontal line drawn to pass through the cardia.

34. **(B)** This is a relatively rare gastric malignancy and can cause confusion, because the overlying gastric mucosa may remain intact. It grows slowly, invades locally, and is not responsive to radiation or chemotherapy. Eosinophilic gastroenteritis is an infiltrative lesion that usually involves the gastric antrum. It is of unknown etiology and differs from Menetrier's disease where the mucosal folds of the proximal part of the stomach are initially involved

35. **(D)** The stomach is the most common site of involvement in extranodal non-Hodgkins lymphoma. The 5-year survival rate following curative resection even when the disease is transmural, is over 70% when chemotherapy and/or radiotherapy is added to gastric resection. At times, the lymphoma may be missed if the overlying mucosal biopsy is reported as normal.

36. (D) Leiomyoma can occur in any part of the stomach. Most commonly, they are found to be in the submucosa and grow toward the lumen. Ulceration may occur and give rise to the characteristic "doughnut sign" on barium radiographs. Hematemesis and/or melena may sometimes be massive. Local resection is curative.

37. (C) Hyperplastic polyps are unlikely to contain carcinoma. Multiplicity of hyperplastic polyps does not seem to enhance the change to cancer. Adenomatous polyps occur more commonly in the antrum; whereas, hyperplastic polyps are distributed more evenly throughout the stomach. For this reason, antral polyps should be removed first.

38. (C) Adenomatous polyps resemble colon polyps. Coexisting carcinoma may be present in 20% of cases. The incidence of carcinoma is increased if lesions are larger than 2 cm. Both hyperplastic and adenomatous polyps are more common in long-term follow-up in patients treated successfully for familial polyposis. All adenomatous polyps should be removed.

39. (E) Gastric volvulus is often associated with a large paraesophageal hiatal hernia. The twist causes cut-off at the cardia above and the pylorus below, leading to distension and ischemia, which may occasionally lead to gangrene and the need for resection. Organ axial volvulus is more common, and rotation occurs along the axis between the cardia and the pylorus. In the less common type of gastric volvulus, rotation occurs through an axis that is at a right angle described as organo-axial above.

40. (C) Treatment consists of nasogastric aspiration for 24–48 hours to allow normal gastric tone to return. Appropriate parenteral fluids are administered.

41. (B) This condition is associated with achlorhydria, parietal cell antibodies, high gastrin levels, and gastric carcinoma. Other premalignant conditions include adenomatous polyps, gastric ulcer, previous (more than 15 years) gastric resection, chronic atrophic gastritis and histological changes showing intestinal metaplasia and dysplasia.

42. (D) If the patient is unconscious, a feeding gastrostomy (or nasogastric tube) will increase the likelihood of aspiration. Feeding jejunostomy would be the preferable procedure. The balloon of a Foley catheter should not be used, because it may be driven distally by peristalsis and occlude the duodenum. A Malecot-type catheter has luminal perforations and does not induce this complication.

43. (A) In 1948, Dragstedt introduced a gastric drainage procedure to overcome stasis occurring in over 30–40% of cases following vagotomy. Pyloroplasty, gastrojejunostomy, and antrectomy are the three recognized drainage procedures from which to choose, when a vagotomy is performed. A drainage procedure is indicated only if a truncal or selective vagotomy is performed. In supraselective vagotomy, the drainage procedure is not required.

44. (D) In general, operation for peptic ulcer bleeding is indicated at an earlier stage in an older patient (>65–70 years of age), because the vessels are atherosclerotic and thus less likely to close spontaneously. In addition, diminished perfusion of heart, brain, and kidneys is less well tolerated in the elderly patient. At surgery, the gastroduodenal artery in the floor of the ulcer is oversewn, and a vagotomy (with gastric drainage) procedure (or partial gastrectomy) is performed.

45. (C) Mainly the G cells in the antrum produce gastrin. Gastrin is also produced in the duodenum (20%) and smaller amounts in the proximal small bowel. Following distal gastrectomy or antrectomy, the major source of gastrin is removed, and effective reduction in acid production occurs. If the antrum is retained, then continuous acid secretion occurs, and peptic ulcer disease may ensue.

46. (C) The scan will fail to visualize the gallbladder if acute cholecystitis is present. In a patient with cholelithiasis, the incidence of cholecystitis and associated biliary complications is increased following vagotomy In a patient with known gallbladder disease, consent for possible cholecystectomy should be obtained before a planned vagotomy operation.

47. **(B)** The stomach is the most common site of GI sarcomas (47%), followed by small intestine (35%), colon and rectum (12%), and esophagus (5%). Nearly all GI sarcomas arise from smooth muscle (leiomyosarcomas).

48. **(B)** Small gastric sarcomas may be treated with less radical procedures, but larger tumors require gastrectomy. The 5-year survival rate exceeds 40%. In this condition, patients present with bleeding rather than pain or a palpable mass.

49. **(C)** Patients with pernicious anemia have achlorhydria and an increased risk (about 5%) of developing gastric carcinoma. There is a deficiency in vitamin B_{12}, which leads to the megaloblastic anemia and neurologic involvement (subacute combined degeneration of the spinal cord).

50. **(D)** Pharyngoesophageal (Zenker's) diverticulum is a mucosal outpouching occurring through the triangular bare area between the cricopharyngeus muscle and the inferior constrictor muscle of the pharynx (Killian's triangle). Most present on the left side of the neck. They are more commonly encountered in elderly men.

51. **(E)** Current surgical treatment for large, symptomatic pharyngoesophageal diverticula is myotomy and diverticulectomy. Small, asymptomatic diverticula require no treatment. Attention has been paid to the role of failure of relaxation of the cricopharyngeus muscle as a cause of the diverticulum. For this reason, myotomy, either alone for smaller diverticula or with diverticulectomy, has become the standard surgical therapy.

52. **(E)** An epiphrenic diverticulum is a pulsion diverticulum and is associated with no obvious lesion (35%), hiatal hernia (30%), diffuse esophageal spasm (20%), achalasia (10%), and miscellaneous causes (5%). It is located within 10 cm of the cardia. An epiphrenic diverticulum is commonly asymptomatic and should not be treated surgically on its own unless symptoms clearly are related to it. Parabronchial lymphadenopathy can cause a traction diverticulum, which is situated at a higher level.

53. **(A)** The appearance of unexplained dysphagia in adults requires urgent barium-swallow study. Carcinoma is particularly prevalent in certain parts of Africa and Asia, but its incidence is increasing in Western countries. In achalasia, there is initially an improved tolerance for solids over liquids. In carcinoma, dysphagia for solids is noted initially, and later there is difficulty in swallowing liquids as well. Esophagoscopy is required in the workup of different causes of dysphagia to exclude the possibility of an underlying carcinoma.

54. **(B)** In addition to the presence of an upper esophageal web leading to dysphagia, the Plummer–Vinson syndrome is characterized by atrophic oral mucosa, spoon-shaped brittle fingernails (koilonychia), and iron-deficiency anemia. Endoscopy reveals a fibrous area just below the cricopharyngeus muscle. There is an increased risk of developing cancer of the esophagus.

55. **(D)** Nonoperative therapy is indicated initially. The treatment for patients with GERD is to lose weight, avoid fatty meals, cigarette smoking, alcohol, lying flat, certain foods such as chocolates, and drugs such as theophyline, anticholinergic agents, and alpha adrenergic antagonists. Dysphagia requires special attention to rule out stricture, cancer, or motility disorder. Poor results in patients who have developed a stricture are more likely where previous dilatation or surgery has failed and patients with scleroderma,

56. **(B)** The cardia is displaced into the posterior mediastinum. The term *sliding hernia* (Figure 3–8) indicates that part of the peritoneum slips or slides with the hernia into the posterior mediastinum. The wall of the sac is formed medially by the stomach and laterally by the peritoneum. Reflux esophagitis is most likely

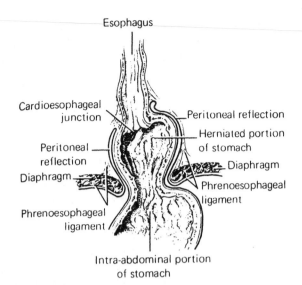

Figure 3–8. Sliding esophageal hiatal hernia; correlate with x-ray in Figure 3–2. (Reproduced, with permission, from Way, LW: Current Surgical Diagnosis & Treatment, 10th ed., Appleton & Lange, 1994.)

to occur with this type of hernia. The sliding hiatal hernia may be entirely asymptomatic or lead to reflux esophagitis and possibly an esophageal stricture.

57. **(C)** Benign peptic strictures are submucosal fibrotic rings that narrow the lumen and obstruct the passage of food. They present with dysphagia. They tend to measure between 1 and 4 cm in length. GERD is the common cause, and other associated motility disorders frequently occur. As reflux esophagitis develops, heartburn may improve because of obstruction to the flow of refluxed material.

58. **(B)** Treatment of benign stricture is controversial. Surgical success is inversely proportional to the number of preoperative dilations performed, and many surgeons believe that strictures secondary to GERD represent failure of conservative therapy. If surgery is undertaken, the correct procedure is an antireflux operation with pre- and postoperative dilations. This succeeds in about 90% of patients.

59. **(D)** The present treatment is aimed at preventing esophagitis. Barret's esophagus is regarded as a premalignant condition and is characterized by columnar metapalsia of the normal squamous epithelial lining of the esophagus. The cancer risk is increased 20- to 50-fold.

About one-third of patients with Barret's esophagus present with malignancy, and many cases of adenocarcinoma of the esophagus arise from Barret's mucosa. Recent evidence also suggests an increased risk for the development of squamous carcinoma. It is found in 8–10% of patients with longstanding reflux.

60. **(D)** This is a type 4 hiatal hernia (Figure 3–9). In the classic case of paraesophageal "rolling" hernia, the gastroesophageal junction remains below the hiatus, allowing the stomach—and sometimes other viscera—to migrate upward into the chest, alongside the esophagus. Paraesophageal hernias are prone to obstruction, bleeding, and volvulus from mesoaxial or organoaxial rotation. Chronic symptoms are pain and postprandial fullness, with heartburn in 90% of cases. Gastric ulcers develop in as many as 30% of cases and may cause acute or chronic blood loss. There is no effective medical treatment for this disease. Surgical treatment is indicated and effective to cure symptoms and to prevent complications, which may be catastrophic.

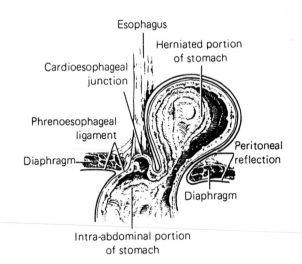

Figure 3–9. Paraesophageal hernia; correlate with x-ray in Figure 3–3. (Reproduced, with permission, from Way, LW: Current Surgical Diagnosis & Treatment, 10th ed., Appleton & Lange, 1994.)

61. **(B)** Endoscopic dilation is the usual treatment. Schatzki's ring is a thin, circumferential scar in the lower esophagus, more common in men (65%). It is acquired and probably results from repeated trauma to the mucosa with chronic inflammation and fibrosis. Endoscopic dilation

is usually successful, but antireflux surgery is occasionally necessary for severe GERD, especially if worsened by dilation. Associated hiatal hernia is very common.

62. **(A)** Dysphagia in esophageal achalasia is described as paradoxical, in that it is more pronounced for liquids than for solids. There are numerous reports of increased incidence of carcinoma in achalasia, varying from 3–10%. In 1975, Belsey reported a 10% incidence in 81 patients in whom symptoms tended to occur at a younger age. Recurrent lung infections from aspiration of esophageal contents are a troublesome complication. Treatment is by cardimyotomy or tube dilation.

63. **(D)** Mallory–Weiss tear, characterized by acute and sometimes massive upper GI hemorrhage, accounts for as many as 15% of upper GI bleeds. It is due to arterial bleeding following repeated vomiting, which causes mucosal tears at the gastroesophageal junction. The cause is the same as that for spontaneous rupture of the esophagus (i.e., an acute increase in intra-abdominal pressure against a closed glottis). Causes other than vomiting, such as paroxysmal coughing or retching, may sometimes lead to this condition. Upper endoscopy confirms the diagnosis. Surgery may occasionally be necessary to stop the bleeding.

64. **(B)** Spontaneous rupture of the esophagus, or Boerhaave syndrome, is most common in men between 35 and 55 years of age. The usual presentation is with extremely severe pain in the precordium, lower thorax, or epigastrium. Classically, it follows an episode of violent vomiting. Chest film shows hydropneumothorax—usually on the left side, but it may be on the right or bilateral. Free air below the diaphragm is not a usual finding. The tear is usually located above the diaphragm and is longitudinal on the left posterolateral wall. Air passes upward around the esophagus in the posterior mediastinum to cause subcutaneous emphysema.

65. **(D)** Spontaneous rupture of the esophagus is an acute emergency that requires immediate efforts to establish the diagnosis, as rapidly as possible, and to perform an emergency operation. Rapid resuscitation is instituted. Shock is not a contraindication to operation, because it is unlikely that the patient's condition will improve until surgery has been performed. The surgical approach is usually thoracic, but the abdominal approach may also be used.

66. **(E)** The esophagus is, essentially, a posterior mediastinal structure in much of its course. The thymus gland is located in the anterior mediastinum. The recurrent laryngeal nerves run between the trachea and esophagus. The aorta loops backward over the left side of the esophagus; at this level, the thoracic duct is on the left side of the esophagus. The brachiocephalic vein is the most anterior positioned vascular structure in the superior mediastinum.

67. **(A)** Most are compatible with life. Practically all can be corrected by appropriate surgical procedures. In the majority of cases, the distal esophagus communicates with the trachea or, less commonly, the bronchus. The fistula from the bronchus or trachea may occur without the presence of an esophageal abnormality.

68. **(D)** Leiomyoma is by far the most common benign tumor encountered in the esophagus. Malignant transformation is thought to be rare. Leiomyomas are the most common benign tumor of the esophagus, but less than 10% of alimentary tract leiomyomas are found in the esophagus. They are composed of spindle cells and grow slowly and may cause progressively obstructive symptoms. Other tumors are congenital or acquired cysts, adenomatous polyps, papillomata, lipomata, neurofibromas, and hemangiomas.

69. **(C)** The gastroesophageal zone of elevated pressure is 3–4 cm long with a resting pressure of 15 cm H_2O. Pregnancy, obesity, and gastric dilation cause a rise in pressure and may result in reflux. Gastric alkalinization of the stomach, gastrin, epinephrine, cholinergic agents (bethanecol), α adrenergic agent (metoclopromide) increase the resting pressure of the lower esophageal sphincter, and anticholinergic agent (atropine), glucagon and secretin decrease it.

70. **(B)** Barret's esophagus, corrosive esophagitis, achalasia, smoking, and alcoholism are associated with increased risk of developing cancer of the esophagus. Lye stricture and long-standing achalasia are also associated with increased incidence of esophageal cancers. Adenocarcinoma is increasing in incidence and now constitutes about 40% of cases in Western countries. The remainder are squamous. Mallory–Weiss tears result in acute upper GI bleeding. They are not premalignant.

71. **(E)** The history of GERD with these findings is highly suggestive of an adenocarcinoma arising in a Barret's esophagus. Squamous carcinoma is more likely to occur higher up in the middle third of the esophagus. Endoscopy and biopsy prove the diagnosis. The patient should be treated surgically by esophagectomy if carcinoma is confirmed.

72. **(D)** Surgical resection of the esophagus remains the standard treatment for patients with carcinoma in the lower esophagus, provided that there is no known metastatic disease, and the medical condition allows surgical intervention. This offers the best palliation and hope of cure; 5-year survival rates vary between 15 and 25%. Radiation and chemotherapy, in combination with surgery in selected patients, may improve these statistics. Management of carcinoma in the middle third of the esophagus may be either surgical resection or radiotherapy, and in the upper third, radiotherapy is often preferred.

73. **(B)** The pericardioperitoneal foramen (of Bochdalek) is a defect due to failure of closure of the pleuroperitoneal folds. This anomaly is more frequent on the left side. Intrauterine diagnosis at 15 weeks is positive by ultrasound. Following delivery, the bowel fills with air and the mediastinum shifts to the opposite side, compromising the better of the two lungs. Chest x-rays show bowel in the chest. Only in 5% do symptoms present after 6 months of age. Early detection of polyhydramnios in utero has resulted in successful prenatal intervention and survival in highly specialized neonatal units.

74. **(A)** Blunt trauma is the most common cause of diaphragmatic rupture. There are often associated injuries. The left hemidiaphragm is ruptured more frequently by blunt trauma than the right, the ratio being 9:1. Stomach, spleen, colon, and omentum may enter the pleural cavity. Early surgery is indicated.

75. **(B)** The lower esophagus drains to the azygos system but has an important communicating anastomosis to the portal system via the left gastric (coronary) vein. The upper part of the esophagus drains into the brachycephalic vein. The esophagus is innervated in its upper part by the recurrent laryngeal nerves and in its lower part by the vagi.

76. **(C)** Pseudomyxoma peritonei may also arise from an appendiceal mucocele. There are no malignant cells in the histological sections. The lesion, however, spreads locally and causes severe local complications.

77. **(B)** Subhepatic (infrahepatic) space infection usually occurs after surgery or peritonitis in the supracolic compartment. It is an unlikely complication of biliary pancreatitis. Infections in the subhepatic space may extend to the infracolic compartment via the paracolic gutter (of Morrison). In addition to the stomach, the subhepatic space may become a source of fluid collection secondarily to perforation of the gallbladder, first part of the duodenum, and inflammatory fluid collections arising from pancreatic or hepatic disease.

78. **(D)** Oral fluid and solid feeds can usually be commenced several days after the injury. Feeding at this stage is encouraged if the patient continues to show favorable improvement. If the caustic burn is superficial, then stricture formation usually does not occur. Endoscopy to the proximal part of the lesion is recommended after admission unless perforation is suspected. No attempt should be made to pass the scope beyond the involved inflammatory segment

79. **(B)** Esophageal perforation has occurred. Alkali caustic ingestion results in a liquefaction

necrosis; whereas, acid solutions usually cause coagulation necrosis. Other features on x-ray indicating esophageal perforation would include pneumothorax, pneumomediastinum, and pleural effusion. After hospital admission, a nasogastric tube should be avoided, because the impact of the alkaline caustic entering the acid stomach is more likely to result in liquefactive necrosis and possible perforation of the stomach.

80. **(B)** The hepatic artery is on the left of the common bile duct and anterior to the portal vein. The inferior vena cava passes behind the foramen of Winslow (epiploic), where it lies behind the portal vein. The foramen represents the only natural communication between the lesser and greater peritoneal bursa (sac).

81. **(E)** This test is a useful method of determining if a mass is due to an intra-abdominal wall lesion rather than being of abdominal origin. Attempts by the patient to sit up will make the anterior abdominal wall muscles taut and thus reduce the clarity of definition of an intra-abdominal mass; an intra-abdominal wall lesion will still be palpable after this maneuver.

82. **(B)** Malignant fibrous histiosarcoma, the most common histologic type of sarcoma, was first described in 1961. Previously, liposarcoma had been considered the most frequent sarcoma. Liposarcoma occurs more commonly in patients between 30 and 50 years of age. It is of interest that the commonly encountered lipoma rarely undergoes malignant change. In general, sarcomas are only minimally sensitive to radiotherapy.

83. **(C, F)** The rise in acid secretion after injection of gastrin is known as the augmented value. Basal acid output is usually 0.5–15 mEq/h. It is lower among women. It also is lower in gastric ulcer and low or absent in gastric cancer patients. The wide range, however, prevents one from being able to use this measurement to distinguish various gastric conditions. After gastrin or histamine administration, there is an increase in acid secretion to between 20 and 60 mEq/h, with a mean value in this group significantly higher than in normal individuals or gastric ulcer patients.

84. **(B, E, K)** Patients with gastric remnant following distal gastrectomy, pernicious anemia, and adenomatous gastric polyps should be investigated at appropriate intervals to exclude malignant change. Gastric ulcer and individuals with group A also have an increased predisposition to develop gastric cancer.

85. **(J)** Acute gastric dilation may result in vasovagal response characterized by typical symptoms associated with marked gastric abdominal distension which is clearly demonstrable in a nonsedated patient. Unfortunately, the syndrome may occur after anesthesia and may pass unrecognized and cause vomiting, aspiration, hypoxia, or bleeding from erosive gastritis due to stress.

86. **(D, H)** Lipoma of the stomach and ectopic pancreas may cause some difficulty in the differentiation from other gastric lesions. Although interesting, they are usually not of clinical significance as they are encountered relatively infrequently.

87. **(L)** Patients with familial adenomatous polyposis, although protected by total colectomy from colonic lesions, are at high risk for development of carcinoma of the stomach and duodenum in adenomatous polyp of those organs. Ampullary and bile duct carcinomas will cause jaundice.

88. **(G)** Distant metastasis is late, and prolonged survival follows resection, including adjacent organs if necessary (e.g., colon, pancreas). Hemorrhage can result when the tumor breaks through the gastric mucosa. Malnutrition results from compromise of the gastric capacity of the stomach.

89. **(H)** Secretors have an excess of blood group antigen that is absent in nonsecretors. The secretor antigen on the RBC appears in body fluids as well. Nonsecretors are more prone than secretors to develop duodenal ulcers.

90. **(H)** Patients in the hospital who have multiple or serious organ involvement from trauma or other disease are at higher risk of developing bleeding from erosive gastritis. Patients in this high-risk category require prophylactic measures to increase the pH of gastric secretion.

91. **(A, D, G)** In addition to these three factors, the rate of back diffusion H^+ ions and the presence of submucosal buffers are relevant to the pathogenesis of erosive gastritis.

92. **(C, I, J)** It is important to monitor the gastric pH to determine whether the method of acid secretion suppression is adequate.

93. **(A, C)** Gastric ulcer (33%) and duodenal ulcer (33%) are the most common causes of upper GI bleeding in patients admitted to an emergency department. Although duodenal ulcers are more common than gastric ulcers, the latter are more likely to cause bleeding. This explains the similar incidence of bleeding occurring from gastric and duodenal ulcers in some reviews. Other causes of bleeding include gastric erosions, carcinoma of the stomach, Mallory–Weiss tear, esophageal ulcer, and esophagitis of the stomach.

94. **(H)** Prostaglandin E (misoprostol [Cytotec]) has not been useful in the management of erosive gastritis, because diarrhea has been a troublesome side effect.

95. **(A, B)** Gastrinoma, Zollinger-Ellison (ZE) syndrome, should always be excluded in patients presenting with severe peptic ulcer disease failing to respond to treatment. Acid secretion tests, which may reveal whether the vagotomy was adequate, are used less frequently since the availability of other tests. In ZE, basal acid is increased above 15 mEq/h.

96. **(D, N)** H_2 blockers and triple therapy with antibiotics (e.g., Biaxin or tetracycline, metronidazole, and bismuth subsalicylate)

97. **(A, I)** The incidence of duodenal ulcer disease has dropped markedly in the United States and other Western countries over the past 20–30 years.

98. **(M)** If medical measures have failed to control bleeding, surgical intervention is indicated where feasible, because it will lower mortality. Knowledge of the exact source of bleeding is important in the planning management.

99. **(C, E)** The 5-year survival rate is about 12%, and there is an increased rate in patients with gastric ulcer. The 5-year survival rate for all types of gastric carcinoma is about 12%, but it is 35% if the nodes are clear and 7% if the nodes are involved. It is important that the cut edges are clear of tumor; otherwise, recurrence will almost certainly occur at the site of tumor resection.

100. **(C)** Gastrostomy performed by percutaneous means via an endoscopy is a more rapid and probably safer method of gastroscopy than conventional surgical measures. It should be considered in any patient who is likely to require a feeding nasogastric tube for prolonged periods. The procedure is performed under local anesthesia, and the tube should not be changed during the first 10-day period that the tract is forming.

CHAPTER 4

Small and Large Intestines and Appendix
Questions

Nicholas A. Balsano, Rao R. Ivatury, and C. Gene Cayten

1. A male neonate develops small-bowel obstruction due to malrotation of the midgut segment. An x-ray of the abdomen confirms the presence of small bowel obstruction (Figure 4–1). He undergoes an emergency laparotomy, untwisting of the malrotated intestines, and partial small-bowel resection for intestinal infarction. Which of the following statements is true of the small intestine (jejunum and ileum)?

   (A) It is derived entirely from the midgut.
   (B) In the fetus, it enters the physiologic umbilical hernia in the the fifth month.
   (C) It remains in the physiologic hernia for 4 months.
   (D) It is attached to the urachus.
   (E) It drains into the lymph nodes around the iliac arteries.

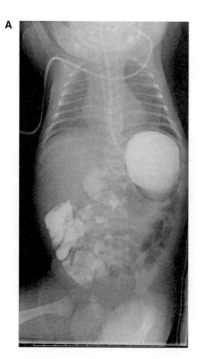
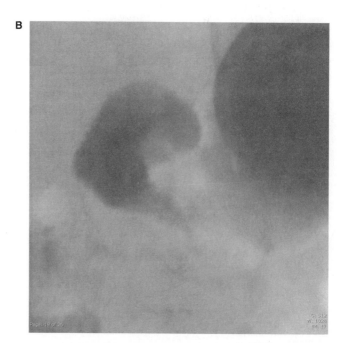

Figure 4–1. A, Upper GI shows dilation of the bowel secondary to volvulus. **B.** Distension of duodenum with beaking of the second portion of the duodenum due to volvulus.

2. A 64-year-old man with mitral stenosis develops mesenteric infarction due to an embolus. At operation and on subsequent pathologic examination, what is noted regarding the small intestine (jejunum and ileum)?

    (A) It commences at the right of the midline.
    (B) It contains crypts but not villi on histologic examination.
    (C) It has a mesentery (parietal) attachment extending 61 cm along the posterior abdominal wall.
    (D) It measures approximately 6 m in length.
    (E) It is supplied by the inferior mesenteric vessels.

Questions 3 and 4

A 43-year-old woman undergoes investigations for colitis. In her history, it is noted that 20 years earlier she underwent a surgical procedure on the large intestine.

3. The diagnosis is more likely to be Crohn's disease rather than ulcerative colitis because the previous operation was which of the following?

    (A) performed in a young patient
    (B) confined to the colon
    (C) followed by improvement after bypass of the diseased segment
    (D) followed by improvement because steroids were prescribed

4. The diagnosis is more likely to be ulcerative colitis rather than Crohn's disease because at the previous operation

    (A) all layers of the bowel wall were involved
    (B) there was evidence of fistula formation
    (C) the serosa appeared normal on inspection, but the colon mucosa was extensively involved
    (D) skip lesions were noted
    (E) the preoperative gastrointestinal (GI) series showed a narrowing stringlike stricture in the ileum (String sign)

Questions 5 and 6

A 64-year-old woman with a known history of cardiac disease is admitted to the hospital with severe abdominal pain. Her blood pressure is 150/95 mmHg, and her pulse rate is 84 beats per minute (bpm). There are minimal signs of intravascular depletion.

5. The possibility of small-bowel infarction is characterized by which of the following?

    (A) the stack-of-coins sign
    (B) marked distention of loops of bowel
    (C) air in the biliary tree
    (D) air in the bowel wall (intramural)
    (E) air below the left diaphragm

6. At operation, 2.5 m of distal ileum is found to be gangrenous. There is, however, pulsation in the superior mesenteric artery and its main branches. Small-bowel gangrene in this patient is caused by which of the following?

    (A) arterial thrombosis
    (B) embolus
    (C) nonocclusive ischemic disease
    (D) von Willebrand's disease
    (E) idiopathic thrombocytopenic purpura

7. A 48-year-old man undergoes a supine abdominal x-ray for epigastric discomfort. He has been on intravenous hyperalimentation since an operative procedure performed 5 days previously. Gas is consistently absent from the alimentary tract because he has previously undergone which of the following?

    (A) appendectomy
    (B) gastrostomy
    (C) ligation of the esophagus and cervical esophagostomy
    (D) lysis of adhesions
    (E) colostomy for large-bowel obstruction

8. A 10-month-old boy has recently been weaned and placed on solid food. He develops colicky abdominal pain with vomiting. Examination of the abdomen shows emptiness in the right iliac fossa and a mass in the epigastrium. Intussusception is suspected. Following adequate hydration, this condition should be treated by which of the following?

    (A) laxatives
    (B) gastrojejunostomy

(C) laparotomy and manual reduction

(D) radiologic reduction by barium with measured pressure control of column of barium

Questions 9 and 10

A 64-year-old woman is admitted to the hospital with abdominal pain, vomiting, and abdominal distention. Bowel sounds are increased on auscultation, and a plain film shows marked distention of loops of bowel with a "featureless" pattern.

9. The most likely diagnosis is which of the following?

   (A) sigmoid volvulus
   (B) cecal volvulus
   (C) jejunal obstruction
   (D) ileal obstruction
   (E) pyloric obstruction

10. Management, following rehydration and electrolyte imbalance correction, should initially involve which of the following?

   (A) nasogastric suction, rehydration and observation
   (B) anticholinergic drugs
   (C) laxatives
   (D) emergency surgery and bowel resection
   (E) appendectomy

11. A 42-year-old woman is admitted to the emergency department with severe colicky pain, vomiting, and abdominal distention. She has not passed stools or flatus for 48 hours. X-rays of the abdomen confirm the presence of small-bowel obstruction. What is the most likely cause of small-bowel obstruction in this patient?

   (A) adenocarcinoma
   (B) adhesions
   (C) Crohn's disease
   (D) ulcerative colitis
   (E) gallstone ileus

12. An 80-year-old woman with a known history of femoral hernia is admitted to the hospital be-

cause of strangulation of the hernia. There is a tender swelling in the right femoral region immediately below and lateral to the pubic tubercle. She has had multiple bowel movements without relief of symptoms. What is the most likely diagnosis?

   (A) lymphadenitis
   (B) diverticulitis
   (C) volvulus
   (D) Richter's hernia
   (E) gastroenteritis

13. A 63-year-old man from Miami presents to the emergency department with abdominal pain due to intestinal obstruction. A diagnosis of small-bowel volvulus is established. Primary small-bowel volvulus is differentiated from secondary small-bowel volvulus in that in the latter there is a secondary cause, such as adhesions, that accounts for the volvulus. Which is true of primary small-bowel volvulus?

   (A) It does not lead to gangrene of bowel.
   (B) It is common in the United States.
   (C) It occurs nearly exclusively in women.
   (D) It usually involves the jejunum.
   (E) It may require a limited resection of small intestine.

Questions 14 and 15

A 44-year-old man is stabbed in the abdomen. The injury penetrates the root of the small-bowel mesentery. At laparotomy, resection of 2 m of ileum is removed.

14. The complication that is more likely to occur after resection of the ileum rather than of an equivalent length of jejunum is the failure to absorb which of the following?

   (A) iron
   (B) zinc
   (C) bile salts
   (D) medium-chain triglycerides
   (E) amylase

15. Why is distal resection, as compared to proximal resection, poorly tolerated?

   (A) Transit time in the ileum is slower than that in the jejunum.
   (B) Transit time in the jejunum is slower than that in the ileum.
   (C) The greater bulk of food is absorbed in the ileum.
   (D) Water absorption is mainly in the ileum.
   (E) All minerals are absorbed preferentially in the ileum.

16. A 66-year-old woman is admitted for hyperalimentation due to malnutrition consequent to massive small-bowel resection. What is the most likely condition that leads to the need to perform a massive resection?

   (A) autoimmune disease
   (B) mesenteric ischemia
   (C) mesenteric adenitis
   (D) cancer
   (E) pseudomyxoma peritonei

Questions 17 and 18

A premature infant is noted at birth to have mild abdominal distention. There are no abnormal pulmonary findings on auscultation.

17. A plain x-ray of the abdomen shows intramural air (Figure 4–2) which is attributed to which of the following?

   (A) choledochojejunal fistula
   (B) perforation of bowel caused by colon cancer
   (C) perforated gastric ulcer
   (D) gangrene of the small bowel
   (E) pneumatosis cystoides intestinalis

18. What is the most appropriate treatment?

   (A) urgent laparotomy
   (B) treatment for *Escherichia coli* sepsis
   (C) treatment for intestinal gangrene
   (D) reassurance and no intervention, in most cases
   (E) charcoal X

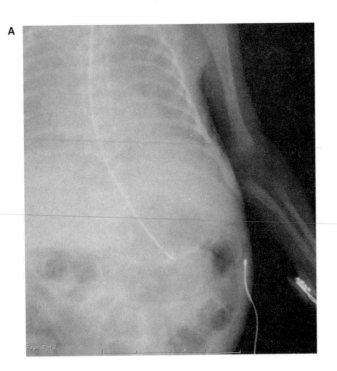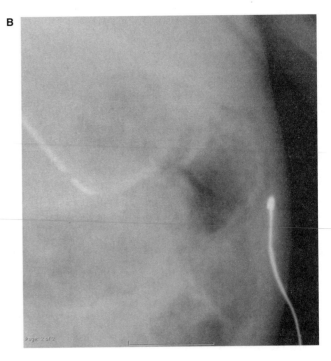

Figure 4–2. Abdominal x-ray of premature infant. Intramural air is evident.

19. A 68-year-old female is known to have had surgery several years previously for a bowel lesion. Her surgeon had told her that she suffers from the blind loop syndrome. In which condition can one anticipate the blind loop syndrome to occur?

   (A) intestinal bypass
   (B) enterocolic fistula
   (C) inflammatory bowel surgery disease
   (D) scleroderma
   (E) all of the above

20. A 33-year-old woman is noted to have a Meckel's diverticulum when she undergoes an emergency appendectomy. The diverticulum is approximately 60 cm from the ileocecal valve and measures 2–3 cm in length. What is the most common complication of Meckel's diverticulum among adults?

   (A) bleeding
   (B) perforation
   (C) intestinal obstruction
   (D) ulceration
   (E) carcinoma

21. In Peutz–Jeghers syndrome, small-bowel polyps are characterized by which of the following?

   (A) adenomas
   (B) hamartomas
   (C) adenomatous polyps
   (D) villoglandular polyps
   (E) villotubular polyps

Questions 22 through 24

A 38-year-old male is admitted to hospital with symptoms suggestive of small bowel obstruction. Examination reveals multiple loops of distended bowel with increased bowel sounds. Treatment with intravenous fluids and nasogastric suction fails to correct symptoms. Laparotomy is performed. Following surgery, copious volumes of fluid occur through the incision. A diagnosis of intestinal fistula is established.

22. What is true of intestinal fistulas?

   (A) They may occur as a complication after an operation to divide adhesions.

   (B) They are rare after irradiation.
   (C) As a result of Crohn's disease, they almost always close spontaneously.
   (D) They should not be treated with a central venous line for fear of sepsis.
   (E) They most commonly arise from the distal colon.

23. Radiologic investigation reveals that the fistula arises from the proximal small intestine which of the following statements is true concerning this fistula?

   (A) If internal, it occurs mainly from iatrogenic causes.
   (B) It occurs more commonly after an anastomosis than spontaneously.
   (C) If internal, it always causes serious complications.
   (D) If external, it closes spontaneously in 10% of cases.
   (E) If external, it requires immediate closure in most cases.

24. Intestinal fistula is least likely to close spontaneously when it occurs

   (A) jejunocutaneously
   (B) ileocutaneously
   (C) colocutaneously
   (D) colocolic

Questions 25 and 26

A 68-year-old retired female plastic surgeon underwent laparotomy through a midline abdominal incision. Intestinal infarction was found and a distal 60% small bowel resection was performed with ileocecal anastomosis. She was placed on hyperalimentation. Seven days after the operation, she underwent a second operation through the same incision.

25. Wound healing is further impaired by which of the following?

   (A) incision through the same abdominal wall scar
   (B) vitamin A administration
   (C) zinc deficiency
   (D) increased local oxygen tension

26. At the second operation an advanced carcinoma of the colon is detected. Wound healing will be further impaired if

   (A) the antimetabolite 5-fluorouracil is given
   (B) doxorubium is given
   (C) chemotherapeutic agents are prescribed 2 weeks after surgery
   (D) oral antibiotics were prescribed before surgery
   (E) denervation of bowel and/or skin incision occurs

27. A 79-year-old man has had abdominal pain for 4 days. An operation is performed, and a gangrenous appendix is removed. The stump is inverted. Why does acute appendicitis in elderly patients and in children have a worse prognosis?

   (A) The appendix is retrocecal.
   (B) The appendix is in the preileal position.
   (C) The appendix is in the pelvic position.
   (D) The omentum and peritoneal cavity appear to be less efficient in localizing the disease in these age groups.

Questions 28 through 31

A 12-year-old boy complains of pain in the lower abdomen (mainly on the right side). Symptoms commenced 12 hours before admission. He had noted anorexia during this period. Examination revealed tenderness in the right iliac fossa, which was maximal 1 cm below Mc Burney's point.

28. In appendicitis, where does the pain frequently commence?

   (A) in the right iliac fossa and remains there
   (B) in the back and moves to the right iliac fossa
   (C) In the rectal region and moves to the right iliac fossa
   (D) In the umbilical region and then moves to the right iliac fossa
   (E) In the right flank

29. On examination, patients presenting with appendicitis typically show maximal tenderness over which of the following?

   (A) inguinal region
   (B) immediately above the umbilicus
   (C) at a point between the outer one-third and inner two-thirds of a line between the umbilicus and the anterior superior iliac spine
   (D) At a point between the outer two-thirds and inner one-third of a line between the umbilicus and the anterior superior iliac spine
   (E) At the midpoint of a line between the umbilicus and the anterior superior iliac spine

30. Which of the following statements about appendicitis is true?

   (A) It occurs equally as often in men as in women.
   (B) With perforation, it will show fecalith in more than 90% of cases.
   (C) Without perforation, it will show fecalith in more than 70% of cases.
   (D) It has increased in frequency in the past 20 years.
   (E) It never presents as recurrent attacks.

31. What is the mortality rate from acute appendicitis?

   (A) In the general population, it is 4/10,000.
   (B) After rupture, appendicitis is 4–5%.
   (C) For nonruptured appendicitis, it is 2%.
   (D) It is 80% if an abscess has formed.
   (E) It has increased in the past 40 years.

32. A 29-year-old woman presents to her physician's office with pain in the right iliac fossa. Examination reveals tenderness in this region. Her last menstrual cycle was 2 weeks previously and findings on gynecologic examination and leukocyte count are normal. A provisional diagnosis of acute appendicitis is made. She should be informed that operations to treat this condition reveal acute appendicitis in what percentage of cases?

   (A) a small percentage of cases
   (B) 50–89% of cases

(C) 90–99% of cases

(D) more than 99% of cases

(E) no reliable statistics are available

33. A 28-year-old man is admitted to the emergency department complaining of pain in the umbilical region that moves to the right iliac fossa. All are corroborative signs of acute appendicitis EXCEPT

(A) referred pain in the right side with pressure on the left (Rovsing sign)

(B) relief of pain with elevation of testicle (Prehn sign)

(C) production of pain in right lower abdomen with extension of thigh (psoas sign)

(D) pain in right lower abdomen with internal rotation of flexed thigh (obturator sign)

(E) hyperanesthesia in the right lower abdomen (Sherren sign)

34. A 28-old-male from Kosovo, who lives alone, presents with diarrhea. On examination he manifests clear wasting and malnutrition. His HCT is 28%, serum albumin reduced to 2.8 g%, and the blood analysis shows a macrocytic anemia. The emergency department physician is unable to secure an accurate history of the nature of multiple previous operations he had undergone before his arrival in the United States several months previously. What is the likely diagnosis that explains these features?

(A) blind loop syndrome

(B) diverticulitis of the sigmoid colon

(C) carcinoma of the left colon

(D) gastric ulcer

(E) carcinoid syndrome

Questions 35 and 36

A 74-year-old patient has a biopsy of the prostate that shows malignancy. He is considering radical prostatectomy or radiation therapy.

35. He is concerned about enterocolitis, which is likely to occur when?

(A) after local treatment with 15 Gy

(B) after local treatment with 35 Gy

(C) after local treatment with 55 Gy

(D) less frequently after previous surgery

(E) less frequently in the presence of adhesions

36. What complication should be anticipated in this patient?

(A) diverticulitis

(B) hemorrhoids

(C) complete occlusion of superior mesenteric artery

(D) complete occlusion of inferior mesenteric artery

(E) rectal bleeding

37. A 49-year-old computer technician receives irradiation to the pelvis for cervical cancer. Three months after irradiation, severe rectal proctitis may be shown by the presence of which of the following?

(A) ulcers

(B) strictures at anal verge

(C) mucosa prolapse

(D) multiple telangiectases and polypoid tumor

(E) free air under the diaphragm

Questions 38 and 39

A 63-year-old man is admitted to the hospital for abdominal pain and diarrhea of 6 days' duration. X-ray of the abdomen shows "thumbprinting" and gaseous distention suggestive of ischemic colitis.

38. What is true of colonic ischemia?

(A) It occurs in a younger age group (40–60 years of age).

(B) In most cases, it occurs in patients with cardiac failure.

(C) It usually causes severe abdominal pain.

(D) It may have a predisposing associated colonic lesion in 20% of patients.

(E) It results in the patient's appearing seriously ill.

39. To confirm the diagnosis of ischemic colitis, what test should be requested?

(A) selective angiogram of inferior mesenteric artery

(B) angiogram of superior and inferior mesenteric arteries

(C) computed tomography (CT) scan of the abdomen

(D) barium enema after 2 weeks

(E) barium enema as soon as possible

40. A 54-year-old man with diarrhea is found to have ulcerative colitis. Colectomy should be advised in patients with ulcerative colitis who have symptoms that persist for more than which of the following?

(A) 1 month

(B) 6 months

(C) 1–5 years

(D) 10–20 years

(E) more than 25 years

41. A 48-year-old woman develops colon cancer. She is known to have a long history of ulcerative colitis. In ulcerative colitis, colon cancer

(A) occurs more frequently than in the rest of the population

(B) is more likely to occur when the ulcerative disease is confined to the left colon

(C) occurs equally in the right and left side

(D) has a synchronous carcinoma in 4–5% of cases

(E) has an excellent prognosis because of physician awareness

42. A 56-year-old man is scheduled to have a left indirect hernia repaired. He is asymptomatic. Before surgical treatment, he should have which of the following?

(A) rectal examination alone

(B) rectal examination and sigmoidoscopy

(C) barium enema

(D) colonoscopy

(E) none of the above

43. A 64-year-old train conductor is diagnosed as having carcinoma confined to the descending colon. Before operation, what should be told?

(A) He will most likely require a colostomy.

(B) He should have the cancer excised by cautery.

(C) He should undergo left hemicolectomy.

(D) Radiotherapy is the treatment of choice.

(E) Forty percent of colorectal cancer involves the colon.

44. A 72-year-old woman is scheduled to undergo right hemicolectomy for cancer of the cecum. In this condition, she can anticipate subsequent recurrence

(A) of 20–30% if confined to the mucosa

(B) close to 100% if there is lymph node involvement

(C) which will not result in small-bowel obstruction

(D) which will not result in hydronephrosis

(E) which with microscopic lymph node metastasis would have a lower rate than that with macroscopic spread

45. A pathology specimen indicates that synchronous lesions are present. Which of the following statements are true regarding colon cancer with synchronous lesions?

(A) Cancer occurs in 20% of patients.

(B) Benign lesions occur in 20–30%.

(C) Malignant lesions are usually adjacent to the primary cancer.

(D) Benign lesions are usually adjacent to the primary cancer.

(E) Lesions occur much less frequently than metachronous lesions.

Questions 46 and 47

A 68-year-old dentist undergoes anterior resection (sigmoid resection) for cancer at the rectosigmoid junction. The tests performed before her surgery were flexible sigmoidoscopy and biopsy. There were no other lesions detected with sigmoidoscopy or in the pathology specimen.

46. Following operation, she requires which of the following within 2–3 months?

(A) repeat rectal examination and sigmoidoscopy

(B) colonoscopy

(C) CT scan of the abdomen

(D) angiography

(E) bone scan

47. The patient requests information from her surgeon as to her subsequent prognosis. She is informed that the prognosis for colon and rectal cancer is favorably affected by which of the following?

(A) minimal serosal extension

(B) minimal lymph node involvement

(C) confinement to the mucosa

(D) right-sided obstructing lesions

(E) elevated carcinoembryonic antigen (CEA) levels

48. An 83-year-old man is diagnosed on colonoscopy to have cancer of the colon. He refuses surgical intervention and after a 3-month follow-up period is admitted to the emergency department with large-bowel obstruction. Carcinoma of the colon is most likely to obstruct if found in the

(A) cecum

(B) ascending colon

(C) splenic flexure

(D) rectum

(E) transverse colon

49. A 43-year-old man is seen in his physician's office for severe pain in the perineum. Examination reveals exquisite tenderness in the area to the right side of the anal verge due to a perianal abscess. Rectal examination is refused. What should be the next step in management?

(A) drainage of the abscess in the office under local anesthesia

(B) excision of the vertical fold of Morgagni

(C) drainage under general anesthesia and immediate colonoscopy

(D) CT scan of the abdomen

(E) insertion of a rectal tube

50. A 64-year-old man undergoes CEA surveillance for cancer, because his brother and father both had colon cancer. He should be informed that

(A) CEA is highly sensitive for diagnosis

(B) if CEA is elevated preoperatively, it implies unresectable disease

(C) increases in CEA after resection may indicate tumor recurrence

(D) CEA is highly specific for the presence of colon cancer

(E) CEA is present in normal adult colonic mucosa

51. A 40-year-old man presents with pallor and breathlessness on exertion. He does not complain of abdominal pain. He has microcytic, hypochromic anemia. What is the most probable cause?

(A) diverticulosis of the colon

(B) peptic ulcer disease

(C) Crohn's disease

(D) ulcerative colitis

(E) carcinoma of the right colon

52. A 25-year-old man has recurrent, indolent fistula in ano. He also complains of weight loss, recurrent attacks of diarrhea with blood mixed in the stool, and tenesmus. Proctoscopy revealed a healthy, normal-appearing rectum. What is the most likely diagnosis?

(A) Crohn's colitis

(B) ulcerative colitis

(C) amoebic colitis

(D) ischemic colitis

(E) Colitis associated with acquired immunodeficiency syndrome (AIDS)

53. A 65-year-old man presents with chronic constipation and abdominal distention of 5 days' duration. He complains of lack of appetite and general malaise. Findings on physical examination are positive for a large distended abdomen with hyperactive bowel sounds. Rectal examination shows minimal stool that is guaiac-positive. Sigmoidoscopy does not reveal any further findings. Abdominal x-rays show a large 15-cm cecum and dilated, fluid-filled transverse and descending colon with very little gas in the rectum. What is the most probable cause of this condition?

(A) volvulus of the sigmoid colon

(B) pseudo-obstruction of the colon

(C) ischemic colitis

(D) carcinoma of the colon

(E) diverticulitis of the colon

54. A 27-year-old homosexual male presents with a foreign body in the rectum. During the extraction of the foreign body, a large tear in the sigmoid colon with extensive devitalization and contamination is observed. What is the preferred method of treatment?

(A) observation

(B) proctoscopic repair

(C) laparotomy and closure of sigmoid colon tear

(D) laparotomy, closure of sigmoid, and proximal colostomy or exteriorization of perforation as a colostomy

(E) laparotomy, resection of sigmoid colon, and colocolostomy

55. A 65-year-old woman with a history of chronic constipation is transferred from a nursing home because of abdominal pain and marked abdominal distention. On examination, her abdomen is found to be distended and tender in the left lower quadrant (LLQ). What is the most likely diagnosis?

(A) appendicitis

(B) carcinoma of the colon

(C) volvulus of the sigmoid colon

(D) volvulus of the cecum

(E) small-bowel obstruction

56. A 40-year-old man with a long history of bloody diarrhea presents with increased abdominal pain, vomiting, and fever. On examination, he is found to be dehydrated and shows tachycardia and hypotension. The abdomen is markedly tender with guarding and rigidity. What is the most likely cause?

(A) toxic megacolon in ulcerative colitis

(B) small-bowel perforation from regional enteritis

(C) perforated carcinoma of the sigmoid colon

(D) volvulus of the sigmoid colon

(E) acute perforated diverticulitis

57. Three days after undergoing an operation for an abdominal aortic aneurysm, a patient has moderate fever, abdominal pain, and rectal bleeding. What is the most helpful investigation?

(A) angiography

(B) upper GI endoscopy

(C) abdominal ultrasound

(D) sigmoidoscopy

(E) abdominal CT scan

58. A 55-year-old woman presents with pain in the LLQ of the abdomen and fever of 102°F. On examination, she is found to be dehydrated and has tenderness in the LLQ. A CT scan shows a mass in the LLQ involving the sigmoid colon. There is a minimal amount of free fluid and no free air. What should the initial treatment of this patient include?

(A) intravenous fluids, penicillin, and steroids

(B) intravenous fluids, cefoxitin, and nasogastric drainage

(C) intravenous fluids, blood transfusion, and laparotomy

(D) immediate laparotomy

(E) bowel preparation followed by laparotomy

Questions 59 and 60

A 72-year-old woman presents with bright red rectal bleeding, not associated with abdominal pain, of 2 day's duration. She had had previous similar episodes but was never hospitalized. Examination reveals a pale but alert individual with no significant abdominal findings. Findings on rectal examination are positive for bright red rectal bleeding. Her vital signs are stable and her hemoglobin is 9.5 g.

59. What is the most probable cause of her bleeding?

(A) diverticulitis of the colon

(B) carcinoma of the sigmoid colon

(C) Meckel's diverticulitis

(D) adenomatous polyp of the colon

(E) diverticulosis of the colon

60. The patient continues to bleed per rectum and becomes hypotensive to a systolic pressure of 60 mmHg despite blood transfusion. What is the optimal management plan?

(A) emergency colonoscopy and cauterization of bleeding vessels

(B) mesenteric angiography and embolization of the bleeder

(C) bleeding scan to localize the bleeder

(D) laparotomy and right colon resection

(E) blood transfusion laparotomy and sub-total colectomy with or without ileoproctostomy

61. A 45-year-old man complains of recurrent attacks of painless rectal bleeding. Colonoscopy reveals normal mucosa between the cecum and the anal verge. What is the most helpful test to determine the cause of bleeding?

(A) angiography to look for angiodysplasia

(B) technetium scan for Meckel's diverticulum

(C) upper GI endoscopy for peptic ulcer

(D) small-bowel series for tumor

(E) ultrasound for abdominal aortic aneurysm

62. The small intestine is characterized by basal crypts and superficial villi (Figure 4–3). Where does cell division take place?

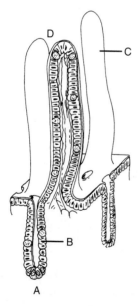

Figure 4–3. Schematic representation of villi and crypts of Lieberkühn. (Reproduced, with permission, from Way, LW: Current Surgical Diagnosis & Treatment, 10th ed., Appleton & Lange, 1994.)

(A) submucosa

(B) crypts

(C) villi

(D) small-bowel lumen

(E) all of the above

63. A 64-year-old man has a benign lesion of the colon. He is informed that the lesion does not predispose to colon cancer. What is the lesion he has?

(A) ulcerative colitis

(B) villous adenoma

(C) hyperplastic polyp

(D) adenoma in familial polyposis

(E) colon mucosa in a patient with colon carcinoma

64. A 25-year-old man complains of rectal bleeding, weight loss, and abdominal pain. He gives a history of similar complaints in his siblings as well as his mother. Findings on physical examination are unremarkable except for guaiac-positive stool. What is the most likely diagnosis?

(A) Peutz–Jegher syndrome

(B) familial polyposis of the colon

(C) ulcerative colitis

(D) carcinoma of the stomach

(E) Crohn's colitis

65. A 55-year-old man has had previous hemicolectomy for a carcinoma of the right colon. At this time, 3 years after the primary resection, a CT scan shows a solitary lesion in the right lobe of the liver. What is the next step in management?

(A) laser cauterization

(B) radiotherapy

(C) hepatic artery catheterization and local chemotherapy

(D) symptomatic treatment with analgesics, because the colon disease is now stage IV

(E) exploratory laparotomy and resection of the tumor

66. Following an appendectomy, a 28-year-old man is placed on ceftizoxime sodium (Cefizox). This antibiotic is unlikely to be effective against which of the following?

(A) *Pseudomonas*

(B) *Staphylococcus aureus*

(C) *Neisseria gonorrhoeae*

(D) *Bacteroides fragilis*

(E) *Haemophilus influenza*

67. A 68-year-old man presents with crampy abdominal pain and distention with vomiting. Findings on physical examination are positive for healed abdominal scars. X-rays reveal multiple gas fluid levels. The white blood cell (WBC) count is 12,000. What is the most likely diagnosis?

    (A) small-bowel intestinal obstruction due to adhesions
    (B) a hernia
    (C) appendicitis
    (D) inflammatory bowel disease
    (E) gallstones and ascites

68. A 55-year-old woman presents with vague right lower quadrant (RLQ) abdominal pain. A palpable mass is noted on abdominal examination. The mass is painless, well defined, mobile, and nonpulsatile. What is the most likely diagnosis?

    (A) a mesenteric cyst
    (B) appendix mass
    (C) perforated tubo-ovarian abscess
    (D) cholecystitis
    (E) Meckel's diverticulum

69. A 74-year-old woman complains of vomiting and intermittent colicky abdominal pain. X-rays reveal fluid levels and air in the biliary tree. What is the likely cause?

    (A) abdominal adhesions
    (B) gallstone ileus
    (C) carcinoma of the right colon
    (D) abdominal lymphosarcoma
    (E) previous choledochoduodenostomy

Questions 70 and 71

A 40-year-old woman experiences flushing, diarrhea, and wheezing. On physical examination, she is found to have tricuspid valve insufficiency.

70. What is the most likely diagnosis?

    (A) appendiceal carcinoid
    (B) ileal carcinoid
    (C) gastric lymphoma
    (D) small-bowel adenocarcinoma

71. The most useful diagnostic finding is which of the following?

    (A) elevated 5-hydroxyindoleacetic acid (5-HIAA) levels
    (B) elevated blood sugar levels
    (C) elevated serum gastrin levels
    (D) elevated amylase levels
    (E) elevated norepinephrine levels

72. A 56-year-old man has suffered from intermittent claudication for 5 years. He has recently developed cramping abdominal pain that is made worse by eating. He has a history of a 15 lb weight loss. What is the most likely diagnosis?

    (A) chronic intestinal ischemia (intestinal angina)
    (B) chronic cholecystitis
    (C) esophageal diverticulum
    (D) peptic ulcer
    (E) abdominal aortic aneurysm

73. A 68-year-old male musician presents to the emergency department with a sudden onset of colicky abdominal pain and massive vomiting of 4 hours' duration. Examination shows an elevated WBC of 13,200 with a HCT of 45%. Electrolytes and BUN are normal. An erect film of the abdomen reveals dilatation of the stomach with distended loops of bowel. What is his clinical diagnosis?

    (A) complete proximal intestinal obstruction
    (B) incomplete proximal intestinal obstruction
    (C) complete ileal obstruction
    (D) incomplete ileal obstruction
    (E) small bowel perforation

74. What is true with reference to small-bowel physiology migrating motor complexes?

    (A) They are increased after feeding.
    (B) They occur once every 10 minutes.
    (C) They continue throughout laparotomy.
    (D) They inhibit nutrient absorption.
    (E) They may explain diarrhea that occurs following vagotomy.

75. A 38-year-old man with a history of fever associated with abdominal pain of 3 weeks' duration presents now with a sudden onset of explosive abdominal pain and vomiting. Plain abdominal x-rays reveal air under a diaphragm. A CT scan shows mesenteric lymphadenopathy and splenomegaly is found. Laparotomy is performed and 3 feet of ileum resected. The luminal aspect of the resected bowel shows marked ulceration of Peyer's patches. What is the most likely diagnosis?

(A) typhoid enteritis
(B) tuberculosis enteritis
(C) Crohn's disease
(D) primary peritonitis
(E) ulcerative colitis

76. Gastrin is a hormone that is

(A) found mainly in the appendix and colon
(B) inhibited by ingestion of protein
(C) increased by vagus stimulation
(D) inhibited by fats
(E) inhibited by calcium salts

Questions 77 and 78

A 48-year-old man is admitted to hospital because of a 3-day history of mild abdominal pain, repeated vomiting, and marked abdominal distension. Immediately after the pain commenced, he had one small bowel movement but no further passage of stool or flatus. An abdominal flat plate revealed marked distension of loops of bowel confined to the small bowel.

77. A plain abdominal film shows loops of bowel that all extensively show valvulae conniventes. What is the most likely site of obstruction in Figure 4–4?

(A) high small bowel
(B) mid-small bowel
(C) distal small bowel
(D) colon
(E) none of the above

78. Following insertion of a nasogastric tube and appropriate rehydration and electrolyte correction, there is no change in clinical presentation. What should the next step involve?

(A) barium reduction with controlled hydrostatic pressure
(B) laparoscopy
(C) colostomy
(D) needle tap to deflate bowel
(E) exploratory laparotomy

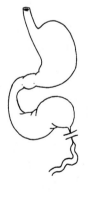 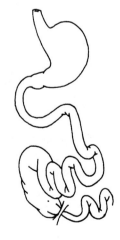 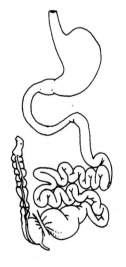 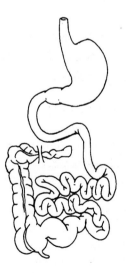

(A) High small bowel   (B) Mid-small bowel   (C) Distal small bowel   (D) Colon

Figure 4–4. Intestinal obstruction. (Reproduced, with permission, from Way, LW: Current Surgical Diagnosis & Treatment, 10th ed., Appleton & Lange, 1994.)

79. Following resection of the left colon, a 67-year-old obese woman develops left-sided leg edema due to deep-vein thrombosis. She is placed on anticoagulants, but after 2 weeks of warfarin (coumadin), she develops a pulmonary embolus with slight hypoxemia. What should the next step in management involve?

    (A) increasing the dose of anticoagulants
    (B) discontinuing anticoagulants
    (C) use of an inferior vena cava (IVC) filter
    (D) CT scan of the leg and abdomen
    (E) femoral vein ligation

Questions 80 and 81

A 44-year-old female immigrant from India and now resident in the US, has been treated for partial intestinal obstruction due to tuberculosis. There is no evidence of intestinal perforation.

80. What should the next step in treatment involve?

    (A) laparoscopy
    (B) laparotomy and bowel resection
    (C) a full course of antituberculous drugs
    (D) steroids
    (E) radiation therapy to the abdomen

81. What is the most likely outcome for the patient?

    (A) full recovery
    (B) rapid deterioration and possible death
    (C) pneumonia
    (D) empyema
    (E) scrofula

82. A 64-year-old woman presents with a strangulated femoral hernia. At operation, what is the criterion used to determine the viability of a loop of bowel?

    (A) increased peristalsis
    (B) absent arterial pulsation
    (C) venous engorgement
    (D) intraoperative CT scan
    (E) serum amylase

DIRECTIONS (Questions 83 through 93): Each set of matching questions in this section consists of a list of lettered options followed by several numbered items. For each numbered item, select the appropriate lettered option(s). Each lettered option may be selected once, more than once, or not at all. EACH ITEM WILL STATE THE NUMBER OF OPTIONS TO SELECT. CHOOSE EXACTLY THIS NUMBER.

Questions 83 through 85

    (A) vitamin A
    (B) vitamin C
    (C) vitamin D
    (D) vitamin E
    (E) vitamin K
    (F) vitamin B_1
    (G) chyle
    (H) sympathetic denervation
    (I) failure of rectal muscles to contract
    (J) gluten
    (K) peptides
    (L) bile salts
    (M) Meissner and Auerbach plexus deficiency
    (N) vagus nerve excess
    (O) inferior mesenteric ischemia

83. Steatorrhea and megaloblastic anemia occurring in a patient after bowel resection is caused by a failure to absorb what? SELECT TWO.

84. Nutritional deficiency in a patient with obstructive jaundice due to pancreatic cancer causing failure to absorb what? SELECT SIX.

85. What does Hirschsprung's disease involve? SELECT ONE.

Questions 86 through 88

    (A) Spigelian hernia
    (B) direct inguinal hernia
    (C) indirect inguinal hernia
    (D) femoral hernia
    (E) Richter's hernia

(F) appendix

(G) hydrocele

(H) sliding hernia

(I) bladder

(J) liver

(K) seminal vesicle

(L) an adrenal metastasis

(M) ureter

(N) prostate

(O) pubic bone

(P) Cowper's (bulbourethral) glands

86. An 84-year-old man has had a reducible hernia in the right groin for 17 years. One day before admission to the hospital, he complains of abdominal pain; because of the swelling, the hernia has become irreducible. At operation, part of the wall of the cecum is noted to form a portion of the hernia sac. What is the hernia? SELECT TWO.

87. Inside the contents of the swelling described in Question 86, what organs may be found? SELECT TWO.

88. A 56-year-old man underwent surgery for removal of cancer of the rectum. It was noted to have extended anteriorly to involve other viscera (Figure 4–5). SELECT FOUR.

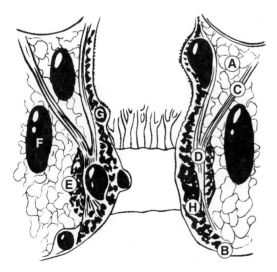

Figure 4–5. The ischioanal (ischiorectal fossa) and surrounding structures. (Reproduced, with permission, from Way, LW: Current Surgical Diagnosis & Treatment, 10th ed., Appleton & Lange, 1994.)

Questions 89 through 91

(A) pelvirectal space

(B) perianal space

(C) levator ani muscle

(D) intermuscular space

(E) external sphincter

(F) ischioanal (ischiorectal) space

(G) submucous space above the levator ani muscle

(H) marginal (mucocutaneous) space

89. Abscess located in which space causes extreme pain? SELECT ONE.

90. What does submucosal abscess involve? SELECT TWO.

91. This space may extend forward to pass superior to the urogenital diaphragm and enter the deep pouch where the external sphincter of the bladder is located. Fat tissue in this space is very loosely arranged and located below the levator ani muscle. What space is this? SELECT ONE.

Questions 92 and 93

(A) pilonidal sinus

(B) posterior perianal sinus

(C) single anterior perianal sinus

(D) multiple anterior perianal sinus

(E) periurethral abscess

(F) bartholin gland abscess

(G) prostatic abscess

(H) rectovaginal fistula

92. Which opens into the anal mucosa in the midline? SELECT ONE.

93. What has hair inside? SELECT ONE.

Answers and Explanations

1. **(A)** The small intestine arises from the midgut segment. The midgut segment extends between the ampulla of Vater and the distal transverse colon. It enters the physiological umbilical hernia at 6 weeks and returns to the peritoneal cavity by the tenth week. The vitellointestinal tract (site from which Meckel's diverticulum arises) is attached to the antimesenteric margin of the distal ileum. The urachus is attached to the bladder. The intestinal lymphatic drainage is directed to the preaortic glands.

2. **(D)** The small intestine commences to the *left* of the midline at Treitz's ligament and ends at the ileocecal junction. The mesenteric attachment is only 15 cm in length. It is supplied by the midgut vessel (superior mesenteric). The sympathetic and parasympathetic (vagus) nerves enter the mesentery to supply the vessels and gut wall.

3. **(C)** Crohn's disease differs from ulcerative coitis in that clinical improvement usually occurs when a diseased segment is excluded from the fecal stream. Crohn's disease involves the distal ileum in most patients, but almost any part of the alimentary tract could be affected. Steroids frequently result in improvement in patients with Crohn's disease and ulcerative colitis. In Crohn's disease, steroids are a double-edged sword, because they clearly allow initial improvement, but eventually their benefit is counteracted by adverse complications of steroids.

4. **(C)** The serosa appeared normal on inspection, but the colon mucosa was extensively involved. In ulcerative colitis, the distal rectum and colon are primarily involved in continuity to the proximal extent of the lesion. In Crohn's disease, a similar pattern may be found on rare occasions, but other features, such as small-intestinal disease, transmural involvement, skip lesions, and fistula formation, favor Crohn's disease. The small bowel is not primarily involved in ulcerative colitis, but a "backwash" ileitis may be encountered.

5. **(D)** Gangrene of the bowel occurs before the ominous sign of intramural air can be detected. The stack-of-coins sign is seen in intestinal obstruction where the proximal small intestine folds are stacked to provide this characteristic feature on a plain x-ray of the abdomen.

6. **(C)** In a patient with small intestine infarction, the possibility of nonocclusive ischemic disease should be excluded by angiography. If there is no evidence of gangrene, then fluid resuscitation and intra-arterial superior mesenteric papaverine administration may be adequate, and surgical intervention may be avoided. Von Willebrand's disease is characterized by a mild to moderate fall in factor VIII levels (pseudohemophilia) but with a much milder bleeding tendency than in true hemophilia. It affects males and females equally.

7. **(C)** Most air that reaches the stomach and intestines arises from swallowed air. Air is nearly always seen in the small intestine on a plain film of the abdomen. Gas in the stomach is derived mainly from swallowed air, which has an oxygen content of 20% and nitrogen content of 80%. CO_2 is formed by organic fermentation and comprises 40% of the gases in the distal bowel.

Nitrogen is absorbed so that it is reduced below 50% distally. Methane and hydrogen sulfide gases are added in the distal bowel.

8. **(D)** Treatment in infants is by controlled radiologic reduction initially, with surgery reserved for cases in which ischemia is expected or reduction is unsuccessful. The leading part of the intussusception is the apex. The outer sheath is the intussuscipiens, which receives the inner intussusceptum. The outer intussuscipiens elicits peristalsis, which forces the intussusceptum to extend distally.

9. **(D)** A plain film of the abdomen shows valvulae conniventes in jejunal (proximal) obstruction a featureless bowel pattern in distal ileal obstruction and haustra in colon obstruction.

10. **(A)** The initial management of intestinal obstruction is to correct fluid and electrolyte imbalance. Surgery is indicated if strangulation is anticipated or if the obstruction fails to respond to conservative management. Nasogastric suction is often effective in obstruction because of adhesions but is contraindicated when the obstruction is caused by a hernia and/or strangulation is suspected.

11. **(B)** In patients presenting with small bowel obstruction, clinical examination can usually identify a groin swelling attributable to strangulated hernia. If external groin hernia is excluded, the presence of an abdominal scar would highly suggest that intestinal obstruction is caused by adhesions. Peritoneal metastasis and primary tumors, bands, Crohn's disease, and gallstone ileus must be excluded. The distention is mainly a result of swallowed air. If the obstruction is proximal, the onset is usually more severe and rapid.

12. **(D)** In a Richter hernia, only part of the circumference of the bowel wall has become trapped in the hernia sac, and normal bowel movements may still occur. In the presence of a reducible groin hernia, it is important on clinic examination to be certain that other pathologic conditions are not overlooked.

13. **(E)** Primary small bowel volvulus is common in countries where the diet is high in bulk. Except for the neonatal variety (associated with malrotation), it is rare in the United States. Small-bowel volvulus secondary to adhesions is more common here. The ileum is more frequently involved than the jejunum. If a small bowel resection is required, it is usually of a limited nature.

14. **(C)** The ileum is the exclusive site of bile salt absorption, and failure of its absorption contributes to the steatorrhea. Ileal resection, which at times includes the ileocecal valve, is more commonly performed than is proximal resection. Over a longer period of time (2–3 years), megaloblastic anemia occurs.

15. **(A)** Transit time in the ileum is slower than that in the jejunum. Resection of equal lengths of intestine results in greater deterioration after ileal resection as the site of slower (and therefore more complete) absorption is removed. Jejunal resection is followed by hypertrophy of the residual villi in the ileum and functional compensation to a degree greater than in the jejunum after ileal resection.

16. **(B)** Massive resection occurs if more than 75–80% is resected (leaving less than 1 m of small bowel). The most common indications for major bowel resection are ischemia, Crohn's disease, volvulus, and trauma.

17. **(E)** Pneumotosis cystoides intestinalis results from diverse causes. In most instances it does not in itself indicate a serious complication. In premature infants, initial feeding results in mucosal damage with tracking of intramural air (Pneumotosis cystoides intestinalis). In adults, it may result from emphysema or rupture of a pulmonary bulla, which tracts below the diaphragm and encircles the bowel wall.

18. **(D)** Pneumatosis cystoides intestinalis may be associated with other conditions in the intestines or elsewhere. The finding of this condition as an incidental finding requires no further treatment other than that of the underlying cause. In newborns pneumotosis cystoides intestinalis must be differentiated from the more serious and critical entity of necrotizing enterocolitis

19. (E) In the blind loop syndrome, bacteria proliferate in an affected segment that fails to show appropriate peristaltic activity. It may be seen in surgery requiring jejunal or ileal bypass, small intestinal diverticular disease, scleroderma, diabetes mellitus and intestinal carcinoma. Macrocytic anemia caused by malabsorption of Vitamin B_{12} and folic acid and is a key diagnostic feature in its diagnosis.

20. (C) Intestinal obstruction in a Meckel's diverticulum may result from a volvulus, band obstruction, or intussusception. Among children, bleeding and inflammation are seen more frequently. Meckel's diverticulum is a remnant of the vitellointestinal duct.

21. (B) Peutz–Jeghers syndrome is rare but should be considered if pigmented spots are found on the lips, mouth, or hands. Hamartomas are not neoplasms; the name is derived from the Greek *hamartos,* which refers to the misfiring of a javelin. The tissues appropriate to the site misfire and are arranged in an irregular order.

22. (A) Unfortunately, in most series, division of adhesions accounts for as much as 25% of postoperative intestinal fistulas. These cases usually involve sites that are not recognized at the time of operation. The fistulas occurring after resection of the bowel in Crohn's disease are less likely to heal without surgical intervention. The small intestine is the most common site of intestinal fistula formation.

23. (B) Internal small-bowel fistulas are caused almost exclusively by small-bowel disease or surrounding visceral disease involving the small bowel. Crohn's disease is the most common cause of internal small-bowel fistulas, but neoplasia, lymphoma, and tuberculosis must be excluded. Internal fistula may be asymptomatic or cause serious malabsorption (proximal to distal fistulas) or infection (enterovesical fistulas).

24. (A) In general, treatment is geared initially for placement of an intestinal tube proximally, appropriate antibiotics if infection is present, and central hyperalimentation. Surgical intervention is required early if a clear-cut focus of infection exists or distal obstruction is present. In general,

if there is no healing of the fistula in 4–6 weeks, surgical intervention should be considered.

25. (D) Both zinc and vitamin C (ascarbate) deficiency, impair wound healing. Incision through the same incision actually promotes wound healing, because the initial lag interval after creation of the wound is avoided (unless the whole scar of the incision is removed). Increase in local oxygen tension actually promotes wound healing.

26. (B) Fluorouracil does not interfere with wound healing. Appropriate antibiotics improve healing of bowel anastomis by reducing local intraluminal bacteria count. The presence of minimal bacteria growth has a favorable effect on wound healing. Denervation of tissue surrounding the incision does not influence wound healing.

27. (D) The omentum and peritoneal cavity seem to be less efficient in localizing the disease in these age groups. Appendicitis has a particularly high complication rate in infants and the elderly. Delay in establishing the accurate diagnosis in these two age groups also contributes to a worse prognosis.

28. (D) In appendicitis, patients frequently note that the pain commences in the umbilical region and moves later to the iliac fossa. Pain in the iliac fossa occurs when the overlying parietal peritoneum is involved. Patients with appendicitis typically indicate that they have anorexia. Seventy to 80% of patients with appendicitis have vomiting.

29. (C) This is McBurney's point and often indicates the region where maximal tenderness can be elicited. In addition to tenderness, guarding and percussion tenderness should be sought to verify whether localized and/or general peritonitis exists.

30. (B) Appendicitis is 1.5 times more common in males than in females. Appendicitis occurs with equal incidence before puberty, but thereafter it is more frequent in men. The diagnosis may be difficult in women because of multiple gynecologic problems that are encountered in the differential diagnosis. There appears to be a drop in incidence of appendicitis during the past 20 years. Fecalith occurs in nearly all patients

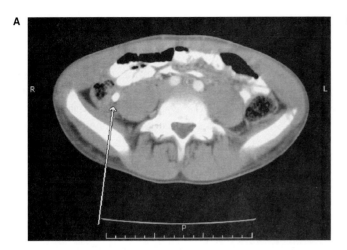
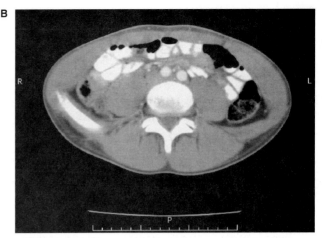

Figure 4–6. A, CT scan shows a fecolith in the appendix. **B,** CT scan shows a dilated appendix with fluid.

with perforation of a gangrenous appendicitis and in 30–40% of those without perforation.

31. **(B)** The mortality rate from appendicitis is 4/1,000,000 in the general population, which is a 20-fold decline from that reported 50 years ago. The mortality rate for ruptured appendicitis is 4–5% but increases to 9% in infants and 15% in patients above 65 years of age and those with serious underlying medical illness. The high rate of perforation is partly due to physician delay in establishing the diagnosis of acute appendicitis. The mortality rate of 0.1% in patients with non-ruptured appendicitis highlights the fact that the condition remains a potentially lethal disease. The diagnosis of acute appendicitis is nearly always determined on clinical grounds without need to request a CT scan (Figure 4–6).

32. **(C)** If the surgeon's records indicate that all operations on the appendix are abnormal, there is a real danger that a true appendicitis will be missed and that the criteria chosen are too rigid. On the other hand, if the rate of normal appendices removed is increased, the criteria selected for operation require further defining. Good clinical observation and appropriate laparoscopy in female patients will help achieve the goal of optimal incidence of accuracy with emergency appendectomy. After unwarranted appendectomy, complications include persistent pain from adhesions, inadvertent visceral trauma at operation, and small bowel obstruction. In older patients in particular, the usual diverse complications of operations occur.

33. **(B)** Relief of pain brought about by elevation of the testicle is characteristic of epididymo-orchitis. Prehn sign is useful to differentiate epididymo-orchitis from torsion of the testis, because elevation of the test will relieve pain only in the inflammatory condition. The other signs are corroborative of appendicitis. Hyperesthesia is a useful sign provided that it is performed objectively. The area of hyperesthesia is a triangular area (base placed upward) in the right lower abdomen.

34. **(A)** The presence of a blind loop leads to malabsorption with steatorrhea, macrocytic anemia, and malabsorption. A blind loop is likely to occur if an antiperistaltic loop is created, and it is more than three to six inches in length. The antiperistaltic loop causes failure of adequate emptying of intestinal contents; this leads to stasis and overgrowth of bacteria.

35. **(C)** Irradiation of the abdominal cavity of more than 50 Gy is associated with a higher rate of complications. The incidence of symptomatic sigmoiditis may be as high as 75%, and histologically abnormal rectal biopsy findings occur in 11% of patients undergoing treatment for pelvic malignancy. Previous surgery with possible adhesion formation increases the risk of irradiation damage.

36. **(E)** In most patients, ischemic colitis is a self-limiting illness that usually resolves within 7–10 days. Patients may manifest pyrexia and peritonitis, have persistent symptoms, and

develop complications, such as stricture formation, perforation, and bleeding. Unlike small bowel ischemia, the main vessels are characteristically patent.

37. **(A)** The mucosa is friable and bleeds readily. Ulcers vary in size and often tend to be transverse in position and surrounded by telangiectases. They are often more prominent on the anterior wall around the anal verge. Rectal strictures usually are located about 8–12 cm above the anal verge. Rectovaginal fistula may develop in female patients. On barium enema, a narrow stricture is difficult to differentiate from a carcinoma.

38. **(D)** In 90% of cases with colonic ischemia, the patient is over 65 years of age. Precipitating causes, such as cardiac disease, are much less frequently encountered than in small-bowel ischemia. In 20% of patients, an underlying obstructive lesion of the colon is noted. Unlike small-bowel ischemia, the pain is often insidious in onset, and there is only minimal tenderness on examination.

39. **(E)** The classic finding of thumbprinting may be missed if the barium enema study is deferred for more than 10 days after onset of symptoms. Unlike small-bowel ischemia, the main vessels are patent in most cases.

40. **(D)** After 10 years with ulcerative colitis, the chances of developing carcinoma increase fourfold. After 20 years, the cumulative risk is 12%, and at 25 years, it is 25%. Malignancy is often detected at a late stage and has a larger percentage of synchronous lesions as compared to that seen in patients with cancer who do not have ulcerative colitis. Patients with extensive disease and those in whom the disease occurs at an earlier age must undergo careful surveillance.

41. **(A)** Occurs more frequently than in the rest of the population. The cumulative risk of developing cancer in patients with extensive ulcerative colitis is greater than in those with more localized disease (42% at 25 years). Children are more likely to have extensive disease. Colon cancer occurs more frequently in the sigmoid and rectum in ulcerative colitis, but cancer is more likely to occur in patients who have universal disease.

Synchronous carcinomas in patients without ulcerative colitis occur in 4%, compared to 25% in those with colitis. Lesions usually are flat, are frequently missed at examination, and have a worse prognosis than other types of cancer. Adults developing cancer under the age of 45 have a poorer prognosis than those who develop it later.

42. **(B)** Patients who have symptoms suggestive of change in bowel habits will require a barium enema or colonoscopy. It is important not to overlook an underlying carcinoma, which could cause the patient to strain and induce a hernia. Carcinoma and/or polyps may be overlooked if this approach is ignored.

43. **(C)** There has been an increase in incidence of colon cancer relative to that of the rectum in recent years. This observation may be related to the improved diagnostic techniques now available with colonoscopy. The higher mortality of some rectal cancer patients may be attributed to an incomplete resection of the tumor when it is close to the cut edge. Each year, 14,000 new cases are diagnosed and over 6,000 deaths occur.

44. **(E)** Just under half of patients with local disease will also have associated metastatic disease. The Aster–Coller classification for colon cancer is as follows: A, mucosal; B1, muscle; B2, external to serosa; C1 and C2, same as B1 and B2 but with lymph node involvement. Patients with microscopic lymph node metastasis—adjacent as opposed to remote—and with one to three lymph nodes involved have a better prognosis than patients with more extensive disease.

45. **(B)** Synchronous malignant lesions (present in 4–5%) refer to those present at the time of surgery or found in investigations carried out within 6 months after operation. Metachronous lesions are those not detected during this period but subsequently identified. Metachronous carcinomas occur in about 5% of cases.

46. **(B)** Both synchronous carcinomas and benign polyps occur mainly at sites in the colon that would not be included in the definite resection for the primary carcinoma. Thus, it is important to try, whenever possible, to perform colonoscopy before colon resection to facilitate planning of the operation should a synchronous lesion be

detected. If this study is omitted, it is advisable to have a complete colonoscopy performed within the first 2–3 months after resection.

47. **(C)** Dukes A lesions have an excellent prognosis of 90% 5-year survival compared to that with serosal extension (B2), particularly if lymph nodes are heavily involved. Seventy percent of obstructing lesions occur on the left side and 30% at or proximal to the hepatic flexure. The CEA level correlates with the extent of encirclement of the tumor, Dukes classification, and the likelihood of recurrence.

48. **(C)** The most common sites of obstruction are descending colon (21%), sigmoid (17%), and splenic flexure (15%). The percentages for cases with obstruction at a particular site are splenic flexure, 37%; sigmoid, 16%; and right colon, 14%.

49. **(A)** The ducts of the anal glands drain into the anus and are covered by the vertical columns of Morgagni. Infection of these glands may account for some cases of perianal abscess. The folds end distally at about the level of the dentate line. The lower third of the anus receives its nerve supply from the pudendal nerve (somatic). In order to minimize spread of infection, the local anesthetic should be confined to the skin immediately overlying the abscess.

50. **(C)** CEA is useful in the follow-up care of patients with colon carcinoma after resection. The levels of this antigen usually come to normal after complete resection of the tumor. A subsequent elevation may suggest a recurrence of the tumor either at the resection margin or at distant sites. The sensitivity and specificity of CEA for diagnosis of colon carcinoma is poor. It has no implications for resectability of the lesion.

51. **(E)** Insidious development of a microcytic, hypochromic anemia is an important clue for the diagnosis of carcinoma of the right colon. Guaiac-positive stool with or without a palpable mass in the right lower quadrant should raise the possibility. All the other possibilities listed may also cause lower GI bleeding but are characteristically associated with abdominal pain (peptic ulcer disease, Crohn's disease, ulcerative colitis). Bleeding in sigmoid diverticulosis usually is bright red and painless.

52. **(A)** Recurrent fistulas in ano are a feature of Crohn's colitis. The absence in the rectum eliminates the possibility of ulcerative colitis. Amebic colitis presents with recurrent episodes of diarrhea with bleeding. Ischemic colitis also presents with diarrhea.

53. **(D)** The picture described suggests large-bowel obstruction in a patient with a competent ileocecal valve. The most likely cause is an obstructing carcinoma. The site of obstruction is in the sigmoid colon above the level of sigmoidoscopy. Sigmoid volvulus, ischemic colitis, and diverticulitis will present some findings on sigmoidoscopy. Pseudo-obstruction of the colon will manifest as colonic distention down to the rectum.

54. **(D)** Rectosigmoid injuries should promptly raise a high index of suspicion, warranting immediate sigmoidoscopy to confirm the diagnosis. The treatment is operative and should consist of decompressive colostomy either proximal to the perforation or at the perforation. In the presence of fecal contamination from a perforation in an unprepared bowel, none of the other choices is safe.

55. **(C)** Volvulus of the sigmoid (secondary type) is common in elderly patients who are chronically constipated. Redundancy of the sigmoid and a narrow mesenteric attachment predispose for the twisting. In the large bowel, the sigmoid is the most common site. Abdominal distention and tenderness are the common presenting symptoms. Volvulus of the sigmoid colon can usually be detected on a supine and erect abdominal x-ray. Sigmoidoscopy and contrast barium studies may be helpful to differentiate carcinoma from volvulus.

56. **(A)** The long history of bloody diarrhea should suggest a diagnosis of inflammatory bowel disease. The acute onset of abdominal pain together with the findings of an acute abdomen and systemic manifestations should raise the suspicion of a devastating complication. The picture is characteristic of acute toxic megacolon in ulcerative colitis. All the other possibilities listed may present with an acute abdomen, but the long history should point to ulcerative colitis.

57. **(D)** In a patient with abdominal aortic aneurysm resection, the most worrisome complication is inadequate blood supply to the sigmoid colon through the marginal artery. Sigmoid ischemia should be ruled out by sigmoidoscopy. In the clinical picture described, sigmoidoscopy should be the most important test.

58. **(B)** The findings described on physical examination and CT scan are suggestive of acute diverticulitis of the sigmoid colon. The initial treatment of this condition is expectant with antibiotics with or without nasogastric drainage. An antibiotic with specificity against the *Bacteroides* species (third-generation cephalosporin, metronidazole, or clindamycin) should be part of the regimen. Steroids have no place in the treatment. Laparotomy is indicated only after failure of conservative treatment.

59. **(E)** The clinical picture of recurrent bright rectal bleeding that is not associated with abdominal pain is characteristic of diverticulosis of the colon. The bleeding in sigmoid carcinoma is often microscopic. Diverticulitis of the colon would present with associated pain. Adenomatous polyp may present with painless rectal bleeding, but the most common condition in this elderly age group is diverticulosis of the colon.

60. **(E)** Laparotomy and subtotal colectomy should be the preferred approach in a hypotensive patient. There is no time for trying to localize the site of bleeding by scans, mesenteric angiography, or colonoscopy. Although the common site of massive diverticular hemorrhage is the right colon, a blind right colon resection in an elderly woman with hypotension is fraught with the danger of recurrent bleeding from the left colon. The safest and most expeditious management is subtotal colectomy. The decision for anastomosis or proximal ileostomy will depend on the stability of the patient.

61. **(A)** A common cause of lower GI bleeding that is recurrent and painless is angiodysplasia of the colon. In the absence of diverticula or hemorrhoids, the suspicion is even higher for these lesions. Peptic ulcer and Meckel's diverticulum can cause predominantly lower GI bleeding. However, the bleeding is usually in the form of melena rather than bright red.

62. **(B)** Small-bowel turnover can be measured in rats by autoradiographic studies in which turnover of cells located in the crypts migrate along the villus toward the tip over a 2- to 3-day period. Intestinal villous mucosa undergoes hypertrophy and hyperplasia whenever an increased food load continuously enters the small intestine.

63. **(C)** All the choices listed except hyperplastic polyp are precancerous lesions. The carcinomas in ulcerative colitis and familial polyposis are multicentric. Large villous adenomas may have carcinomatous changes. Any patient with a colon carcinoma is predisposed to develop a metachronous lesion in the remaining colon, hence the importance of regular follow-up examinations in these patients.

64. **(B)** All the clinical features mentioned and the strong family history should raise the possibility of familial polyposis. Although other possibilities listed may also cause rectal bleeding and abdominal pain, the strong familial history should give a clue to the diagnosis. The early onset of invasive carcinoma in these patients makes recognizing familial polyposis very important.

65. **(E)** Many patients who have metastases to the liver or lung have resectable tumors. A reasonable disease-free interval has been reported after such resections, especially with carcinoma of the colon as the primary lesion.

66. **(A)** Cefizox is not effective against many strains of *Pseudomonas*. If the drug is used in pseudomonas infection a higher dosage may be indicated, and the antibiotic should be changed if a quick response does not occur. Complications include cross reactions in patients who are allergic to penicillin. It does not seem to have nephrotoxic side effects.

67. **(A)** The presence of distended loops of bowel indicate bowel obstruction. The clinical features favor mechanical obstruction rather than paralytic ileus due to infection. Obstruction due to adhesions is more common than obstruction due to hernia.

68. **(A)** This is a relatively uncommon lesion. One sign that may be elicited with a mesenteric cyst is that the swelling moves freely in the direction between the left iliac fossa and the right hypochondria (i.e., perpendicular to the small-bowel mesentery axis).

69. **(B)** Gallstone ileus results in "tumbling" intestinal obstruction due to the intermittent nature of the condition. Previous choledochoduodenostomy could give air in the biliary tree but not obstruction.

70. **(B)** The carcinoid syndrome in patients with intestinal carcinoid tumors will occur only in the presence of hepatic metastasis. Approximately 40% of patients with hepatic metastasis from an ileal carcinoid will develop the syndrome.

71. **(A)** Patients with carcinoid tumor due to ovarian dermoid or pulmonary lesion may develop the syndrome with an elevated 5-HIAA, although hepatic metastases are absent. The liver does not counteract the hormone in this instance, because the portal system is bypassed.

72. **(A)** Patients with underlying ischemic disease may develop acute intestinal infarction or intestinal angina, which is aggravated by eating.

73. **(A)** Mechanical obstruction implies a barrier that impedes progress of intestinal contents. Complete mid- or distal small bowel obstruction presents with colicky abdominal pain, more marked abdominal distention but with vomiting that is less frequent and occurs at a later stage than that of proximal jejunal obstruction.

74. **(E)** Migrating motor complexes (MMC) are isoperistaltic waves and occur approximately once every 90 minutes. Oral feeding inhibits the MMC for as much as 3–4 hours. The inhibition of the MMC in the stomach and intestine may account in part for nausea and vomiting occurring after surgery. The major force that drives chyme aborally is that of segmentation and not the MMC.

75. **(A)** Typhoid fever typically presents with initial symptoms. Small-intestine complications are related to involvement of Peyer's patches of the small intestine, which result in bleeding and/or perforation in the second and third week after symptoms are noted.

76. **(C)** Gastrin is found in the pyloric antrum, duodenum, and small intestine. It is not present in the fundus of the stomach. Vagal stimulation acts in part by increasing gastrin release. Protein and amino acids cause marked stimulation of gastrin. Glucose and fats are less potent than protein as a cause of gastrin release. Gastrin release is stimulated by oral calcium salt intake.

77. **(B)** The absence of loops of colon makes a colonic site most unlikely as a cause of the current clinical presentation. Distention does not occur in high small-bowel obstruction.

78. **(E)** In view of the presence of bowel obstruction, surgery is indicated. In general, patients who have obstruction due to adhesions may undergo an initial short trial period of conservative management. Laparotomy is usually indicated in bowel obstruction due to other causes, where gangrene may be evident, and in all cases in which an initial period of conservative treatment fails.

79. **(C)** In general, failure (or inability) to continue anticoagulants is an indication to insert an IVC filter to minimize the possibility of serious and possibly fatal pulmonary embolus.

80. **(C)** Tuberculosis is the great mimicker of disease and, therefore, should always be considered in the differential diagnosis of different abdominal conditions. Surgical intervention will be required if the obstruction should become complete.

81. **(A)** Although intestinal tuberculosis still remains relatively uncommon in the United States, it should be particularly excluded in the AIDS population. In these patients, the rarity of the condition may make its clinical detection particularly difficult. Always suspect tuberculosis in the differential diagnosis of fever without a clearly defined cause.

82. **(B)** The blood supply to a loop of ischemic bowel is determined by the presence or absence of arterial pulsation, peristalsis, and color of the bowel after resuscitation and relief of obstruction.

83. **(H, L)** The jejunum is the first part of the alimentary tract and, therefore, is the primary site

of absorption of nearly all nutrients. It is unable to absorb vitamin B$_{12}$ and bile salts, which are absorbed exclusively in the ileum. If the ileum is transposed between the duodenum and the jejunum, it undergoes compensatory hypertrophy and takes over the function of the jejunum and becomes the primary site of nutrient absorption.

84. **(A, C, D, E, K, L)** In obstructive jaundice and major small-bowel resection, there will be failure to absorb the fat-soluble vitamins and bile salts. Vitamin K deficiency is an important clinical problem in such patients and requires appropriate parenteral replacement before a surgical procedure is undertaken.

85. **(M)** In Hirschsprung's disease, there is an absence of myenteric plexus in the upper anal segment (i.e., the most distal portion of the cloaca). In 15%, the myenteric plexus involves only the upper anus; in 70%, the rectum is also involved; and in 15%, part of the colon is also involved. The abnormal segment is contracted; whereas, the dilated bowel is proximal to the diseased segment.

86. **(C, H)** In this variety, the hernia does not have a complete covering of peritoneum. It is important that the surgeon does not attempt to remove peritoneum from the circumference bowel wall where it does not exist, because the bowel will become devascularized.

87. **(F, J)** Care must be taken to avoid injury to the bladder. In general, the bowel is less likely to undergo gangrenous changes as compared to other types of indirect inguinal hernias.

88. **(I, K, M, N)** In resection of the rectum for cancer, the tumor may have invaded these structures anteriorly. These organs may be included in the resected specimen in selected cases to improve survival.

89. **(B)** The perianal space is below (i.e., external to) the perianal fascia. The perianal fascia separates the more superficial subcutaneous (tightly compact) fat from the more internal (superior) fat in the ischioanal (ischiorectal) fossa, in which the

fat is less dense. Ischioanal abscess may be potentially more serious, because the clinical presentation is less acute, and the patient may seek medical assistance at a very late stage.

90. **(G, H)** The submucous space is in the mucous membrane and, therefore, internal to the double layer of smooth muscle (circular and longitudinal muscles). The innervation of the mucosa of the distal anus is somatic (proctadeum); that from the upper two-thirds of the anus (and rectum) is visceral from the hindgut.

91. **(F)** The inferior rectal nerve and vessels travel here to supply the rectum. An abscess in this space may extend posteriorly and form a horseshoe connection with the opposite side. The anterior extension of an ischioanal (ischiorectal) abscess may extend anteriorly toward the deep pouch.

92. **(B)** A single or multiple sinus that has an external opening in the posterior half of the skin that surrounds the anus will have an internal opening in the midline on the distal anus if a fistula has formed (Figure 4–7).

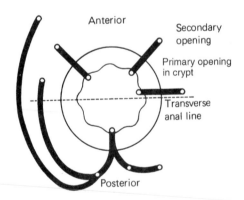

Figure 4–7. Salmon–Goodsall rule. The usual relation of the primary and secondary openings of fistulas. When the external opening of a fistula is anteriorly situated, the internal opening is found internal to it in the same radial position; when the external opening of a fistula is posteriorly situated, the internal opening is found in the midline posteriorly. Note the exception to this rule of the far lateral (anterior) fistula. (Reproduced, with permission, from Way, LW: Current Surgical Diagnosis & Treatment, 10th ed., Appleton & Lange, 1994.)

93. **(A)** The most common site for a pilonidal abscess to develop is in the midline posteriorly in the natal cleft posterior to the sacrum.

CHAPTER 5

Pancreas, Biliary Tract, Liver, and Spleen
Questions

Khawaja Azimuddin and C. Gene Cayten

DIRECTIONS (Questions 1 through 81): Each of the numbered items or incomplete statements in this section are followed by answers or by completions of the statement. Select the ONE lettered answer or completion that is BEST in each case.

1. A 42-year-old man who consumed more than 3 bottles of vodka weekly over the past 20 years is admitted with upper abdominal pain radiating to the back, nausea, and vomiting. Serum amylase and lipase are elevated, and a diagnosis of pancreatitis is made. In determining his prognosis, which of the following factors would cause the greatest concern?

   (A) hypercalcemia (Ca >12 mg/dL)
   (B) age over 40 years
   (C) hypoxemia
   (D) hyperamylasemia (>600 U)
   (E) elevated lipase

2. A 62-year-old man with a chronic history of alcohol abuse is admitted to the hospital with abdominal pain. Examination of the abdomen reveals epigastric fullness. Which test will most likely elucidate the cause of the swelling?

   (A) serum amylase
   (B) amylase–creatinine clearance ratio
   (C) endoscopy
   (D) ultrasound
   (E) technetium scan

3. A 24-year-old college student recovers from a bout of severe pancreatitis. He has mild epigastric discomfort, sensation of bloating, and loss of appetite. Examination reveals an epigastric fullness that on ultrasound is confirmed to be a pseudocyst. The swelling increases in size over a 3-week period of observation. What should be the next step in management?

   (A) percutaneous drainage of the cyst
   (B) laparotomy and internal drainage of the cyst
   (C) excision of pseudocyst
   (D) total pancreatectomy
   (E) administration of pancreatic enzymes

4. A 40-year-old alcoholic male is admitted with severe epigastric pain radiating to the back. Serum amylase level is reported as normal, but serum lipase is elevated. The serum is noted to be milky in appearance. A diagnosis of pancreatitis is made. The serum amylase is normal because

   (A) the patient has chronic renal failure
   (B) the patient has hyperlipidemia
   (C) the patient has alcoholic cirrhosis
   (D) the patient has alcoholic hepatitis
   (E) the diagnosis of pancreatitis is incorrect

5. A 52-year-old woman is admitted to the hospital with abdominal pain. She reports that she drinks alcohol only at social occasions. The amylase is elevated to 340 U. Which following x-ray finding would support a diagnosis of idiopathic pancreatitis?

(A) hepatic lesion on computed tomography (CT) scan
(B) choledocholithiasis on ultrasound
(C) anterior displacement of the stomach on barium upper gastrointestinal (GI) series
(D) trefoil sign in the first part of the duodenum
(E) irregular cutoff of the common bile duct on cholangiogram

6. A 67-year-old woman is noted to have a gradual increase in the size of the abdomen. A CT scan reveals a large pancreatic mass. The lesion was excised; on pathology examination, it is shown to be a true cyst. Which statement is correct regarding true cysts?

(A) They are commonly seen in alcoholic pancreatitis.
(B) They commonly occur after trauma.
(C) They are frequently malignant.
(D) They are associated commonly with choledochocele.
(E) They have an epithelial lining.

7. A 40-year-old man with a history of alcohol consumption of 25 years' duration is admitted with a history of a 6-lb weight loss and upper abdominal pain of 3 weeks' duration. Examination reveals fullness in the epigastrium. His temperature is 99°F, and his white blood cell (WBC) count is 10,000. Which is the most likely diagnosis?

(A) pancreatic pseudocyst
(B) subhepatic abscess
(C) biliary pancreatitis
(D) cirrhosis
(E) splenic vein thrombosis

8. A 58-year-old man with a 30-year history of alcoholism and pancreatitis is admitted to the hospital with an elevated bilirubin level of 5 mg/dL,

alcoholic stools, and an amylase level of 600 U. Obstructive jaundice in chronic pancreatitis usually results from which of the following?

(A) sclerosing cholangitis
(B) common bile duct (CBD) compression caused by inflammation
(C) alcoholic hepatitis
(D) biliary dyskinesia
(E) splenic vein thrombosis

9. A 48-year-old woman is admitted with acute cholecystitis. The bilirubin level is elevated, as are the serum and urinary amylase levels. Which radiologic sign indicates biliary obstruction in pancreatitis?

(A) pancreatic intraductal calcification
(B) smooth narrowing of the distal CBD
(C) stomach displaced anteriorly
(D) calcified gallstone
(E) air in the biliary tree

10. A 62-year-old man is admitted with abdominal pain and weight loss of 5 lb over the past month. He has continued to consume large amounts of rum. Examination reveals icteric sclera. The indirect bilirubin level is 5.6 mg/dL with a total bilirubin of 6 mg/dL. An ultrasound shows a 4-cm pseudocyst. What is the most likely cause of jaundice in a patient with alcoholic pancreatitis?

(A) alcoholic hepatitis
(B) carcinoma of pancreas
(C) intrahepatic cyst
(D) pancreatic pseudocyst
(E) hemolytic anemia

11. A 42-year-old woman with a history of chronic alcoholism is admitted to the hospital because of acute pancreatitis. The bilirubin and amylase levels are in the normal range. An ultrasound reveals cholelithiasis. The symptoms abate on the 5th day after admission. How should she be advised?

(A) to start on a low-fat diet
(B) to increase the fat content of her diet
(C) to undergo immediate cholecystectomy

(D) to undergo cholecystectomy during the same hospital stay

(E) that she will be discharged and now should undergo elective cholecystectomy after 3 months

12. Following a motor vehicle accident a truck driver complains of severe abdominal pain. Serum amylase level is markedly increased to 800 U. Grey Turner sign is seen in the flanks. Pancreatic trauma is suspected. Which statement is true of pancreatic trauma?

(A) It is mainly caused by blunt injuries.

(B) It is usually an isolated single-organ injury.

(C) It often requires a total pancreatectomy.

(D) It may easily be overlooked at operation.

(E) It is proved by the elevated amylase level.

13. The highest mortality can be anticipated when pancreatitis occurs after which of the following?

(A) beer ingestion

(B) wine ingestion

(C) trauma and operation

(D) hemolytic anemia

(E) parotitis

14. A 40-year-old woman with severe chronic pancreatitis is scheduled to undergo an operation, because other forms of treatment have failed. The ultrasound shows no evidence of pseudocyst formation or cholelithiasis and endoscopic retrograde cholangiopancreatogram (ERCP) demonstrates dilated pancreatic ducts with multiple stricture formation. Which operation is suitable to treat this condition?

(A) pancreaticojejunostomy (Puestow)

(B) gastrojejunostomy

(C) cholecystectomy

(D) splenectomy

(E) subtotal pancreatectomy

15. A 26-year-old woman with a known history of chronic alcoholism is admitted to the hospital with severe abdominal pain due to acute pancreatitis. The serum and urinary amylase levels are normal. On the day following admission to the hospital, there is no improvement, and she has a mild cough and and slight dyspnea. What is the most likely complication?

(A) pulmonary atelectasis

(B) bronchitis

(C) pulmonary embolus

(D) afferent loop syndrome

(E) pneumonia

16. A 30-year-old male is admitted with frequent episodes of hypoglycemia. Biochemical investigations confirmed an insulinoma. Localization studies were carried out. A CT scan and MRI of the abdomen failed to reveal a tumor in the pancreas. An endoscopic ultrasound, however, localized a 2-cm insulinoma in the tail of the pancreas. What should be the next step in the management of this patient?

(A) somatostatin receptor scintigraphy (SRS) to confirm the insulinoma

(B) exploratory laparotomy and total pancreatectomy

(C) distal pancreatectomy

(D) whipple pancreaticoduodenectomy

(E) enucleation of the tumor

17. A 66-year-old man with obstructive jaundice is found on ERCP to have periampullary carcinoma. He is otherwise in excellent physical shape and there is no evidence of metastasis. What is the most appropriate treatment?

(A) radical excision (Whipple procedure) where possible

(B) local excision and radiotherapy

(C) external radiotherapy

(D) internal radiation seeds via catheter

(E) stent and chemotherapy

A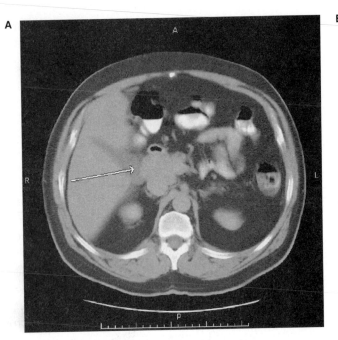

B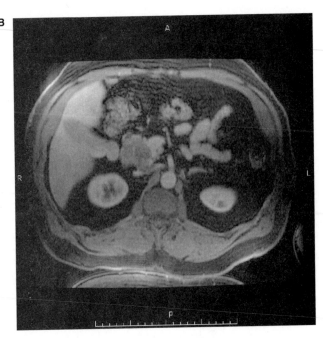

Figure 5–1. A, CT scan shows dilated gallbladder, which in obstructive jaundice, suggests the presence of an underlying malignancy (Courvoisier's sign). **B,** MRI at a lower level than **A** shows tumor (anterior and medial to that of the right kidney).

18. A 74-year-old man complains of epigastric discomfort. There is no jaundice evident, but an enlarged gallbladder is palpated. The bilirubin level is 13 mg/dL, the alkaline phosphatase level is 410 U, and the hematocrit is 35%. CT scan and MRI findings are shown in Fig. 5–1. What is the most likely malignant tumor causing extrahepatic obstructive jaundice?

   (A) gallbladder
   (B) common hepatic duct
   (C) cystic duct
   (D) periampullary area
   (E) head of the pancreas

19. A 25-year-old female presents with episodes of bizarre behavior, memory lapse, and unconsciousness. She also demonstrated previously episodes of extreme hunger, sweating, and tachycardia. During one of these episodes, her blood sugar was tested and was found to be 40 mg/dL. Which would suggest a diagnosis of insulinoma?

   (A) demonstration of insulin antibodies in blood
   (B) abnormal glucagen level

   (C) CT of the pancreas
   (D) hypoglycemia during a symptomatic episode with relief of symptoms by intravenous glucose.
   (E) decreased circulating P peptide in the blood

20. A 41-year-old woman is known to have multiple endocrine neoplasia syndrome. She has multiple family members who have had adenoma tumors removed from the parathyroid, pancreas, and/or pituitary glands. She has severe diarrhea associated with low gastric acid secretion and a normal gastrin level. Which of the following serum assays would be best to evaluate the possible cause of the diarrhea?

   (A) gastrin
   (B) vasoactive intestinal peptide (VIP)
   (C) cholecystokinin
   (D) serotonin
   (E) norepinephrine

21. A 45-year-old patient with chronic pancreatitis is suffering from malnutrition and weight loss secondary to inadequate pancreatic exocrine secretions. Which is true regarding pancreatic secretions?

(A) Secretin releases fluid rich in enzymes.

(B) Secretin releases fluid rich mainly in electrolytes and bicarbonate.

(C) Cholecystokinin releases fluid, predominantly rich in electrolytes, and bicarbonate.

(D) All pancreatic enzymes are secreted in an inactive form.

(E) The pancreas produces proteolytic enzymes only.

Questions 22 and 23

A 48-year old woman presents with severe recurrent peptic ulcer located in the proximal jejunum. Five years previously she underwent parathyroidectomy for hypercalcemia. Her brother was previously diagnosed as having Zollinger–Ellison syndrome.

22. To confirm the diagnosis of Zollinger–Ellison syndrome, blood should be tested for levels of which of the following?

(A) parathyroid hormone
(B) histamine
(C) pepsin
(D) gastrin
(E) secretin

23. The patient develops severe peptic ulcer disease that recurs despite gastric resection and vagotomy operations. She now presents with melena from a peptic ulcer located in the third part of the duodenum. To localize the gastrin-producing tumor, she should have which of the following?

(A) CT scan of the abdomen
(B) ultrasound of the abdomen
(C) somatostatin receptor scintigraphy (SRS)
(D) MRI of the abdomen
(E) barium meal and follow through

24. A 42-year-old accountant presents with recurrent right upper quadrant pain of 3 years' duration. He had undergone a laparoscopic cholecystectomy 2 years ago for presumed symptomatic cholelithiasis, but the pain persisted. An upper GI endoscopy is normal. A sonogram and CT scan of the abdomen are normal. An ERCP is performed, and the pressure in the CBD is 45 cm

saline (normal bile duct pressure is 10–18 cm saline). What is the most likely diagnosis?

(A) acalculous cholecystitis
(B) emphysematous cholecystitis
(C) biliary dyskinesia
(D) cancer of the gallbladder
(E) myasthenia gravis

25. In the emergency department, blood is taken from a 42-year-old man who presents with central abdominal pain of 12 hours' duration. There is no history of alcohol abuse or gallstones. The serum is noted to be lactescent (milky appearance). To help elucidate the significance of the abdominal pain, which of the following tests should be requested?

(A) cholesterol
(B) triglycerides
(C) creatinine kinase MB (CK-MB)
(D) hemoglobin S (Hbs) electrophoresis
(E) calcium

26. A 67-year-old woman is evaluated for obstructive jaundice. The cholangiographic findings indicate that she has a cancer of the lower end of the common bile duct. Clinical examination would most likely reveal which of the following?

(A) enlarged gallbladder
(B) shrunken gallbladder
(C) enlarged pancreas
(D) shrunken pancreas
(E) palpable tumor

27. A 73-year-old woman is evaluated for obstructive jaundice consequent to an injury to the CBD 7 months previously at laparoscopic cholecystectomy. The alkaline phosphatase is elevated. In obstructive jaundice, what is alkaline phosphatase likely to do?

(A) Its level increases before that of bilirubin.
(B) Its level is unlikely to be increased in pancreatic malignancy.
(C) Its elevation indicates bone metastasis.
(D) Its elevation excludes hepatic metastasis.
(E) Its level falls after that of the bilirubin following surgical intervention.

28. A recently arrived emigrant from China develops jaundice, rigors, and high fever. Investigations revealed that he is suffering from Oriental cholangiohepatitis. This condition is confirmed by detecting which of the following?

    (A) schistosomiasis (*Bilharzia*) parasite
    (B) ameba
    (C) *Opisthorchis (Clonorchis) sinensis*
    (D) hydatid cyst (*Echinococcus*)
    (E) hookworm

29. A 48-year-old female travel agent presents with jaundice. Radiological findings confirm the presence of sclerosing cholangitis. She gives a long history of diarrhea for which she has received steroids on several occasions. She is likely to suffer from which of the following?

    (A) pernicious anemia
    (B) ulcerative colitis
    (C) celiac disease
    (D) liver cirrhosis
    (E) Crohn's disease

30. A 55-year-old obese woman undergoes laparoscopic cholecystectomy for symptomatic cholelithiasis. The operation is proceeding well, and boundaries of the Calot's triangle are identified easily. There is no evidence of obstructive jaundice. Cystic duct cholangiogram should be performed if the diameter of the CBD is which of the following?

    (A) Smaller than 0.1 cm
    (B) 0.1–0.2 cm
    (C) 0.3–1 cm
    (D) 1.1–2.5 cm
    (E) Greater than 2.5 cm

31. A 40-year-old man underwent laparoscopic cholecystectomy 2 years earlier. He remains asymptomatic until 1 week before admission, when he complains of right upper quadrant (RUQ) pain and jaundice. He develops a fever and has several rigor attacks on the day of admission. An ultrasound confirms the presence of gallstones in the distal common bile duct. The patient should be given antibiotics. Which of the following should be undertaken?

    (A) should be discharged home under observation
    (B) should be observed in the hospital
    (C) undergo surgical exploration of the common bile duct (CBD)
    (D) ERCP with sphincterotomy and stone removal
    (E) anticoagulants

32. A 43-year-old woman undergoes open cholecystectomy. Intraoperative cholangiogram revealed multiple stones in the CBD. Exploration of the CBD was performed to extract gallstones. The CBD was drained with a #18 T-tube After 10 days, a T-tube cholangiogram reveals a retained CBD stone. This should be treated by which of the following?

    (A) laparotomy and CBD exploration
    (B) subcutaneous heparinization
    (C) antibiotic therapy for 6 months and then re-evaluation
    (D) extraction of the stone through the pathway created by the T-tube (after 6 weeks)
    (E) ultrasound crushing of the CBD stone

Questions 33 through 35

A 62-year-old woman who underwent cholecystectomy and choledochoduodenostomy (CBD duodenal anastomosis) 5 years previously is admitted to the hospital with a 3-day history of upper abdominal pain, chills, fever, and dark urine. These symptoms are suggestive of ascending cholangitis.

33. What is the most likely laboratory finding?

    (A) amylase elevation with normal findings on liver studies
    (B) alkaline phosphatase elevation with normal or elevated normal bilirubin levels
    (C) elevated serum glutamic oxaloacetic transaminase (SGOT) levels
    (D) altered urea/creatinine ratio
    (E) urobilin in urine

34. What should be the initial test to determine patency of the choledocho-duodenostomy?

    (A) ERCP

(B) percutaneous transhepatic cholangiogram (PTC)

(C) HIDA scan

(D) CT scan of the abdomen

(E) ultrasound of the abdomen

35. Which organism is most likely involved in the pathogenesis of ascending cholangitis?

(A) *Clonorchis sinensis*

(B) *Escherichia coli*

(C) *Salmonella*

(D) *Staphylococcus aureus*

(E) *clostridia*

36. Following admission to the hospital for intestinal obstruction, a 48-year-old woman states that she previously had undergone cholecystectomy and choledochoduodenostomy. The presence of a previously constructed choledochoduodenostomy indicates which of the following?

(A) Hepatic metastases were present.

(B) Multiple stones were present in the gallbladder at the previous operation.

(C) Multiple stones were present in the CBD at the previous operation.

(D) The common hepatic duct had a stricture.

(E) The small intestine was occluded.

37. In attempting to minimize complications during cholecystectomy, the surgeon defines the triangle of Calot during the operation. The boundaries of the triangle of Calot (modified) are the common hepatic duct medially, the cystic duct inferiorly, and the liver superiorly. In this triangle, injury is most likely to occur to which of the following?

(A) left hepatic artery

(B) right renal vein

(C) right hepatic artery

(D) duodenum

(E) superior mesenteric vein

38. A 64- year-old man complains of abdominal pain, pruritus, 4-lb weight loss, and anorexia.

There are multiple scratch marks on the skin of the extremities and flank. The bilirubin is 1.0 mg/dL. To determine if the condition is due to cholestasis, blood should be tested for which of the following?

(A) direct and indirect bilirubin

(B) alkaline phosphatase

(C) serum glutamic-oxaloacetic transaminase (SGOT)

(D) serum glutamic-pyruvic transaminase (SGPT)

(E) bile pigments

39. A 49-year-old African American woman born in New York is admitted with right upper quadrant pain, fever, and jaundice (Charcot's triad). A diagnosis of ascending cholangitis is made. With regard to the etiology of ascending cholangitis, which of the following is true?

(A) It usually occurs in the absence of jaundice.

(B) It usually occurs secondary to CBD stones.

(C) It occurs frequently after choledochoduodenostomy.

(D) It does not occur in patients with cholangiocarcinoma.

(E) It is mainly caused by the liver fluke.

40. A 43-year-old man is admitted with jaundice of 6 weeks duration. An ultrasound shows multiple small stones in the gallbladder and the presence of a CBD stone. A preoperative ERCP followed by a laparoscopic cholecystectomy is planned. The INR (international normalization ratio) is elevated to 3.1 What is the next step in management?

(A) infusion of cryoprecipitate

(B) oral vitamin K tablets to decrease prolonged INR

(C) parenteral vitamin K to decrease prolonged INR

(D) demonstration that urobilinogen is increased in the urine

(E) demonstration that stercobilinogen is increased in the stools

41. A 65-year-old woman is admitted with right upper quadrant pain radiating to the right shoulder, accompanied by nausea and vomiting. Examination reveals tenderness in the right upper quadrant and a positive Murphy's sign. A diagnosis of acute cholecystitis is made. What is the most likely finding?

    (A) Serum bilirubin levels may be elevated.
    (B) Cholelithiasis is present in 40–60%.
    (C) Bacteria are rarely found at operation.
    (D) An elevated amylase level excludes this diagnosis.
    (E) Contraction of the gallbladder is noted on ultrasound.

42. A surgeon is removing the gallbladder of a 35-year-old obese man. One week previously the patient had recovered from obstructive jaundice and at operation, numerous small stones are present in the gallbladder. In addition to cholecystectomy, the surgeon should also perform which of the following?

    (A) intraoperative cystic duct cholangiogram
    (B) liver biopsy
    (C) no further treatment
    (D) removal of the head of the pancreas
    (E) common bile duct exploration

43. A 42-year-old man presents with recurrent right upper quadrant pain for 2 years. A sonogram is negative for gallstones, and the CBD is normal. An upper GI endoscopy is also normal, and there is no peptic ulcer disease. Biliary dyskinesia is suspected, and the patient undergoes further evaluation. Which of the following will stimulate contraction of the gallbladder?

    (A) cholecystokinin
    (B) vagal section
    (C) secretin
    (D) epinephrine
    (E) gastrin

44. A 57-year-old previously healthy business executive presents with gradually increasing obstructive jaundice. An ultrasound of the liver shows dilated intrahepatic ducts, but the common bile duct is normal. An ERCP shows a filling defect at the level of the common hepatic duct. Endoscopic brush biopsies are taken, and histology confirms cholangiocarcinoma. In discussing these findings, the surgeon should inform the patient that

    (A) this tumor affects men more commonly than women
    (B) the tumor is a result of gallstones
    (C) the tumor is best treated with a stent to relieve obstructive jaundice
    (D) weight loss is common in this condition
    (E) the most common location of these tumors is at the ampulla of Vater

45. A 38-year-old male lawyer develops abdominal pain after having a fatty meal. Examination reveals tenderness in the right hypochondrium and a positive Murphy's sign. Which test is most likely to reveal acute cholecystitis?

    (A) HIDA scan
    (B) oral cholecystogram
    (C) intravenous cholangiogram
    (D) CT scan of the abdomen
    (E) ERCP

46. A 55-year-old white female undergoes a laparoscopic cholecystectomy for symptomatic cholelithiasis. The operation went well, and the patient was discharged home. One week later, she comes to your office for a routine postoperative follow-up. The final pathology report shows an incidental finding of a gallbladder carcinoma confined to the mucosa. In further advising the patient, you should inform her that

    (A) She should undergo radiation therapy
    (B) She should undergo right hepatectomy to remove locally infiltrating disease
    (C) She should undergo regional lymphadenectomy
    (D) She requires systemic chemotherapy
    (E) She does not require any further therapy

47. A 49-year-old man who recovered 7 years ago from acute viral hepatitis develops chronic active hepatitis and liver cirrhosis. He is seen in

the office without any abdominal symptoms. An ultrasound reveals cholelithiasis and ascites. What treatment should be instituted?

(A) He should undergo percutaneous dissolution of stones.

(B) He should undergo cholecystectomy.

(C) He should undergo cholecystostomy.

(D) He should be placed on a diet that avoids fatty foods and discouraged from undergoing elective cholecystectomy.

(E) He should be treated with ursodeoxycholic acid.

48. A 48-year-old man is admitted to the hospital with severe abdominal pain, tenderness in the right hypochondrium, and a WBC count of 12,000. A HIDA scan fails to show the gallbladder after 4 hours. Acute cholecystitis is established. After diagnosis, cholecystectomy should be performed within which of the following?

(A) 3–60 minutes

(B) the first 2–3 days following hospital admission

(C) 8 days

(D) 3 weeks

(E) 3 months

49. A 60-year-old diabetic man is admitted to the hospital with a diagnosis of acute cholecystitis. The WBC count is 28,000, and a plain film of the abdomen and CT scan show evidence of intramural gas in the gallbladder. What is the most likely diagnosis?

(A) emphysematous gallbladder

(B) acalculous cholecystitis

(C) cholangiohepatitis

(D) sclerosing cholangitis

(E) gallstone ileus

50. A 60-year-old woman is recovering from a major pelvic cancer operation and develops severe abdominal pain and sepsis. Following a positive HIDA scan, laparotomy is performed. The gallbladder is severely inflamed and removed. There is no evidence of gallbladder stones (acalculous cholecystitis). Cholecystectomy is performed. Which is true of acalculous cholecystitis?

(A) It is usually associated with stones CBD.

(B) It occurs in 10–20% of cases of cholecystitis.

(C) It has a more favorable prognosis than calculous cholecystitis.

(D) It is increased in frequency after trauma or operation.

(E) It is characterized on HIDA scan by filling of the gallbladder.

51. Following recovery in the hospital from a fracture of the femur, a 70-year-old nursing home female patient develops RUQ abdominal pain and fever. She has tenderness in the right subcostal region. There is evidence of progressive sepsis and hemodynamic instability. The WBC count is 24,000. A bedside sonogram confirms the presence of calculous cholecystitis. What should treatment involve?

(A) intravenous antibiotics alone

(B) ERCP

(C) percutaneous drainage of the gallbladder

(D) urgent cholecystectomy

(E) elective cholecystectomy after 3 months

52. In designing a study related to gallbladder function, it should be noted that the healthy gallbladder mucosa selectively absorbs which of the following?

(A) bile pigment

(B) bile salts

(C) cholesterol

(D) sodium

(E) none of the above

Question 53 and 54

On a recent safari in Africa, a 39-year-old male engineer developed an acute diarrhea state requiring hospitalization and treatment with flagyl. Six weeks after his return, he developed right upper quadrant pain fever and chills. A chest x-ray showed elevation of the right hemidiaphragm, and sonogram showed a large abscess in the right lobe of the liver.

53. One characteristic of this condition is which of the following?

    (A) Satisfactory treatment is not readily available.
    (B) Diagnosis is easily made by finding *Entamoeba histolytica* in stools in nearly all patients.
    (C) Bloody diarrhea is always present.
    (D) Anchovy-paste pus is usually present in the abscess cavity.
    (E) Extensive surgical drainage is usually indicated.

54. Serum bilirubin is mildly elevated. The WBC is 11,000 but there is eosinophilia. The initial line of treatment involves which of the following?

    (A) cortisone
    (B) metronidazol (Flagyl)
    (C) surgical excision
    (D) sulfonamides and penicillin
    (E) colon resection

55. In performing hepatic resection, a knowledge of the different lobes and segments of the liver is mandatory. The right and left lobes of the liver are separated by an imaginary plane (Cantlie's line) that passes between the the inferior vena cava (IVC) and which of the following?

    (A) portal vein
    (B) falciform ligament
    (C) left margin of the quadrate lobe
    (D) gallbladder
    (E) left margin of the caudate lobe

56. A 32-year-old diabetic woman who has taken contraceptive pills for 12 years develops right upper quadrant pain. CT scan of the abdomen reveals a 5-cm hypodense lesion in the right lobe of the liver consistent with a hepatic adenoma. What should the patient be advised to do?

    (A) undergo excision of the adenoma
    (B) stop oral contraceptives only
    (C) stop oral hypoglycemic medication
    (D) undergo right hepatectomy
    (E) have serial CT scans every 6 months

57. A 35-year-old woman is seen in the office with focal nodular hyperplasia. This condition is similar to hepatic adenoma in that it does what?

    (A) frequently causes symptoms
    (B) tends to lead to liver rupture
    (C) tends to undergo malignant changes
    (D) is easily detected by CT scan of the liver
    (E) none of the above

58. A 64-year-old man has mild upper abdominal pain. On contrast CT scan, a 5-cm lesion in the left lobe of the liver enhances and then decreases over a 10-minute period from without to within. The most likely lesion is which of the following?

    (A) congenital cyst
    (B) hemangioma
    (C) fungal abscess
    (D) focal nodular hyperplasia
    (E) hepatic adenoma

59. A 16-year-old previously healthy male fell off his bicycle while riding back home from school. On examination there was mild tenderness in the right upper quadrant. No other abnormality was detected. A sonogram showed a large solitary hypoechogenic cyst in the liver. The liver function tests are normal, and there is no family history of cystic disease involving solid organs. What is the most likely cause?

    (A) fungal abscess
    (B) trauma
    (C) developmental
    (D) neoplastic
    (E) pyogenic abscess

60. A healthy 64-year-old woman had a cancer of the left colon resected 4 years previously. Dur-

ing follow-up, an increased carcino-embryonic antigen (CEA) level lead to a CT scan of the abdomen, which revealed two discrete lesions in the left lateral lobe of the liver. Liver biopsy confirms that this is metastatic colon cancer. What is the most appropriate plan?

(A) Inform the patient that there is no treatment, and that her expectation of life is limited.
(B) Irradiation is recommended.
(C) Local cauterization of the cancer is recommended.
(D) Liver resection is recommended.
(E) Chemotherapy is recommended.

61. A 42-year-old man undergoes a liver transplantation. There is rapid deterioration after the completion of the graft, and the patient dies within 12 hours. What is the most likely cause of death?

(A) massive pulmonary embolus
(B) graft rejection
(C) fat embolus
(D) massive hemorrhage
(E) subphrenic abscess

62. In discussing the treatment of a 42-year-old man with severe liver cirrhosis, the possibility of heterotopic transplantation is considered. Which statement about heterotopic liver transplantation is true?

(A) It implies removal of the recipient's liver.
(B) It is preferable to orthotopic liver transplantation.
(C) It should be done in the iliac vessels.
(D) It is rarely associated with long-term survival.
(E) none of the above

63. A 43-year-old man develops chronic hepatitis, which was attributed to a complication resulting from multiple blood transfusions for sickle cell anemia. He complains of chronic sweating, palpitation, and hunger attacks. What would be the most likely cause of these symptoms?

(A) hepatogenic hypoglycemia
(B) hemolytic anemia
(C) jaundice

(D) spontaneous hyperglycemia
(E) elevated bile salts in the blood

64. A 55-year-old man has lost weight and has severe hypoglycemia. Examination of the upper abdomen reveals a large mass. The CT scan shows that the pancreas is normal. A biopsy reveals that the tumor is malignant. What is the most likely histologic feature of a tumor in a patient with a normal pancreas?

(A) hepatoma
(B) nephroblastoma
(C) carcinoid
(D) ileum
(E) sarcoma

65. A 42-year-old man is admitted with bleeding from esophageal varices. Investigation reveals that he has an occlusion of the portal vein. There is no evidence of liver cirrhosis. Which test will most likely reveal an underlying predisposing factor for this condition?

(A) hepatitis screening
(B) isoamylase
(C) intravenous pyelogram to exclude hydronephrosis
(D) coagulation tests to include antithrombin III
(E) none of the above

66. A 9-year-old girl had multiple episodes of upper gastrointestinal bleeding. Contrast enhanced CT scan showed multiple cavernous malformation surrounding the portal vein (Figure 5-2). She is admitted with severe hematemesis and melena. At birth, she had developed an infection around the umbilicus. What is the most likely site of bleeding?

(A) Meckel's diverticulum
(B) esophageal varices
(C) peptic ulcer
(D) duodenal varices
(E) Mallory–Weiss tear of the lower end of the esophagus

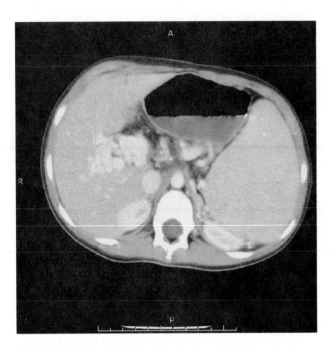

Figure 5–2. Following portal vein thrombosis, massive cavernous malformations around the portal vein is demonstrated. Note large spleen.

67. A 49-year-old man with a history of cirrhosis is admitted with significant hematemesis. There is jaundice and clubbing of the fingers. His extremities are cold and clammy, and the systolic blood pressure drops to 84 mmHg. The initial step in the management is to proceed with which of the following?

    (A) urgent endoscopy and sclerotherapy
    (B) Sengstaken–Blakemore tube
    (C) infusion of intravenous crystalloids
    (D) intravenous pitressin
    (E) surgery to stop bleeding

68. A 42-year-old woman with a known history of esophageal varices secondary to hepatitis and cirrhosis is admitted with severe hematemesis from esophageal varices. Bleeding persists after pitressin therapy. What would the next step in management involve?

    (A) emergency portacaval shunt
    (B) emergency lienorenal shunt
    (C) insertion of Sengstaken–Blakemore tube
    (D) vagotomy
    (E) TIPS (transjugular intrahepatic porta-systemic shunt)

69. A 12-year-old boy who underwent a previous splenectomy for thalasemia presents to the emergency room with fever, chills, and septic shock. The parents give a history of seemingly minor sore throat, which started only a few hours previously. The child is hypotensive and appears moribund. A diagnosis of overwhelming post-splenectomy infection (OPSI) is made. Which of the following statements about OPSI are true?

    (A) The condition is more common in children.
    (B) The condition is more common after splenectomy for trauma.
    (C) Prophylactic antibiotics have not been shown to improve outcome in children.
    (D) Prophylactic vaccination against *Enterococcus* should be performed.
    (E) The condition is very common after splenectomy.

70. A 43-year-old man with chronic hepatitis and liver cirrhosis is admitted with upper gastrointestinal bleeding. He has marked ascites and shows multiple telangectasias, liver palmar erythema, and clubbing. A diagnosis of bleeding esophageal varices secondary to portal hypertension is made. Portal pressure is considered elevated when it is above which of the following?

    (A) 0.15 mmHg
    (B) 1.5 mmHg
    (C) 12 mmHg
    (D) 40 mmHg
    (E) 105 mmHg

71. A 23-year-old male college student has a history of liver cirrhosis due to Kimmelstiel–Wilson syndrome (abnormality in copper metabolism). He should be treated with which of the following?

    (A) penicillamine as soon as the diagnosis is established
    (B) penicillamine after variceal bleeding has occurred
    (C) a portocaval shunt
    (D) sclerosis of the esophageal varices as a prophylactic measure

Questions 72 and 73

A 24-year-old woman presents with mennorhagia, an easy tendency toward bruising, and a history of prolonged bleeding after extraction of an impacted molar several years previously. A diagnosis of idiopathic thrombocytopenic purpura (ITP) is made after appropriate investigations. Her disease has failed to respond to steroid and immunoglobin therapy.

72. She is scheduled to undergo splenectomy in 1 week, but her platelet count is 22,000. What should be the treatment of choice?

   (A) She should be given platelets daily and be scheduled for splenectomy when her platelet count is more than 75,000.
   (B) She should undergo bone marrow transplantation.
   (C) She should be treated with steroids only, and the operation should be canceled.
   (D) She should receive transfusion with 3 U of packed cells.
   (E) She should not be given platelets routinely before surgery.

73. Following a successful splenectomy, she noted that she was no longer prone to excessive bleeding. Her platelet count had become elevated. However, 2 years later, she developed further skin purpura, and her platelet count was reduced to 45,000. What should she undergo?

   (A) radioactive technetium (^{99}Tc) scan to see if a splenunculus is present
   (B) radioactive (I^{135}) to see if a splenunculus is present
   (C) exploratory laparotomy
   (D) platelet transfusion
   (E) red blood cell fragility test

74. A 28-year-old woman is diagnosed with thrombotic thrombocytopenic purpura (TTP). In addition to purpura and thrombocytopenia, studies will show which of the following?

   (A) normal arterioles on biopsy of the spleen
   (B) absence of infarction on biopsy of the spleen
   (C) leukopenia

   (D) elevated urea and creatinine levels
   (E) suppression of reticulocytes

75. A 24-year-old African American man has sickle cell disease. He is admitted to the hospital because of a sickle cell crisis. His hemoglobin is 10 g%, and he complains of pain in the lower chest wall and legs. His further course of management should include which of the following?

   (A) emergency splenectomy
   (B) elective splenectomy
   (C) admission to the hospital for hydration and given dehydromorphine as required
   (D) administer steroids
   (E) exchange transfusions to keep his hemoglobin at a normal level

76. A 24-year-old woman from the Caribbean is admitted to the hospital for severe lower chest and upper abdominal pain. Her hemoglobin is 9 g%. The findings on ultrasound of the abdomen and chest x-ray are normal. Her father has sickle cell disease. For her physician to establish the diagnosis of sickle cell trait or disease, she must undergo which procedure?

   (A) a bone marrow study
   (B) injection of radioactive RBCs
   (C) red cell fragility studies
   (D) studies to determine her response to erythropoietin
   (E) blood smear and electrophoresis

77. Splenectomy is often indicated in the management of which of the following?

   (A) hereditary spherocytosis
   (B) hereditary neurofibromatosis
   (C) aplastic anemia
   (D) pheochromocytoma
   (E) Hashimoto's disease

78. A 2-year-old African-American boy is diagnosed as having hereditary spherocytosis. His parents should be informed that this condition is which of the following?

   (A) It is not associated with a marked increase in gallstones.
   (B) It is transmitted as a recessive trait.
   (C) It is diagnosed by showing RBCs undergo lysis at a higher osmotic pressure.
   (D) It is characterized by a low reticulocyte count.
   (E) It is infrequently treated by splenectomy.

79. A 67-year-old man is admitted to hospital with a diagnosis of polycythemia vera. He has considerable back pain and is diagnosed as having myeloid metaplasia. This condition is characterized by which of the following?

   (A) decrease of the connective tissue in the spleen
   (B) decrease in the blood elements of the spleen
   (C) aplastic anemia
   (D) deterioration after splenectomy
   (E) a favorable response to alkylating agents

80. A 24-year-old woman with rheumatoid arthritis involving the sacroiliac joint and fingers is noted to have splenomegaly and neutropenia (Felty's syndrome). She is advised to have splenectomy, but she should be informed that

   (A) large-joint disease symptoms will lessen
   (B) small-joint disease symptoms will lessen
   (C) neutropenia responds to splenectomy
   (D) the joint symptoms will become worse
   (E) all symptoms will lessen

81. A 10-year-old boy is hit by a truck while riding his bicycle home from school. A CT scan shows a tear of the spleen. His hematocrit is 32%, and he is in pain, although fully alert and oriented. His blood pressure is 110/60 mmHg, and his heart rate is 104/min. The next step in management should be which of the following?

   (A) Cross-match blood and transfuse appropriately.
   (B) Perform splenectomy as soon as possible.

   (C) Perform laparotomy, and suture the tear where possible.
   (D) Perform angiographic embolization of the spleen.
   (E) Avoid surgery, even if bleeding continues profusely after transfusion.

DIRECTIONS (Questions 82 through 96): Each set of matching questions in this section consists of a list of lettered options followed by several numbered items. For each numbered item, select the appropriate lettered option(s). Each lettered option may be selected once, more than once, or not at all. EACH ITEM WILL STATE THE NUMBER OF OPTIONS TO SELECT. CHOOSE EXACTLY THIS NUMBER.

Question 82

   (A) injury to Santorini's (accessory pancreatic) duct
   (B) pancreas division
   (C) hyperthyroidism
   (D) hyperlipidemia
   (E) hyperparathyroidism
   (F) Hashimoto subacute thyroiditis
   (G) strangulated groin hernia
   (H) injury to Wharton's duct

82. Where does acute pancreatitis occur more commonly? SELECT ONLY FOUR.

Question 83

   (A) obstructive jaundice
   (B) pseudocysts
   (C) abscess
   (D) acute edematous pancreatitis
   (E) splenic vein thrombosis
   (F) pancreatic ascites
   (G) choledocholithiasis
   (H) cholecystitis

83. Surgical intervention is not usually recommended to treat complications in patients with pancreatitis presenting with what? SELECT ONLY ONE.

Question 84

(A) lowered basal acid output (<5mEq/L)

(B) islet cells of the pancreas

(C) duodenum

(D) adrenal cortex

(E) pituitary gland tumor

(F) pheochromocytoma

(G) severe peptic ulcer disease

(H) multiple endocrine neoplasia

84. What does Zollinger–Ellison syndrome involves? SELECT ONLY FOUR.

Question 85

(A) pleural effusion

(B) string sign in small intestine

(C) pancreatic calcification

(D) distended inner curve of duodenum (on GI series)

(E) air in the portal vein

(F) apple-core lesion in the colon

(G) Free air below left diaphragm

(H) colon cut-off sign

85. A 42-year-old man with a known history of chronic pancreatitis presents with malnutrition and abdominal pain. What radiologic changes may be present? SELECT ONLY FOUR.

Question 86

(A) cancer of the tail of the pancreas

(B) acute cholecystitis

(C) chronic cholecystitis

(D) hepatocyte evaluation

(E) hepatic abscess

(F) parasystemic shunt

(G) biliary dyskinesia

86. A 62-year-old man is admitted with upper abdominal pain, nausea, and vomiting. An HIDA scan is helpful in establishing the diagnosis of what? SELECT ONLY THREE.

Question 87

(A) splenic cyst

(B) diabetes mellitus

(C) hypertension

(D) nitroglycerin

(E) trauma

(F) renal disease

(G) duodenal ulcer disease

(H) hiatal hernia

87. Acalculous cholecystitis is found in the presence of what SELECT ONLY TWO.

Question 88

(A) routine cholecystectomy

(B) carcinoma tail of pancreas

(C) carcinoma head of pancreas

(D) recurrent stone in the common bile duct (CBD)

(E) cancer of the upper end of the common hepatic duct

(F) unresectable cancer of the gallbladder

(G) benign stricture of CBD in a patient with chronic pancreatitis

88. Construction of choledochoduodenostomy is indicated for which SELECT ONLY TWO.

Question 89

(A) accounts for 10% of all cancers

(B) the female/male ratio is 1:4

(C) fails to produce jaundice in the earlier stages

(D) encroaches on the CBD and/or hepatic duct in later stages

(E) gallstones are absent

(F) is of the squamous cell type

(G) associated with porcelain gallbladder

(H) carries a 20% 5-year survival rate

89. In most cases, which are true of cancer of the gallbladder? SELECT ONLY THREE.

Question 90

    (A) hyperthyroidism
    (B) aplastic anemia
    (C) asthma
    (D) sarcoid
    (E) breast metastasis
    (F) inguinal hernia
    (G) ectopic testis
    (H) pharyngeal diverticulum

90. Alkaline phosphatase elevation is associated with which? SELECT ONLY TWO.

Question 91

    (A) common hepatic artery
    (B) right renal artery
    (C) gastroduodenal artery
    (D) inferior epigastric artery
    (E) left adrenal artery
    (F) left hepatic artery
    (G) hypogastric artery

91. The cystic artery may arise from which? SELECT ONLY THREE.

Question 92

    (A) phospholipids
    (B) gastrin
    (C) intrinsic factor
    (D) secretin
    (E) calcium bilirubinate
    (F) cholesterol
    (G) amylase
    (H) trypsinogen
    (I) lipase
    (J) insulin

92. What is found in bile? SELECT ONLY THREE.

Question 93

    (A) mainly unconjugated (indirect) bilirubin
    (B) alkaline phosphatase
    (C) acid phosphatase
    (D) reticulocytes
    (E) bile salts
    (F) platelets
    (G) stercobilinogen

93. A 59-year-old woman presents with obstructive jaundice and pruritis of 2 months' duration. A CT scan of the abdomen reveals cancer of the head of the pancreas. What are the likely abnormalities? SELECT ONLY TWO.

Questions 94 and 95

    (A) metabolic stones in 80% of cases
    (B) mainly of the pigmented variety
    (C) occur mainly in women
    (D) account for most cases of jaundice in cirrhosis
    (E) evidence of encephalopathy
    (F) treated by reducing bile salts
    (G) routine laparoscopic cholecystectomy required
    (H) may lead to choledocholithiasis
    (I) absence of ascites
    (J) evidence of hypoalbuminemia
    (K) evidence of malnutrition
    (L) prolonged PT

94. A 58-year-old chronic alcoholic man presents with liver cirrhosis and gallstones. SELECT ONLY TWO.

95. The chance of complications of major surgery in liver cirrhosis is increased. SELECT ONLY FOUR.

Question 96

(A) cholesterol

(B) high-density lipoprotein

(C) MB isoenzymes

(D) HbS electrophoresis

(E) ultrasound of the chest

(F) chest x-ray

(G) glucose tolerance test

(H) pancreatogram

(I) urine/serum amylase ratio

96. In the emergency department, blood is taken from a 44-year-old man who presents with central abdominal pain of 10 hours duration. The serum amylase level is normal and findings on electrocardiogram (ECG) are abnormal. To distinguish myocardial infarction from an acute abdominal condition, which is the most important and reliable test? SELECT ONLY ONE.

Answers and Explanations

1. **(C)** Ranson's criteria allow for early identification of patients who have severe pancreatitis. Mortality increases with increasing number of Ranson's criteria score. The five criteria of poor prognosis at the time of admission are age >55, WBC >16,000 blood glucose >200 mg/dL, AST >250, LDH >350. During the following 48 hours, six additional criteria may develop. These include hypoxemia with arterial pO_2 <60 mm on room air, base deficit >4, fluid requirement >6 L, hematocrit fall >10%, BUN increase >8 mg/dL, and serum Ca <8 mg/dL. Amylase and lipase elevation may focus attention on the appropriate diagnosis, but amylase levels fail to correlate with prognosis

2. **(D)** After the onset of acute pancreatitis, an area of fluid accumulation may be evident in the lesser sac. In most instances, this finding on ultrasound improves over a few days. Serum amylase and amylase-creatine clearance ratio often point to a diagnosis of pancreatitis but are not sufficiently sensitive as a specific test.

3. **(A)** Pseudocysts frequently are encountered on ultrasound examination early after an acute attack of pancreatitis. In most cases, the pseudocyst resolves, but if it enlarges, it may compress the stomach anteriorly. An enlarging pseudocyst is an indication to attempt percutaneous drainage. If percutaneous drainage is unsuccessful, internal drainage into the stomach should be performed at an appropriate interval to allow the pseudocyst wall to mature (Figure 5-3).

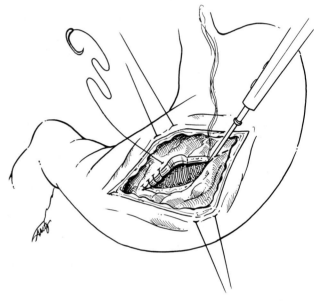

Figure 5–3. After cyst evacuation, the opening is enlarged to 3- to 4-cm diameter. Adherent posterior gastric and anterior cyst wall is sewn with nonabsorbable suture. (Reproduced with permission, from Maingot's Abdominal Operations, 10th ed., p. 2023, Appleton & Lange, 1996.)

4. **(B)** In pancreatitis, the serum amylase level may be normal. The causes include: (a) hyperlipedemia, which interferes with chemical determination of amylase; (b) increased urinary excretion of amylase; and (c) near complete destruction of pancreatic parenchyma as a result of chronic pancreatitis. On the other hand, the serum amylase level may be elevated in the absence of pancreatitis (for example perforated peptic ulcer, gangrenous cholecystitis, small-bowel strangulation or chronic renal failure.)

5. **(C)** If a large pseudocyst is present, it may cause displacement of the transverse colon, duodenum, or stomach (anteriorly). Other radiologic signs in pancreatitis include pseudocyst on ultrasound or CT scan, downward displacement of transverse colon, dilated pancreatic duct on pancreatogram, and smooth tapering of the CBD on cholangiogram (if the head of the pancreas is diseased). Trefoil sign occurs as a result of scarring in duodenal ulcer disease.

6. **(E)** True epithelial-lined cysts in the pancreas are extremely rare. They should not be confused with the more common pseudocyst (no epithelial lining), benign cystadenoma, or malignant cystadenoma of the pancreas. Pseudocysts are more common in men, but cystadenocarcinoma occurs more frequently in women.

7. **(A)** The presence of an epigastric mass 2–3 weeks after the onset of acute pancreatitis strongly favors a pancreatic pseudocyst. The history of alcoholism points to pancreatitis as a possible etiologic factor in the differential diagnosis. Pseudocysts develop in 10% of patients following acute pancreatitis. Most of these, however, resolve spontaneously. They may also develop in patients with chronic pancreatitis or after pancreatic trauma.

8. **(B)** Fibrosis in the head of the pancreas as a result of chronic inflammation may lead to compression of the CBD. In pancreatitis, the narrowing of the CBD is smooth on x-ray studies. There is no association with pancreatitis and sclerosing cholangitis. Alcoholic hepatitis is the most common cause of jaundice, but it most frequently is not of an obstructive nature. Pseudocysts and carcinoma of the head of the pancreas are other recognized causes of obstructive jaundice in patients with chronic pancreatitis.

9. **(B)** The passage of small stones through Vater's ampulla often results in pancreatitis. It is important to perform cholecystectomy after pancreatitis has subsided but during the same hospital stay in patients with documented gallstone pancreatitis (to avoid recurrence of symptoms). Pancreatic calcification, smooth narrowing of the distal CBD, and a pseudocyst are features of chronic pancreatitis caused by alcohol consumption.

10. **(A)** A recent increase in alcohol consumption explains the jaundice secondary to alcoholic hepatitis in the majority of such patients. Carcinoma of the pancreas is relatively rare but often causes difficulty in the differentiation from pancreatitis. A pseudocyst measuring 4 cm is not associated with nonobstructive jaundice in this patient.

11. **(D)** Patients who develop acute pancreatitis as a result of cholelithiasis should have gallbladder surgery performed during the same hospital stay to avoid recurrence. Elective cholecystectomy should be avoided during the actual phase of pancreatitis.

12. **(D)** Because of its protected retroperitoneal location, pancreatic injury occurs with deep penetrating wounds or with significant blunt trauma to upper abdomen. Blunt trauma accounts for less than 20–30% of all pancreatic injuries. The most common site of injury is at the neck of the pancreas where the pancreatic tissue is compressed against the spine. Associated visceral and vascular injuries occur commonly and together with the delay in diagnosis account for the high morbidity and mortality. Fistulae, pseudocyst, infection, and secondary (delayed) hemorrhage are common complications. Pancreatic injuries frequently are overlooked initially, and their detection requires a high index of suspicion. Elevation of amylase after trauma is nonspecific.

13. **(C)** Pancreatitis occurring after trauma and operation has a higher mortality rate and often is difficult to diagnose. It is in these circumstances that the possibility of acute pancreatitis is frequently not considered initially in the differential diagnosis.

14. **(A)** If the pancreatic duct is dilated and symptoms persist, a longitudinal pancreaticojejunostomy (Puestow) is performed (Figure 5–4). In this operation, the pancreatic duct is slit open and anastomosed end-to-end to the cut end of the divided jejunum with a Roux-en-Y anastomosis. Resection of the pancreas is reserved for patients

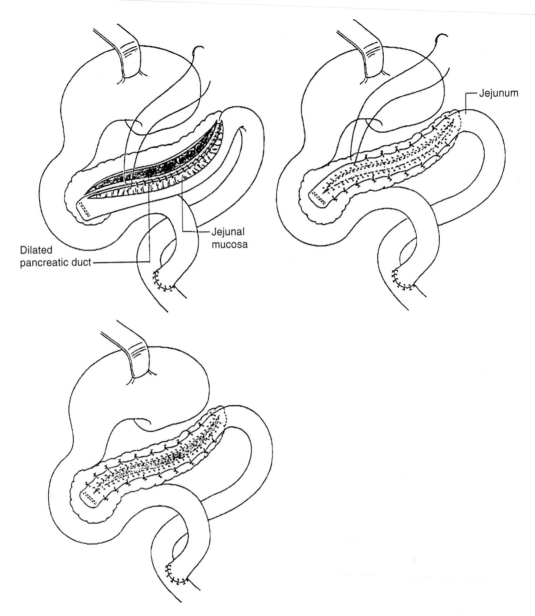

Figure 5–4. Performance of lateral pancreaticojejunostomy (Puestow) for chronic pancreatitus. (Reproduced, with permission, from Greenfield, Surgery: Scientific Principles & Practice, 2nd ed., p. 812, J.B. Lippincott Company, 1996.)

without a dilated duct (<6 mm). In these cases, a distal pancreatectomy is performed when the disease primarily involves the body and tail of the pancreas; whereas, a Whipple operation is performed when the disease is confined to the head.

15. **(A)** Atelectasis is partly due to a factor released from the pancreas that alters pulmonary surfactant. The other conditions listed are not specifically related to pancreatitis.

16. **(E)** Most insulinomas are small (<2 cm), solitary and benign. Therefore, simple enucleation is adequate. Less than 10% of cases are malignant and require resection in the form of either pancreaticoduodenectomy or distal pancreatectomy (depending upon the location of the tumor). Ten percent of insulinomas are associated with MEN I syndrome, and in these cases, the tumors are multiple. Partial pancreatic resection may be required for these patients. Total pancreatectomy is almost never required for the removal of insuli-

nomas. Somatostatin receptors are not always present on insulinoma cells, and, therefore, SRS is less useful for localization of this tumor.

17. **(A)** Carcinoma of the head of the pancreas is treated with radical excision of the head of the pancreas along with the duodenum. Continuity of the biliary and GI tract is established by performing hepaticojejunostomy pancreaticojejunostomy and gastrojejunostomy (Figure 5–5). The 5-year survival rate is higher for periampullary carcinoma (30%) than that for pancreatic head lesions (10%). Most centers do not give irradia-

tion routinely before or after surgery, because pancreatic cancers do not respond well to radiotherapy. Endoscopically placed stents alone are used only in palliative circumstances in patients with limited life expectancy.

18. **(E)** Cancer of the head of the pancreas is the most common cause of obstructive jaundice. In cholangiocarcinoma of the common hepatic duct, the gallbladder will be empty and not distended. Anemia may occur as a result of bleeding into the duodenum in periampullary cancer, but this is relatively rare. Carcinoma of the gall-

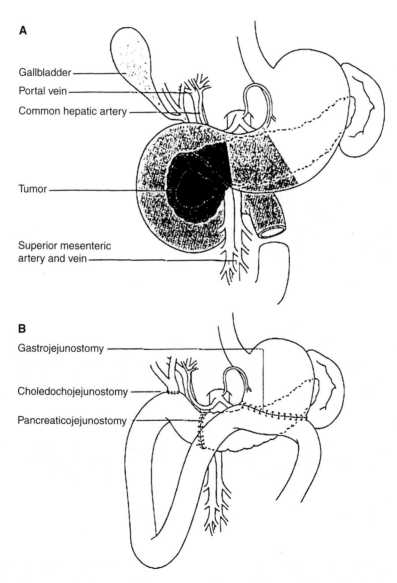

Figure 5–5. Pancreaticoduodenectomy (Whipple procedure). **A,** The tissues to be resected in a standard pancreaticoduodenectomy are indicated. **B,** Reconstruction after standard pancreaticoduodenectomy. (Reproduced, with permission, from Greenfield, Surgery: Scientific Principles & Practice, 2nd ed., p. 824, J.B. Lippincott Company, 1996.)

bladder results in jaundice only after the tumor invades the adjacent biliary tree.

19. **(D)** The characteristic features of insulinomas include: (a) hypoglycemic symptoms; (b) blood glucose <50 mg/dL during the symptomatic episodes; and (c) relief of symptoms by intravenous injection of glucose (Whipple's triad). Diagnosis is confirmed by demonstration of fasting hypoglycemia in the presence of inappropriately elevated levels of insulin in the blood. A ratio of plasma insulin to glucose greater than 0.3 is diagnostic. Circulating levels of C-peptide are usually elevated in patients with insulinoma but not in patients with such other causes of hypoglycemia as tumors of mesenchymal origin and liver tumors. Patients who surreptitiously administer insulin develop insulin antibodies.

20. **(B)** VIP producing tumors (VIPomas) are usually malignant, although benign tumors and hyperplasia may also occur. Increase of VIP results in the watery diarrhea, hypokalemia, and alkalosis (WDHA) syndrome. Diarrhea is severe and results in fluid and electrolyte disturbances. Treatment is directed to removal of the pancreatic tumor. Gastrinoma is more common but is associated with increased gastrin level in the blood.

21. **(B)** Secretin releases fluid rich mainly in electrolytes and bicarbonate. Both cholecystokinin and vagal stimulation result in fluid with a high content of enzymes. Among the pancreatic enzymes, amylase and lipase are released in their active forms; whereas, the proteolytic enzymes (trypsinogen, chymotrypsinogen) are secreted as inactive zymogens. Their activation occurs in the duodenum, where the zymogens are exposed to enterokinase.

22. **(D)** Zollinger–Ellison syndrome is caused by secretion of excessive amounts of gastrin by islet cells of the pancreas (gastrinoma). It should always be thought of in patients with peptic ulcer disease, whose ulcers are severe, refractory to management, recurrent or located distally, beyond the first part of the duodenum. Gastrin levels in the blood are increased markedly and can be raised further by secretin injection (paradoxi-

cal response). The source of gastrin level in the blood may arise from hyperplasia, adenoma, or most commonly carcinoma of the islets. Most gastrinomas are sporadic, but 25% of patients have a family history of multiple endocrine neoplasia.

23. **(C)** Because most gastrinomas are small, preoperative localization of the tumor may be difficult. A nuclear scan may be performed using radiolabeled somatostatin (octreotide) analogue. This binds with the somatostatin receptors present on the gastrin-producing cells which identifies the tumor. Endoscopic (not transcutaneous) ultrasound is also useful in localizing these lesions in the pancreas and in the duodenum. The combined accuracy of SRS and endoscopic ultrasound in preoperative localization of gastrinomas is 93%.

24. **(C)** Patients with biliary dyskinesia present with typical symptoms of gall stone disease, but investigations fail to reveal cholelithiasis or choledocholithiasis. Ironically, many patients will have undergone cholecystectomy for incidentally found gallstones but without relief of pain. ERCP with measurement of sphincter pressure will reveal basal sphincter pressure above 40 cm of water. Calcium channel blockers may be tried initially to relieve the spasm of the sphincter of Oddi, but many patients will require an endoscopic sphincterotomy.

25. **(B)** Latescent serum is sometimes seen soon after an acute attack of pancreatitis. Hypertriglyceridemia artificially towers serum amylase levels. If the blood specimen appears milky, the serum should be diluted; after dilution, serum amylase levels may become elevated. Other uncommon causes of pancreatitis include steroids, thiazide diuretics, lasix, sulphonamides, protein deficiency, hypercalcemia, familial, traumatic, idiopathic, and anatomic anomalies such as stricture, or pancreas divisum of the pancreatic duct.

26. **(A)** The gallbladder is enlarged (Courvoisier's sign) in most cases of obstructive jaundice attributable to malignancy. In obstructive jaundice attributable to gallstones, the gallbladder is usually shrunken, owing to the previous inflammatory condition affecting the gallbladder.

27. **(A)** Alkaline phosphatase level usually is more sensitive than the bilirubin level for indicating cholestatic jaundice. It also is more likely to fall before the bilirubin level when the obstruction has been relieved. If an unexplained alkaline phosphatase elevation exists (even in the presence of a normal bilirubin), biliary pathology must be excluded. Elevation of the alkaline phosphatase from a possible source in bone disease can be excluded by measuring isoenzymes.

28. **(C)** Oriental cholangiohepatitis is thought to be caused by the Chinese liver fluke (*C. sinensis*). It is encountered mainly in China (Canton) and Hong Kong and among Chinese who have emigrated elsewhere. There are multiple strictures in the biliary tree, and the intrahepatic ducts are dilated. Secondary infection supervenes. Schistosomiasis causes liver fibrosis, ameba causes liver abscess. *Echinococcus,* causes hydatid liver cysts, and hookworm causes anemia.

29. **(B)** Sclerosing cholangitis is rare and occurs mainly in the third and fourth decades of life. Unlike most autoimmune disorders, it affects men more commonly. It may occur without any other abnormal pathology or may be associated with ulcerative colitis or retroperitoneal fibrosis. The CBD is converted to a thickened cord whose lumen is almost completely obliterated. The prognosis is guarded, and the mean survival is only 5–6 years.

30. **(D)** The normal diameter of CBD is 0.3–0.5 cm and increases with age to up to 0.8 cm by the 8th decade. The cystic duct cholangiogram will provide information as to the reason for the ductal dilation; e.g., gallstone strictures or carcinoma of the biliary tree or pancreas. The history in this patient suggests the most likely cause of a dilated CBD would be attributed to choledocholithiasis. For Calot's triangle, see question 37.

31. **(D)** The patient described has the features of Charcot's triad-jaundice, abdominal pain, and rigors, which indicates the presence of ascending cholangitis in a patient with obstructive jaundice. The patient should be treated with broad spectrum IV antibiotics and undergo ERCP, sphincterotomy, and stone extraction. If this fails, surgical exploration of the CBD will be required.

32. **(D)** If a stone is detected, the T tube should be left in place for 6 weeks to allow the tract to mature. At this time, the T tube can be removed, and the stone can be extracted by using a Dormia basket under fluoroscopy. This approach is indicated only when a T-tube larger than size 16 has been inserted. If this approach is not feasible, the stone can be extracted by retrograde endoscopic techniques or CBD exploration.

33. **(B)** In the presence of previous gallbladder surgery, the possibility of cholestatic jaundice must be excluded. Elevation of alkaline phosphatase (with normal or elevated bilirubin level) strongly supports this diagnosis. The dark urine results from increase in conjugated bilirubin (regurgitated jaundice). Urobilin is excreted in the urine in hepatocellular jaundice but is absent in the urine in obstructive jaundice, because this pigment forms only if bile reaches the small intestine.

34. **(C)** A HIDA scan will show excretion of the radiolabeled isotope into the biliary tree, but there will be no flow into the duodenum, indicating that the biliary–enteric anastomosis is occluded. If an upper GI study with barium is performed, visualization of the common bile-duct would indicate patency of the choledocho-duodenal anastomosis.

35. **(B)** Gram-negative bacilli including *E. coli, Klebsiella*, and *proteus* are the organisms most commonly involved in ascending cholangitis. Anaerobic bacteroids should also be excluded, especially in elderly patients. Intravenous hydration and early institution of appropriate antibiotics is indicated. The antibiotics selected should be effective against the isolated organisms. Combined therapy with an aminoglycoside, penicillin and an antibiotic targeted specifically against anaerobic organisms should be administered initially until blood culture results are available.

36. **(C)** Multiple stones were present in the CBD at the previous operation, During exploration of the CBD, most stones can be removed by using Desjardin's forceps or under direct vision using a choledochoscope and Dormia basket. However, if there are multiple stones impacted in the

lower part of the CBD, a drainage procedure may be indicated. The CBD must be dilated before considering performing a choledochoduodenostomy at the time of gallbladder surgery (Figure 5–6). If a stone is present in a dilated CBD after previous cholecystectomy, a choledochoduodenostomy is performed, because the rate of recurrent jaundice is high (over 20%). Alternatively ERCP and sphincterotomy could be considered.

37. **(C)** The right hepatic artery may pass horizontal and parallel to the cystic duct in some cases. In addition, other abnormalities of the right hepatic duct and drainage of an aberrant hepatic duct may be located in Calot's triangle. Identification of the boundaries of the triangle at operation will minimize serious complications following injury to these structures as they pass through it. The modified definition of Calot's triangle uses liver as the superior boundary rather than cystic artery in the original description by Calot.

38. **(B)** Pruritus occurs frequently in untreated obstructive jaundice. Bile salt elevation is a possible cause of pruritus. Patients with generalized pruritus should have alkaline phosphatase levels determined; if levels are elevated, the possibility of cholestatic jaundice should be considered. Bilirubin is not always elevated in obstructive jaundice. Increased levels of gamma-glutamyl-transferase (GGT) and 5'-nucleotidase may also be noted in cholestatic jaundice.

39. **(B)** Any obstruction to the biliary tree (stones, and benign, malignant, or anastomotic strictures) can lead to infection and cholangitis. It may also occur after trauma to the biliary tree. In ascending cholangitis, there is fever, jaundice, and rigors (Charcot's triad). Suppurative cholangitis is suspected when additional signs of deterioration in mental status and hypotension are present in addition (Reynold's pentad). This entity requires immediate biliary decompression either endoscopically or surgically. *C. sinensis,* the liver fluke, causes suppurative cholangitis in the Far East.

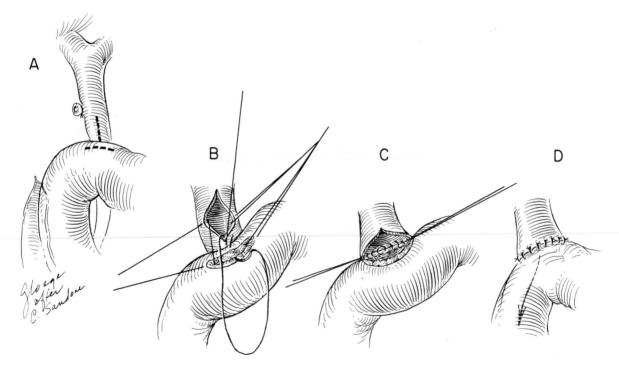

Figure 5–6. Choledochoduodenostomy. **A,** The distal common bile duct is opened longitudinally, as is the duodenum, in preparation for side-to-side anastomosis. **B,** Interrupted sutures are placed between the common bile duct and the duodenum. **C,** The interrupted sutures can have knots on the outside (as shown) or can be done with absorbable sutures and knots on the inside of the duct. **D,** A completed choledochoduodenostomy showing the wide stoma between the duodenum and the common bile duct. (Reproduced, with permission from Schwartz, Principles of Surgery, 6th ed., p. 1464, McGraw-Hill, 1994.)

40. **(C)** Vitamin K requires bile salts for efficient absorption from the gut, as do the other fat-soluble vitamins—A, D, and E. Therefore, the oral route is not suitable to administer to patients with obstructive jaundice. If intramuscular vitamin K is given, correction will occur if there has been no hepatocellular damage. When emergency surgery is required in this circumstance, the coagulation defect due to hepatic disease may be corrected with fresh frozen plasma. Urobilinogen usually is absent in the urine in obstructive jaundice, because its presence depends on a patent biliary–enteric circulation. Stercobilinogen will be absent in fecal examination.

41. **(A)** Stones are found in the gallbladder in over 90% of patients with cholecystitis. Bacteria are cultured in bile in about half the patients undergoing surgery; however, many patients have previously received antibiotics. The gallbladder is usually dilated in patients with acute cholecystitis but contracted in chronic cholecystitis.

42. **(A)** If there is a recent history of jaundice, although the common bile duct is not dilated, cystic duct cholangiography must be performed to exclude CBD stones. Other indications for cystic duct cholangiogram include a recent history of ascending cholangitis, dilated CBD on preoperative sonogram, or suspicion of a "missing" stone in the gallbladder (i.e., as detected by ultrasound or other observations). Elevated bilirubin and alkaline phosphatase are other indications that a CBD stone may be present.

43. **(A)** A cholecystokinin stimulated HIDA scan should be performed. Failure of the gallbladder to contract after stimulation by cholecystokinin may suggest dyskinesia. This is an indication for cholecystectomy, even though stones are not demonstrated. Secretin is the duodenal hormone that stimulates exocrine pancreatic secretion. Gastrin, released mainly from the antrum, increases gastric acid secretion that is high in bicarbonate and electrolytes.

44. **(A)** Unlike most biliary disease conditions, cholangiocarcinoma condition affects men more commonly than women. Primary sclerosing cholangitis, *C. Sinensis,* and choledochal cysts may play an etiological role in some cases, but gallstones are not involved in the pathogenesis of this tumor. Patients present with obstructive jaundice; pain and weight loss are less common. Proximal tumors (Klatskin) are most common, and they require excision of hepatic duct bifurcation and reconstruction with a Roux-en-Y limb of jejunum. Tumors of the distal duct can be resected by performing a Whipple pancreatoduodenectomy. Patients who are not operative candidates (those with advanced disease or those who cannot withstand a major operation) should undergo palliative endoscopic stent placement to relieve the obstruction.

45. **(A)** The HIDA scan is most accurate in establishing a diagnosis of acute cholecystitis. After injection, the technetium-labeled imminodiacetic acid radioisotopes are taken up by the liver and excreted into the biliary tree. If the cystic duct is obstructed (as in patients with acute cholecystitis) the gallbladder will not be visualized. Ultrasound may show ductal dilation, the presence of wall thickening (<3 mm), or pericholecystic fluid, which is highly suggestive of acute cholecystitis.

46. **(E)** She does not require any further therapy. In instances where gallbladder carcinoma is discovered incidentally during cholecystectomy and is shown to have only invaded the mucosa and submucosa it is classified as stage I. The 5-year survival for these patients is 100% and no further treatment is required as for more advanced lesions, i.e., those penetrating the muscular layer or with lymph node involvement (stages II & III). Here there is a higher incidence of local and regional spread to the liver and porta-hepatis lymph nodes, respectively. For these patients an en-bloc resection of segments 4 and 5 of the liver is performed along with dissection of celiac axis and porta hepatis lymph nodes (Figure 5–7). For more advanced lesions (stage IV), the prognosis is very poor, and further resection is not indicated. Gallbladder carcinoma responds poorly to radiotherapy or chemotherapy.

47. **(D)** The morbidity and mortality of cholecystectomy is markedly increased in the presence of cirrhosis. The prognosis is particularly grave in

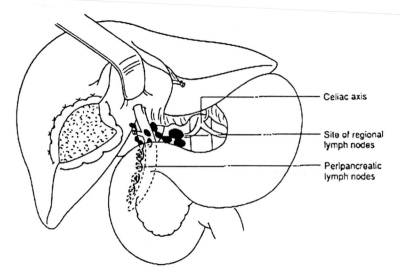

Figure 5–7. Treatment for invasive gallbladder cancer is cholecystectomy and a wedge re-section of the liver along with a regional lymphadenectomy. The wedge resection of the liver is illustrated. Segments 4 and 5 together with the lymph node regions should be removed. (Reproduced, with permission, from Greenfield: Surgery: Scientific Principles & Practice, 2nd. ed., p. 957, J.B. Lippincott Company, 1996.)

patients with decompensated liver disease. Most gallstones in patients with cirrhosis are pigment stones, and hence dissolution with ur-sodeoxycholic acid is not an acceptable option of treatment.

48. **(B)** Early after the onset of acute cholecystitis, the plane of dissection may be facilitated because of early inflammatory response. Between the 7th and 14th day after admission, surgery may be extremely difficult because of resolving infection and adhesions. Where possible surgery should be avoided during this period.

49. **(A)** Emphysematous cholecystitis is caused by gas-forming organisms. On a plain x-ray of the abdomen, gas may be seen within the wall of the gallbladder. Clinically, the patient has rapidly progressive sepsis, RUQ pain, fever, and hemodynamic instability. The disease primarily affects diabetic men. Treatment with laparotomy and cholecystectomy is urgent to avoid complications. Air within the biliary tree (not gallbladder wall) may be seen in gall stone ileus, after biliary–enteric anastomosis or after sphincterotomy.

50. **(D)** Acute acalculous cholecystitis is most commonly encountered in critically ill patients after trauma, other unrelated surgical operations, burns, sepsis, and multiorgan failure. The HIDA scan fails to visualize the gallbladder, and a sonogram may show a distended gallbladder with wall thickening and pericholecystic fluid. Acalculous cholecystitis carries a mortality rate of 10–30%. Delay in diagnosis and hence treatment is accompanied by severe complications, such as gangrene and perforation of the gallbladder in a patient who usually has other debilitating illnesses.

51. **(C)** Obstruction of the cystic duct may be caused by factors other than stones. Acalculous cholecystitis carries a high mortality, because it occurs in patients who are already critically ill. Furthermore, the establishment of the diagnosis is often delayed. Urgent cholecystostomy should be performed. In recent years, percutaneous cholecystostomy under CT or US guidance is performed more commonly than surgical cholecystectomy, because it carries a lower operative mortality rate. In a stable patient, cholecystectomy may be considered.

52. **(D)** Sodium chloride and water are selectively absorbed by the gallbladder mucosa. Bile salts and pigments are concentrated in the bile. Mucus also is secreted into the bile to function in a pro-

tective capacity. The presence of cholesterol crystals in biliary drainage material warrants further investigation, although the biliary system is normal.

53. **(D)** This patient has an amoebic liver abscess. In most patients, the antecedent intestinal phase has subsided by the time patient presents with fever, chills, and a painful, tender enlarged liver. Amoebae are found in examination of fresh stools in 15% of cases, but the indirect hemagglutination test is almost always positive. Amebic abscess responds rapidly to treatment with metronidazol (Flagyl). Surgery should be avoided when possible and is indicated only when medical treatment has failed or complications, such as perforation, have occurred.

54. **(B)** Amebic liver abscess almost always responds to treatment with metronidazole (Flagyl). Occasionally, percutaneous aspiration is required when there is no response to flagyl or if the abscess is secondarily infected. Amebic lever abscess affects mainly middle-aged men. Complications of amebic liver abscess include secondary infection in 20% and rupture into pleural, peritoneal, or pericardial cavity in 10% of cases.

55. **(D)** The hepatic artery, portal vein, and hepatic bile duct are distributed equally between both lobes of the liver divided by Cantlie's line. This line passes between the inferior vena cava posteriorly and the gallbladder fossa anteroinferioly. The falciform ligament does not divide the liver into a right and left lobe; it divides the true left lobe into medial and lateral segments. The caudate and quadrate lobes are part of the left lobe, and, thus, Cantlie's line passes along their right (and not left) margins.

56. **(A)** Hepatic adenomas are associated with an increased incidence in patients receiving oral contraceptives, diabetes, and pregnancy. Most patients are symptomatic with pain and bleeding. Because of the real risk of intraperitoneal or intratumoral bleeding as well as malignant transformation, excision of the adenoma is recommended. Tumors are removed by enucleation or with a narrow rim of normal parenchyma, and major liver resection is not required.

57. **(E)** Unlike hepatic adenomas, these lesions do not usually cause symptoms. Unlike hepatic adenomas, focal nodular hyperplasia does not tend to cause intramural bleeding with rupture into the peritoneal cavity. CT or US scan may frequently miss the lesion, because it is so dense. There is no definite relationship with oral contraceptives. Focal nodular hyperplasia lesions are not well encapsulated and have a central stellate scar. Malignant changes have not been reported.

58. **(B)** Hemangioma is the commonest nodule in the liver. On intravenous contrast CT or MRI, a liver hemangioma shows initial centripetal enhancement followed by decrease in dye over 10 minutes from without to within. Hemangiomas occur more frequently in women. Most lesions are asymptomatic, discovered incidentally, and require no treatment. Larger hemangiomas may cause pain because of stretching of liver capsule or thrombocytopenia due to platelet trapping. These tumors may occasionally require resection.

59. **(C)** Congenital cysts are more frequently encountered than those that are acquired, which are caused by trauma, inflammation, or parasitic disease. Most congenital cysts tend to be asymptomatic and require no treatment. Larger cysts may cause pain and occasionally require radiologically guided percutaneous drainage or operative unroofing to prevent recurrence. Fungal abscesses, encountered mainly in immunosupressed patients, tend to be multiple. Pyogenic abscesses tend to be symptomatic with fever and pain, whereas, tumors are generally not hypoechoeic.

60. **(D)** Before performing the left hepatic lobectomy, any extrahepatic metastasis should be ruled out. If lung, bone, adrenal, or skin metastasis were present, then subjecting the patient to a major operation would not be warranted in most cases. Moreover, before proceeding with surgery, it must be ascertained that control of the primary tumor has been achieved and that the patient's physical condition will allow such a major operation. Surgical excision of hepatic metastasis results in 25%, 5-year survival. Pa-

tients not treated by hepatic resection do not usually survive into the first year after clinical detection. Chemotherapy would be offered if resection were not indicated.

61. **(D)** Massive hemorrhage. Hemorrhage is a major cause of death after liver transplantation. Subphrenic infection and other intraabdominal and intrahepatic infections may occur later in the postoperative period. Graft rejection is mainly a problem at a later period.

62. **(D)** Is rarely associated with long-term survival. Heterotopic (to a remote position) auxiliary transplantation is only occasionally indicated where orthotopic transplantation cannot be carried out. Long-term survival with this procedure is limited (2 of 69 cases). Hetrotropic auxiliary liver transplants require low outflow pressure and are, therefore, most likely to succeed if placed proximally as close to the heart as possible. One advantage of this procedure is that the procedure is technically easier, because the patient's liver is not disturbed.

63. **(A)** The liver plays a role in glucose formation from various glucogenic amino acids and other substances. Hepatic disease removes this source of glucose supply. In insulin hypoglycemia, there is enhanced rapid uptake of glucose by fat tissue and muscle.

64. **(A)** Malignant tumors of the liver may result in severe hepatogenic hypoglycemia. In some cases, a hormone may be secreted from the tumor. Other causes of hypoglycemia include insulinomas and hemangiopericytoma.

65. **(D)** Antithrombin III counteracts excess of thrombin formation. The excess of thrombin facilitates conversion of fibrinogen to fibrin. Portal vein thrombosis will lead to portal hypertension but not hepatic congestion, as seen in Budd–Chiari syndrome. Portal vein thrombosis may occur in cirrhosis, trauma, in patients on contraceptive tablets, and in those who have an increased propensity for thrombus formation. It is also a direct complication of periumbilical infection in the neonate.

66. **(B)** Umbilical infection at birth is associated with ascending infection along the remnant of the left umbilical vein in the round ligament. This vein communicates with the left portal vein. Portal hypertension occurs because of portal vein thrombosis. In general, liver function tests are normal, because the site of portal obstruction is outside the liver. Other causes of portal vein thrombosis include chronic pancreatitis, carcinoma of the pancreas, surgical intervention in this region, and diseases associated with an increased tendency toward clot formation. (See Answer 65.)

67. **(C)** As in any patient with upper gastrointestinal bleeding, the initial intervention following clinical evaluation requires appropriate resuscitation. Blood transfusion may be required. Liver functions must be assessed, and coagulopathy should be corrected with fresh frozen plasma FFP or vitamin K injection. After resuscitation is completed, every attempt should be made to perform an upper GI endoscopy as soon as possible. These patients may be bleeding from varices, portal hypertensive gastropathy, peptic ulcer, or Mallory–Weiss tear, and early endoscopy will provide a higher diagnostic yield as to which lesion is actually bleeding.

68. **(E)** Transjugular intrahepatic portasystemic shunt (TIPS) refers to an implantable, expandable metal stent placed radiologically through the hepatic parenchyma to establish a tract between the hepatic and portal vein. A portal systemic shunt is, therefore, created, and the varices are decompressed. Because of the high incidence of complications (esophageal perforation, aspiration, airway obstruction) associated with the Sengstaken–Blakemore tube, it is only used as a last ditch attempt to control exanguination. In >50% of cases, bleeding recurs after the tube is deflated.

69. **(A)** The condition is more common in children. Splenectomy predisposes the patient to overwhelming postsplenectomy infection characterized by fulminant bacteremia, meningitis, or pneumonia. The mortality of this condition is high. The risk is greatest in children under 4 and for those undergoing splenectomy for thalase-

mia or lymphoma. The risk is lower in adults and those undergoing splenectomy for trauma than for ITP. All patients undergoing elective splenectomy should receive vaccination against pneumococcus and *H. Influenzae* about 2 weeks before surgery. Vaccination should be repeated every 5 years. In addition, children should be given penicillin prophylactically until they are 18 years of age. Postsplenectomy patients should seek medical attention at the first sign of even seemingly mild upper respiratory tract infection and should be advised to wear a Medic Alert tag indicating their asplenic state.

70. **(C)** Portal hypertension is suspected clinically if esophageal varices are detected, hypersplenism occurs, or ascites develop. Normal portal venous pressure is 5–10 mmHg. Pressure may be measured indirectly by using hepatic venous wedge pressure (occlusive hepatic wedge pressure). About two-thirds of patients with portal hypertension will develop varices of which one-third will bleed.

71. **(A)** Penicillamine counteracts the adverse effects of copper on the liver in patients with Kimmelstiel–Wilson syndrome. This has been demonstrated in both humans and animals afflicted with this disease. Portocaval shunt and esophageal varices are not indicated prophylactically.

72. **(E)** Platelets should not be given before splenectomy, but arrangements should be made to have them available immediately before the operation. They should be used only if bleeding occurs and after the spleen has been removed. ITP is a hemorrhagic disorder characterized by a low platelet count with bone marrow findings that show normal or increased megakaryocytes. The female/male ratio is 3:1. This diagnosis implies that no other systemic disease or past history of drug intake could account for these changes. Some cases may be caused by an autoimmune response.

73. **(A)** Radioactive technetium (^{99m}Tc) scan to see if a retained accessory spleen (splenunculus) is present which may account for postoperative thrombocytopenia. Radioactive technetium (not I^{135}) is used to localize splenic tissue. Patients

with ITP have petechiae, ecchymosis, and/or bleeding. Splenectomy performed initially for ITP is likely to be successful in 80% of patients, but is less effective in older patients.

74. **(D)** Features of TTP include fever, thrombocytopenic purpura, hemolytic anemia, neurological manifestations, and renal disease. The exact cause of TTP has not been determined. Histologically, there is diffuse hyalinization of arterioles and capillaries, with occlusion and infarction. The disease may follow a rapid and fulminant course, with death occurring secondary to cerebral hemorrhage or renal failure. Treatment includes steroids, plasmapheresis, and splenectomy. Approximately 1/20 cases occur in pregnancy, but unlike ITP, TTP is not improved by termination of pregnancy.

75. **(C)** Sickle cell disease is relatively common in African-Americans and certain ethnic communities in the United States. Most patients with sickle cell disease respond favorably to rehydration and analgesia for each attack. The patient must avoid unnecessary exposure to infections, hypoxemia, and dehydration. In most patients with sickle cell disease, there is autoinfarction of the spleen. Splenectomy is rarely indicated, except for patients with sickle cell disease with a massively enlarge spleen, where trapping of RBCs is demonstrated.

76. **(E)** Sickle cell disease is diagnosed by peripheral smear showing sickle-shaped red cells and HbS on electrophoresis. The pathogenesis of the disease is characterized by microinfarction in different parts of the body. This can lead to serious (and in some instances fatal) outcome.

77. **(A)** In hereditary spherocytosis, the abnormally shaped erythrocytes fail to pass through the splenic pulp and are more prone to earlier destruction. In hereditary elliptocytosis, the erythrocyte membrane also is abnormal. Children with spherocytosis should undergo splenectomy around their fourth birthday. Other less common hematological indications for splenectomy are thalasemia, sickle cell anemia, autoimmune anemia, and an enlarged spleen that becomes a major site of red cell sequestration.

78. **(C)** Characterized by RBCs that undergo lysis at a higher osmotic pressure. Gallstones are frequently encountered as a result of increased production of bilirubin. Hereditary spherocytosis is transmitted as an autosomal-dominant trait. Because of a fault in the RBC membrane, the cells are smaller and round and undergo lysis in a minor vessel, which results in a relative obstruction to flow.

79. **(E)** Alkalating agents must be given cautiously, because patients with myeloid metaplasia are sensitive to these agents. The connective and hemopoietic tissues in the spleen and liver are increased. Polycythemia vera, myelogenous leukemia, and idiopathic thrombocytosis must be excluded. Splenectomy is often of value.

80. **(C)** Felty's syndrome is characterized by splenomegaly, neutropenia, and rheumatoid arthritis. Steroids are used initially, but their effect usually is transient. Splenectomy favorably alters the leukocyte count; it does not alter the clinical course of rheumatoid arthritis. As with all patients undergoing elective splenectomy, this patient must be given pneumovax, as well as hemophillus and meningiocal vaccines before surgery.

81. **(A)** The risk of infection after removal of the spleen as well as the good results of conserva-tive treatment should encourage a nonoperative approach in children. In adults, surgery is usually recommended, but when possible, the spleen should be repaired and not removed. If the spleen is to be removed on an elective basis, Pneumovax and prophylactic vaccine against *H. influenza* are given about 2 weeks before surgery. (See Answer 69.)

82. **(A, B, D, E)** Santorini's duct is an accessory duct that receives drainage from the head of the pancreas and drains into the duodenum about 1 cm above the main pancreatic duct of Wirsung's duct (Figure 5–8). Injury to this duct may occur during gastrectomy. In pancreas divisum, most of the pancreas drains through the minor duct, and a relative obstruction to the flow develops. Hyperlipidemias may cause pancreatitis. Hypercalcemia caused by hyperparathyroidism may predispose to pancreatitis by precipitation of intraductal stones and by activating pancreatic enzymes. Wharton's duct drains the parotid gland.

83. **(D)** In general, pancreatitis is treated without surgery, because surgical intervention may increase morbidity and mortality. Surgery may be indicated in acute necrotizing pancreatitis. The other specific conditions listed may require surgical intervention.

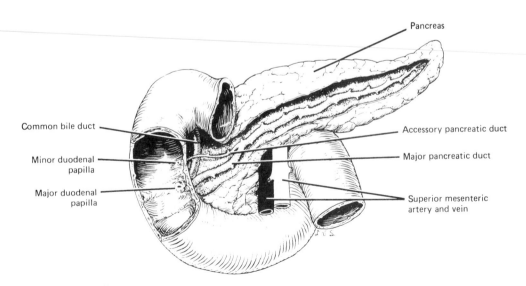

Figure 5–8. The ductal system of the pancreas and the liver. (Reproduced, with permission, from Lindner, HH: Clinical Anatomy, Appleton & Lange, 1989.)

84. **(B, C, G, H)** Neoplasia of the alimentary tract is not a feature of the Zollinger–Ellison syndrome. Basal acid secretion of gastric juice is elevated, and there is severe peptic ulcer disease. In the past, most gastrinomas were thought to arise from the pancreas, but now it is being increasingly recognized that many small gastrinomas occur in the duodenum. MEN 1 involve pituitary, pancreatic, and parathyroid adenomas or hyperplasia. MEN 11 involve medullary carcinoma of the thyroid, pheochromocytoma and hyperparathyroidism.

85. **(A, C, D, H)** Pleural effusion may represent the sole feature of pancreatic ascites. Pancreatic calcification is an important diagnostic feature of chronic pancreatitis. The enlargement of the head of pancreas caused by inflammation will distend the C loop of the duodenum. A colon cut-off sign may be present in both acute and chronic pancreatitis and is due to colonic spasm near the inflamed pancreas. The chain of lakes appearance of pancreatic duct on ERCP is also characteristic of chronic pancreatitis.

86. **(B, C, G)** The HIDA scan is a test frequently used to detect acute cholecystitis to demonstrate delay in filling of the gallbladder. In chronic cholecystitis, the filling of gallbladder occurs after 4 hours. Biliary dyskinesia is diagnosed when the gallbladder fails to empty appropriately (ejection fraction >35%) in response to cholecystokinin stimulation. HIDA scan may also be used to detect biliary leaks following operative bile duct injuries and to verify the free flow of bile from the biliary tree into the duodenum.

87. **(B, E)** Ultrasound may reveal a thickened gallbladder wall, an enlarged (tender) gallbladder, and a collection around the gallbladder. Acalculous cholecystitis may also be encountered in the postoperative period, or can be caused by a tumor or stricture of the cystic duct or diabetes mellitus.

88. **(D, G)** Choledochoduodenostomy is indicated in the management of recurrent stones in the CBD. In a properly constructed choledochoduodenostomy, narrowing of the anastomosis is unlikely to occur. The CBD must be dilated, and the incision must be at least 3 cm long. The CBD is also referred to as the biliary duct. Choledochoduodenostomy is not a good palliative bypass procedure for pancreatic head cancer, because continued growth of the tumor can occlude the anastomosis. Cancer of the pancreatic tail usually does not cause obstruction of the CBD.

89. **(C, D, G)** Gallbladder carcinoma does not usually result in jaundice in the earlier stages. Later, the tumor itself encroaches on the CBD or hepatic duct to produce obstructive jaundice. Porcelain gallbladder is associated with carcinoma in 20% of cases. Gallbladder cancer accounts for 0.3% of all cancers. The female-to-male ratio is 4:1. Treatment is wedge resection of the liver to include gallbladder along with a regional lymphadenectomy if the gallbladder wall is penetrated or lymphnode metastasis is evident. Most cases are detected late, and the 5-year survival is <5%.

90. **(D, E)** Alkaline phosphatase is elevated in bony metastases and bone disease, sarcoid, rickets, a hyperparathyroidism. Isoenzyme studies may be required to distinguish the cause for this elevation from that of a hepatic source. Alkaline phosphatase enzyme may be elevated without a concomitant increase in bilirubin in obstructive jaundice, even when there is major dilation of the CBD.

91. **(A, C, F)** In general, the cystic artery arises from the right hepatic artery. Anomalies of the cystic artery are common and may arise from any of the main visceral arteries in the region. Accurate knowledge of the course and origin of the cystic artery is important in the performance of a safe cholecystectomy.

92. **(A, E, F)** Bile is the major route of excretion of cholesterol. Gallstones are more likely to form when cholesterol and lecithin are increased, and bile salts are relatively decreased in bile. Cholesterol forms in over 50% of mixed and metabolic stones. Calcium bilirubinate constitutes less than 1% of these stones but over 30% of pigmented stones.

93. **(B, E)** Elevation in bile salts accounts in part for the pruritus. Direct bilirubin is predominantly elevated in obstructive jaundice, and indirect bilirubin is increased in hemolytic jaundice. Jaundice is progressive. When the tumor is in the periampullary region, it may slough off into the duodenum and temporarily allow bile to enter the duodenum, thereby causing intermittent jaundice.

94. **(B, H)** Stones are pigmented in 60% of alcoholic liver cirrhosis, as compared to 15% in the rest of the population. The distribution of stones by sex is equal, but in cirrhosis, it is more commonly seen in men. Jaundice in cirrhotic patients is only rarely attributed to stones in the CBD. Cholecystectomy in a patient with cirrhosis carries a high risk and may be complicated by intraoperative bleeding and should be performed only for patients with severe symptoms refractory to medical therapy and when the risk of bleeding can be minimized.

95. **(E, J, K, L)** In liver cirrhosis, mortality and complications are markedly increased in the presence of decompensation (ascites) encephalopathy, jaundice, hypoalbuminemia, malnutrition, or a prolonged PT. Child's classification divides patients into three (A, B, and C) groups based upon these factors. The mortality of patients with Child's C (poor hepatic function) is significantly worse than that of a patient with Child's A (good hepatic reserve).

96. **(C)** If the MB fraction is normal, a recent myocardial infarction can usually be excluded. In acute abdominal emergencies, surgery should be delayed when clinically possible until the results of this test are available.

Cardiac and Vascular
Questions
Zahi E. Nassoura, Mayank Patel, and Simon Wapnick

DIRECTIONS (Questions 1 through 83): Each of the numbered items or incomplete statements in this section is followed by answers or by completions of the statement. Select the ONE lettered answer or completion that is BEST in each case.

1. A 63-year-old man has had a cyanotic painful left fourth toe for 2 days. The dorsalis pedis and posterior tibial arteries are palpable on both sides. There is no history of cardiac or vascular disease. What is the most likely diagnosis?

   (A) cardiac embolus
   (B) atheroembolism
   (C) lupus vasculitis
   (D) digital atherosclerosis
   (E) Raynaud syndrome

2. A 40-year-old chronic smoker presents with ulceration of the tip of the right second, third, and fourth toes. He gives a history of recurrent migratory superficial phlebitis of the feet occurring a few years ago. Physical examination findings are remarkable for absent bilateral posterior tibial and dorsalis pedis pulses with palpable popliteal pulses. What is the single most important step in management?

   (A) multiple toe amputations
   (B) long-term anticoagulant therapy
   (C) immediate operative intervention
   (D) angiography followed by bypass surgery
   (E) cessation of smoking

3. A 60-year-old woman with a 5-cm abdominal aortic aneurysm is referred for surgical repair. The most important preoperative evaluation for use in estimating surgical risk is which of the following?

   (A) renal function
   (B) cardiac evaluation
   (C) pulmonary function tests
   (D) duplex scanning of the carotid arteries
   (E) coagulation profile

4. A middle-aged man is found to have a small pulsating mass at the level of the umbilicus during a routine abdominal examination. What is the best initial test to establish the diagnosis?

   (A) aortography
   (B) ultrasound
   (C) computed tomography (CT)
   (D) magnetic resonance imaging (MRI)
   (E) plain films of the abdomen

5. A 58-year-old woman is found to have a right carotid bruit on routine examination. She is completely asymptomatic. A carotid duplex scan and carotid arteriogram (Figure 6–1) reveals a right carotid stenosis. Which of the following statements is true?

   (A) Operative treatment is indicated if the stenosis is greater than 80%, even if the patient is asymptomatic.
   (B) The incidence of stroke can be decreased by prophylactic carotid endarterectomy in patients with as little as 40% stenosis.
   (C) Aspirin is always a superior treatment to surgery regardless of the degree of stenosis.
   (D) If symptoms eventually develop, they are invariably transient ischemic attacks (TIAs), not stroke.
   (E) Neither surgery nor aspirin is indicated, because the patient is asymptomatic.

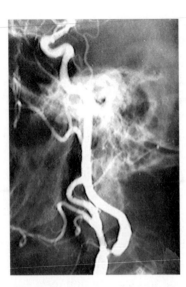

Figure 6–1. Preoperative carotid arteriogram showing stenosis of the proximal internal carotid artery (immediately distal to the bifurcation of common carotid artery). (Reproduced, with permission, from Way, LW: Current Surgical Diagnosis & Treatment, 10th ed., Appleton & Lange, 1994.)

6. A 57-year-old male smoker is referred to you because of two episodes of right upper extremity weakness over the past 6 months, each lasting for 10–15 minutes. Findings on CT scan of the head are negative. An angiogram shows a 75% stenosis of the left carotid artery. What is the most appropriate treatment?

   (A) antiplatelet therapy
   (B) oral anticoagulants
   (C) carotid endarterectomy
   (D) carotid artery bypass to vertebral system
   (E) surgery only if a stroke develops

7. A 24-year-old man complains of progressive intermittent claudication of the left leg. On examination, the popliteal, dorsalis pedis, and posterior tibial pulses are normal; but they disappear on dorsiflexion of the foot. What is the most likely diagnosis?

   (A) embolic occlusion
   (B) thromboangiitis obliterans
   (C) atherosclerosis obliterans
   (D) popliteal artery entrapment syndrome
   (E) cystic degeneration of the popliteal artery

8. Four days after undergoing hysterectomy, a 30-year-old woman develops phlegmasia cerulea dolens over the right lower extremity. What is the most appropriate treatment?

   (A) bed rest and elevation
   (B) systemic heparinization
   (C) venous thrombectomy
   (D) prophylactic vena caval filter
   (E) local urokinase infusion

9. 21-year-old woman is referred to your of office because of multiple lower extremity varicose veins. She has large varicosities in the distribution of the long saphenous vein. What is the next step in management?

   (A) a ligation and stripping operation
   (B) ligation of both the long and short saphenous system
   (C) sclerotherapy
   (D) duplex evaluation along with clinical correlation as an essential initial step
   (E) compression stockings and anticoagulation therapy

10. A 45-year-old woman undergoes cardiac catheterization through a right femoral approach. Two months later, she complains of right lower extremity swelling and notes the appearance of multiple varicosities. On examination, a bruit is heard over the right groin. What is the most likely diagnosis?

   (A) femoral artery thrombosis
   (B) superficial venous insufficiency
   (C) arteriovenous (AV) fistula
   (D) pseudoaneurysm
   (E) deep vein insufficiency

11. A young basketball player develops an acute onset of subclavian vein thrombosis (effort thrombosis) after heavy exercise. What is the next step in management?

   (A) active exercise of the limb
   (B) anti-inflammatory drugs
   (C) thrombolytic therapy
   (D) antibiotics
   (E) first-rib resection

12. A middle-aged man undergoes a left below-knee amputation for left-foot gangrene secondary to arterial occlusive disease. Which of the following statements is true after the below-knee amputation?

   (A) There is less efficient function than after a through-knee amputation.
   (B) Stump prognosis can be judged by transcutaneous oxygen monitoring.
   (C) Poor prognosis is inevitable if Doppler fails to record a pulse at that level.
   (D) The fibula and tibia are of equal length.
   (E) The level of transection is 5 cm above the medial malleolus.

13. A 72-year-old retired banker complains of left-leg intermittent claudication while playing golf. An angiogram shows occlusion of the superficial femoral artery and reconstitution of the popliteal artery below the knee. What is the treatment of choice?

   (A) a vigorous exercise program
   (B) endarterectomy of the superficial femoral artery
   (C) femoropopliteal bypass with expanded polytetrofluoroethylene (PTFE) graft
   (D) in situ femoropopliteal bypass
   (E) femoropopliteal bypass with reversed saphenous vein graft

14. A 40-year-old patient undergoes a CT scan of the abdomen for nonspecific abdominal pain. A splenic artery aneurysm is incidentally identified. What is true of the splenic artery aneurysm?

   (A) It requires splenectomy for optimal treatment.
   (B) It is more common in men.
   (C) It is caused by atherosclerosis in most cases.
   (D) It may rupture during pregnancy.
   (E) It is rarely calcified on an abdominal x-ray.

15. A 70-year-old man with a long-standing history of diabetes develops gangrene of the right second toe. What is true of his diabetic foot?

   (A) Dorsalis pedis and posterior tibial arteries are always absent.
   (B) Gangrene of the toe always requires urgent below-knee amputation.
   (C) Arterial reconstruction is invariably required.
   (D) His right femoral artery is most probably occluded or stenosed.
   (E) Trophic ulcers are sharply demarcated.

16. Eleven years after undergoing right modified radical mastectomy, a 61-year-old woman develops raised red and purple nodules over the right arm. What is the most likely diagnosis?

   (A) lymphangitis
   (B) lymphedema
   (C) lymphangiosarcoma
   (D) hyperkeratosis
   (E) metastatic breast cancer

17. Four days after undergoing subtotal gastrectomy for stomach cancer, a 58-year-old woman complains of right leg and thigh pain, swelling, and redness and has tenderness on examination. The diagnosis of deep vein thrombosis is entertained. What is the initial test to establish the diagnosis?

   (A) venography
   (B) venous duplex ultrasound
   (C) impedance plethysmography
   (D) radio-labeled fibrinogen
   (E) assay of fibrin/fibrinogen products

18. A middle-age woman has right leg and foot nonpitting edema associated with dermatitis and hyperpigmentation. The diagnosis of chronic venous insufficiency is made. What is the treatment of choice?

   (A) vein stripping
   (B) pressure-gradient stockings
   (C) skin grafting
   (D) perforator vein ligation
   (E) valvuloplasty

19. A 55-year-old woman has bilateral leg edema associated with thick, darkly pigmented skin. A Trendelenburg test is done, and results are interpreted as positive/positive. What does this patient have?

    (A) competent varicose veins/competent perforators

    (B) Competent varicose veins/incompetent perforators

    (C) Deep vein thrombosis (DVT)

    (D) Incompetent varicose veins/competent perforators

    (E) incompetent varicose veins/incompetent perforators

20. A middle-aged man known to have peptic ulcer disease is admitted with upper GI bleeding. During his hospital stay, he develops DVT of the left lower extremity. What is the most appropriate management?

    (A) anticoagulation

    (B) observation

    (C) thrombolytic therapy

    (D) inferior vena cava (IVC) filter

    (E) venous thrombectomy

21. A 70-year-old executive is complaining of three-block intermittent claudication of both legs. What is the percentage chance of his developing limb-threatening gangrene?

    (A) less than 10%

    (B) 20%

    (C) 45%

    (D) 60%

    (E) more than 75%

22. Thirty-six hours after undergoing an abdominal aortic aneurysm repair, a 70-year-old woman develops abdominal distension associated with bloody diarrhea. What is the most likely diagnosis?

    (A) aortoduodenal fistulas

    (B) diverticulitis

    (C) pseudomembranous enterocolitis

    (D) ischemic colitis

    (E) acute hepatic failure

23. A 65-year-old man is referred to you because of an incidental finding of a 3-cm left popliteal aneurysm (Figure 6–2). The patient is completely asymptomatic and has normal pulses. How should the aneurysm be treated?

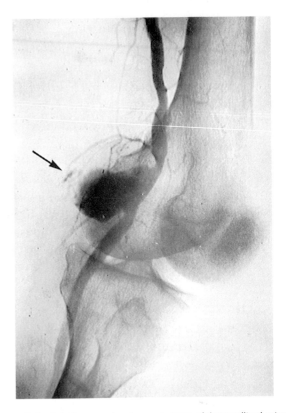

Figure 6–2. Arteriogram showing aneurysm of the popliteal artery (arrow). (Reproduced, with permission, from Way, LW: Current Surgical Diagnosis & Treatment, 10th ed., Appleton & Lange, 1994.)

    (A) It should be observed.

    (B) It should be repaired because it may lead to spontaneous rupture.

    (C) It should be repaired only if it is larger than 5 cm.

    (D) It should be repaired because of its tendency to either undergo thrombosis or embolize distally.

    (E) It should be repaired because of its tendency to cause nerve compression if it enlarges.

24. A 72-year-old woman falls at home after an episode of dizziness. She had been complaining of low back pain for 3 days before the fall. In the emergency department, she is hypotensive and has cold, clammy extremities. A pulsating mass is palpable on abdominal examination. Following resuscitation, the next step in the management should involve which of the following?

(A) peritoneal lavage
(B) immediate abdominal exploration
(C) CT scan of the abdomen
(D) abdominal aortogram
(E) abdominal ultrasound

25. A 60-year-old man complains of dizziness, vertigo, and mild right-arm claudication. On physical examination, there is decreased pulse and blood pressure of the right upper extremity. What is the treatment of choice?

(A) anticoagulation
(B) Repair of coarctation of the aorta
(C) ligation of vertebral artery
(D) carotid endarterectomy
(E) carotid subclavian bypass

26. An 18-year-old man develops a painful swollen leg while training for the New York Marathon. There is tenderness in the calf and ecchymosis is present. What is the most likely diagnosis?

(A) cellulitis
(B) DVT
(C) superficial thrombophlebitis
(D) tear of the plantaris muscle
(E) medical lemniscus tear

Questions 27 and 28

Four days after suffering myocardial infarction, a 78-year-old woman suddenly develops severe diffuse abdominal plain. Her electrocardiogram (ECG) shows atrial fibrillation. On examination, the abdomen is soft, minimally tender, and slightly distended. Hyperactive bowel sounds are present.

27. What is the most likely diagnosis?

(A) mesenteric embolus
(B) nonocclusive ischemic disease

(C) perforated peptic ulcer
(D) congestive heart failure (CHF)
(E) digoxin toxicity

28. The most appropriate initial examination consists of which of the following?

(A) gastrografin upper GI series
(B) white blood cell (WBC) counts and serial abdominal examination
(C) colonoscopy
(D) diagnostic peritoneal lavage
(E) angiography

29. A 28-year-old woman has new-onset hypertension and a bruit on abdominal examination. An arteriogram shows fibromuscular dysplasia (FMD) of the right renal artery. What is the best treatment option?

(A) aortorenal saphenous vein bypass
(B) patch angioplasty of the renal artery
(C) percutaneous transluminal angioplasty (PTA)
(D) transaortic renal endarterectomy
(E) hepatorenal bypass

Questions 30 through 32

A 60-year-old man with a history of atrial fibrillation is found to have a cyanotic, cold right lower extremity.

30. The embolus is most probably originating from which of the following?

(A) an atherosclerotic plaque
(B) an abdominal aortic aneurysm
(C) heart
(D) lungs
(E) paradoxical embolus

31. Which is the most common site at which an arterial embolus lodges?

(A) aortic bifurcation
(B) popliteal artery
(C) tibial arteries
(D) common femoral artery
(E) iliac artery

32. What is the most appropriate management?

    (A) embolectomy
    (B) lumbar sympathectomy
    (C) bypass surgery
    (D) amputation
    (E) arteriography

33. An elderly patient with ischemic rest pain is found to have combined aortoiliac and femoropopliteal occlusive disease. What is the treatment of choice?

    (A) aortofemoral bypass
    (B) femoropopliteal bypass
    (C) aortofemoral and femoropopliteal bypass
    (D) lumbar sympathectomy
    (E) vasodilator therapy

34. A 66-year-old woman has a 5.5-cm infrarenal abdominal aortic aneurysm. What is the most common manifestation of such an aneurysm?

    (A) abdominal or back pain
    (B) acute leak or rupture
    (C) incidental finding on abdominal examination
    (D) atheroembolism
    (E) spontaneous thrombosis

35. A 72-year-old man complains of bilateral thigh and buttock claudication of several months' duration. He was told by his physician that the angiogram revealed findings indicating that he has Leriche syndrome. What does this patient have?

    (A) abdominal aortic aneurysm
    (B) aortoiliac occlusive disease
    (C) iliac artery aneurysm
    (D) femoropopliteal occlusive disease
    (E) tibial occlusive disease

36. A young woman develops a left femoral arteriovenous fistula a few months after a stab wound to the groin. Which of the following physiological changes (Nicoladoni–Branham sign) is elicited on physical examination?

    (A) appearance of CHF when the artery proximal to the fistula is compressed
    (B) slowing of the pulse rate when the fistula is compressed
    (C) a rise in the pulse rate when the artery distal to the fistula is compressed
    (D) a bruit heard only after the fistula is occluded
    (E) absent dorsalis pedis after leg is elevated

37. A young patient sustains blunt trauma to his right knee that results in acute thrombosis of his popliteal artery. Which tissue is most sensitive to ischemia?

    (A) muscle
    (B) nerve
    (C) skin
    (D) fat
    (E) bone

38. Seven years after undergoing resection of an abdominal aortic aneurysm and repair with a Dacron graft, a 65-year-old man develops an aortoenteric fistula. What would be the safest method to treat this patient?

    (A) administration of a prolonged course of antibiotics
    (B) removal of the Dacron graft, closure of the enteric defect, and the insertion of a new aortic graft
    (C) closure of the enteric fistula, removal of the Dacron graft, ligation of the infrarenal aorta, and insertion of an extra-anatomic axillobifemoral bypass graft
    (D) division of the fistula, closure of the aortic and enteric defects, and interposition of omentum in between
    (E) closure of the enteric fistula, removal of the Dacron graft, ligation of the infrarenal aorta, and insertion of an extra-anatomic bypass at a later date

39. A 24-year-old male cyclist undergoes repair of both popliteal artery and vein following a gunshot wound to the right knee. Thirty-six hours postoperatively, there is increasing swelling of

the leg and foot, and the patient complains of increasing foot pain and inability to move his toes. His pedal pulses are palpable. What is the most immediate next step that should be undertaken?

(A) arteriography
(B) leg and foot elevation
(C) fasciotomy
(D) venography
(E) immediate re-exploration of the popliteal space

40. A homeless elderly man is brought to the emergency department after sustaining frostbite to both feet. What is the most appropriate immediate management?

(A) slow rewarming at room temperature
(B) amputation of the gangrenous toes
(C) rapid rewarming with warm water
(D) rapid rewarming with hot water or dry heat
(E) thorough debridement of blisters and devitalized tissue

41. A 55-year-old woman who comes from a high-altitude location is diagnosed as having a carotid body tumor. What is true of these tumors?

(A) They most frequently present as a painless neck mass.
(B) They arise from endothelial cells.
(C) They are usually hypovascular.
(D) They frequently manifest with a stroke.
(E) They are usually treated by embolization.

42. A middle-aged man complains of short-distance claudication in the right thigh. The angiogram shows a right common iliac artery stenosis of 90% over a short segment. What is the treatment of choice?

(A) aortofemoral bypass
(B) left-to-right fermorofemoral bypass
(C) iliofemoral bypass
(D) PTA (percutaneous transluminal angioplasty) and stent placement
(E) axillofemoral bypass

43. A 65-year-old man with hypertension and a blood pressure of 190/105 mmHg has unilateral renal artery stenosis. What is the best diagnostic test to determine the physiologic significance of the lesion?

(A) aortography
(B) renal scan
(C) renal ultrasound
(D) renal vein renin assay
(E) rapid-sequence intravenous pyelogram

44. A young college student injures his left knee while playing football and is unable to bear weight. The provisional x-ray report indicates there are no fractures seen. He is discharged home but presents the next morning to the emergency department with a severely swollen, painful left knee and severe pain in the foot. On examination, the foot is pale, cold, and pulseless. What is the most likely diagnosis?

(A) traumatic deep vein thrombosis
(B) gastrocnemius muscle tear
(C) traumatic arteriovenous fistula
(D) posterior knee dislocation with thrombosed popliteal artery
(E) traumatic sciatic neuropathy

45. An elderly patient complains of recurrent episodes of amaurosis fugax. This is attributable to microembolization of which of the following?

(A) facial artery
(B) retinal artery
(C) occipital artery
(D) posterior auricular artery
(E) superficial temporal artery

46. A 65-year-old woman television technician undergoes femoral embolectomy and leg fasciotomy. Following surgery, she is noted to have oliguria, and her urine is red. What is the most probable diagnosis?

(A) hematuria secondary to heparin
(B) embolus of the renal artery
(C) myoglobinuria
(D) retroperitoneal hematoma
(E) hemoglobinuria

47. A 24-year-old woman on oral contraceptive pills develops an episode of deep vein thrombosis that is adequately treated with anticoagulation. She is at increased risk of developing which of the following?

(A) recurrent foot infections
(B) claudication
(C) pulmonary embolism
(D) postphlebetic syndrome
(E) superficial varicose veins

48. A 72-year-old businessman undergoes a femoral-to-posterior tibial *in situ* bypass graft for a nonhealing foot ulcer. During routine follow-up examination 4 years later, the graft is found to be occluded. The cause of his graft failure is most probably secondary to which of the following?

(A) progression of atherosclerosis
(B) technical error
(C) retained valve in the conduit
(D) venous aneurysm
(E) intimal hyperplasia

49. A 60-year-old woman has an asymptomatic right carotid bruit. A carotid duplex scan shows no evidence of significant carotid bifurcation disease but reveals reversal of flow in the right vertebral artery. What is the most likely diagnosis?

(A) stenosis of the origin of the common carotid artery
(B) stenosis of the vertebral artery
(C) stenosis of the subclavian artery
(D) stenosis of the external carotid artery
(E) stenosis of the intracranial portion of the internal carotid artery

50. A newborn girl with family history of lymphedema is noted to have bilateral lower extremity swelling. What is the diagnosis?

(A) secondary lymphedema
(B) lymphedema praecox
(C) Milroy's disease
(D) lymphedema tarda
(E) Meigs' syndrome

51. During a routine examination of a 30-year-old female actuary seeking life insurance, she is found to have a ventricular septal defect (VSD). She undergoes subsequent studies, including ECG, chest x-ray, echocardiography, and Doppler ultrasound. What is the major determinant of operability in VSD?

(A) age of patient
(B) pulmonary vascular resistance
(C) size of the VSD
(D) location of the VSD
(E) presence of cyanosis

52. At the age of 3 years, a child with a VSD becomes progressively short of breath and requires urgent surgery. What is the most common type of VSD (Figure 6–3)?

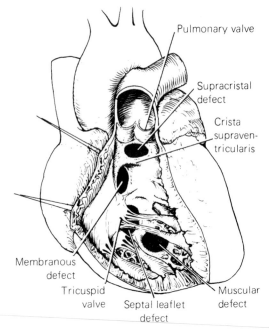

Figure 6–3. Anatomical locations of various ventricular septal defects. The wall of the right ventricle has been excised to expose the ventricular septum. (Reproduced, with permission, from Way, LW: Current Surgical Diagnosis & Treatment, 10th ed., Appleton & Lange, 1994.)

(A) defect anterior to the crista supraventricular
(B) membranous septal defect
(C) posterior septal defect
(D) low muscular defect
(E) right-to-left shunt

53. A 1-year-old girl is found to have a posterior membranous VSD. Peripheral resistance of the pulmonary system is 40% that of the systemic. How should you proceed?

   (A) Observe the child, because most VSDs close spontaneously.
   (B) Band the pulmonary artery and fix the defect at age 6.
   (C) Repair electively at age 14.
   (D) Repair electively between ages 4 and 6 years.
   (E) Repair immediately as an emergency.

54. At birth, the 6 weeks premature infant is noted to have progressive dyspnea. There is a continuous murmur in the pulmonic area (second left intercostal space), and cyanosis is absent. ECG findings are normal. An x-ray of the heart shows cardiomegaly, and the pulse is bounding. Patent ductus arteriosus (PDA) is diagnosed. What does treatment include?

   (A) immediate surgical correction
   (B) administration of indomethacin
   (C) administration of cortisone
   (D) renal dialysis
   (E) endotracheal intubation in all cases

55. During a routine preschool physical examination, the physician notes that a 3-year-old girl has a machinery-type murmur on auscultation of the chest. The pulse is bounding and palpable in the femoral and radial region of both sides of her body. There were no symptoms, and she has excellent exercise performance. Persistent PDA is confirmed on subsequent examination. The parents should be advised that the girl requires which of the following?

   (A) surgical correction and closure of the PDA
   (B) indomethacin
   (C) coronary angiography
   (D) no treatment unless symptoms occur
   (E) CT scan of the heart

56. At age 34, a female long-distance runner notes increasing dyspnea after running more than 10 miles. On inspection and palpation, a prom-

inent right ventricular heave is noted. There is a loud systolic murmur in the left third interspace. The ECG shows right-axis deviation with right bundle branch block. An x-ray of the chest shows a small aortic knob. What sign or test will most likely reveal the cause of the congenital heart abnormality thought to be atrial septal defect?

   (A) beading (scalloping) of the ribs on x-ray
   (B) decreased carotid pulse
   (C) left ventricular hypertrophy on ECG
   (D) elevated sedimentation rate
   (E) increased oxygen saturation gradient between the superior vena cava and the right ventricle

57. A 16-year-old girl was scheduled for cardiac surgery for progressive symptoms. Increased pulmonary vascular resistance was noted on studies. What is the most likely abnormality?

   (A) ostium primum defect
   (B) coronary sinus aneurysm
   (C) persistent right aortic arch
   (D) ostium secundum defect
   (E) atrioventricular (AVA) canal

58. During a routine examination, a 4-year-old girl is noted by her pediatrician to have a murmur that he thinks is attributable to valvular disease. The clinical diagnosis of tricuspid regurgitation disease can be differentiated from mitral valve disease by which of the following?

   (A) appropriate positioning
   (B) time relationship to that of the carotid pulse
   (C) large x descent of the jugular wave
   (D) Decrease in the v (regurgitant systolic) jugular wave
   (E) Harsh left parasternal systolic murmur that is augmented during deep inspiration

59. The only son of a physiology instructor dies suddenly at the age of 12 years following worsening symptoms of tetralogy of Fallot. What would an autopsy reveal?

   (A) dextroposition of the appendix
   (B) brachiocephalic vein draining into the right renal vein
   (C) IVC draining to the superior mesenteric vein
   (D) ASD
   (E) decreased vascularity of the lung field

60. A cyanotic male neonate is born with transposition of the great arteries. The chest x-ray shows a narrow base, and ECG findings are normal. Metabolic acidosis is evident. Life-threatening hypoxemia is treated by prostaglandin E_1 and immediate atrial septotomy. After marked improvement in condition, the infant is scheduled to have a Mustard operation to redirect systemic and pulmonary venous return. However, the baby's condition deteriorates after 2 weeks, and features of heart failure are evident. What is the most sensitive marker of heart failure in children?

   (A) pulmonary congestion
   (B) weak pulses
   (C) ankle edema
   (D) hepatic enlargement
   (E) S3 gallop rhythm

61. After suffering a streptococcal throat infection, a 12-year-old immigrant boy develops cardiac symptoms that are attributed to rheumatic fever. Years later at the age of 34, he is admitted to the hospital with pulmonary edema. Further examination reveals a diastolic murmur at the apex and mitral stenosis is diagnosed. Before surgical evaluation, which of the following findings can be attributed to mitral stenosis?

   (A) large left ventricle
   (B) indentation of the middle third of the esophagus by an enlarged left atrium
   (C) notching of the ribs
   (D) bounding, full pulse
   (E) angina pectoris

62. A 23-year-old ballet dancer is concerned about the recent sudden death on a New York stage of a young famous Russian dancer. The patient seeks advice about his own risk for developing cardiac disease. His father died suddenly from ischemic heart disease at the age of 40. What is the most important risk factor that would further indicate the possibility of coronary artery heart disease?

   (A) diabetes mellitus
   (B) personality type
   (C) elevated high-density lipoprotein
   (D) elevation of total cholesterol/high-density lipoprotein ratio
   (E) obesity

63. In evaluating the risk factors involved in advising elective cholecystectomy in a 52-year-old man with heart disease, which of the following should alert the surgeon to avoid an elective procedure?

   (A) myocardial infarction 9 months earlier
   (B) persistent nonspecific changes on ECG
   (C) increased frequency and severity of attacks of angina
   (D) elevated alkaline phosphatase levels
   (E) hypertension controlled with diuretics

64. Following his first heart attack 3 years ago, a 63-year-old painter complained of central chest pains that radiated to the left arm following exercise. The pain was alleviated by nitroglycerin. Recently, he fell on a steel object and severed the median nerve and flexor tendons at the wrist. The skin was sutured but he is now scheduled to have a second operation that will require anesthesia. What is the best method to diagnose angina pectoris?

   (A) cholesterol/high-density lipid ratio
   (B) isoenzymes
   (C) stress electrocardiography
   (D) echocardiography
   (E) chest x-ray

65. Eight days after undergoing a hysterectomy, a 64-year-old woman complains of chest pain.

After 12 hours, the internist orders tests to exclude myocardial infarction (MI). Which test will most likely support this diagnosis?

(A) serum glutamic oxaloacetic transaminase (SGOT) elevation
(B) increased sedimentation rate
(C) ^{99m}Tc pyrophosphate scintigraphy showing a "hot spot"
(D) thallium 201 (^{201}Tl) scintigraphy showing a "hot spot"
(E) dimethyliminodiacetic acid (HIDA) scan

66. After undergoing repair of a left indirect inguinal hernia, a 72-year-old obese man is admitted to the emergency department with severe retrosternal pain of 1 hour's duration. The pain radiates to the medial aspect of the left hand. The ECG shows Q waves and an elevated ST segment. A diagnosis of acute MI is established 1 hour after admission. Immediate management should include which of the following?

(A) thrombolytic therapy with tPA
(B) vitamin K
(C) ampicillin, 2 mg t.i.d. PO
(D) hydrochlorthiazide, 50 mg/d
(E) sodium, nitroprusside 0.5 µg/kg/min

67. Following recovery from an acute MI, a 44-year-old embryology lecturer is discharged from the hospital with what instructions?

(A) angiogram every 3 months to evaluate the degree of atherosclerosis
(B) nitroglycerin three times a day
(C) digoxin
(D) 325 mg of aspirin on alternate days
(E) pacemaker insertion

68. While crossing the street after her Thursday afternoon bridge game, a 63-year-old woman fell. Attempts at resuscitation for cardiac arrest by the emergency medical service (EMS) team were unsuccessful. The woman had previously been diagnosed as having aortic stenosis and left ventricular hypertrophy. In addition to these factors, which of the following predisposes to sudden cardiac death?

(A) split first heart sound
(B) hypokalemia
(C) soft murmur at left of sternum that varies with inspiration
(D) Failure of the central venous pressure (CVP) to rise more than 1 cm H_2O with 30-second pressure on the liver (hepatojugular reflux)
(E) CVP of –1 cm H_2O

69. A 62-year-old actor has undergone several episodes of myocardial disease. He undergoes cardiac surgery for left anterior descending artery stenosis. What can he anticipate?

(A) mortality of 20–30% in most centers
(B) 95% chance that the graft will become occluded within 12 months
(C) poor outcome if CHF is evident
(D) 5% chance of living 5 years
(E) worst results if saphenous graft is used

70. A 68-year-old male presents with a pulsatile abdominal mass. He has a history of severe COPD, associated with pulmonary hypertension, and advanced CHF. A CT angiogram reveals a 6.5-cm infrarenal aortic aneurysm not involving the iliac arteries. His normal aortic diameter is 23 mm, with an infrarenal neck of 1.5 cm that is angulated at 30%. What should preoperative discussions include?

(A) Because of his high risk history, he is not a candidate for endovascular repair.
(B) Endovascular repair is associated with a lower cardiac morbidity and mortality.
(C) His normal aorta of 23 mm and angulation of the neck precludes endovascular repair.
(D) Laproscopic repair of his aneurysm is associated with the lowest morbidity and mortality.
(E) Endovascular repair could mean a higher rate of secondary procedures with endoleaks being a major morbidity.

71. Advantages of endovascular abdominal aortic aneurysm (EAAA) repair over open repair include which of the following?

    (A) shorter duration of post-operative recovery
    (B) Studies that demonstrate that the technique can be acquired with minimal experience and no learning curve requirements
    (C) markedly decreased morbidity
    (D) markedly decreased operative time
    (E) markedly decreased mortality

72. A 73-year-old female undergoes a EAAA repair, the procedure is a technical success. She is being discharged on the second postoperative day. A routine CT angiogram done before her discharge shows the aneurysm to be of the same size with contrast outside the graft. She is diagnosed as having a type II endoleak. Which of the following is true about her complication?

    (A) immediate return to OR with open repair of her endoleak
    (B) immediate return to the OR with endovascular repair of her endoleak
    (C) continue with her discharge plans with follow-up CT angiogram
    (D) laproscopic repair not an option
    (E) type II endoleaks are secondary to graft failure

73. A 68-year-old retired male nurse undergoes open-heart surgery for occlusive multiple coronary artery disease (CAD). During the procedure, there is a short period of hypotension. The best indication of adequacy of perfusion by a heart/lung machine is measured by which of the following?

    (A) venous oxygen saturation
    (B) arterial oxygen saturation
    (C) arterial pH
    (D) arterial P_{CO_2}
    (E) urine output

74. Two months after undergoing successful open-heart surgery for repair of triple CAD, a 64-year-old man presents with left-sided chest pain, fever, elevated sedimentation rate, and leuko-cytosis. Pericardial effusion and pleural effusion are evident on chest x-ray. What is the most likely diagnosis?

    (A) tuberculosis
    (B) metastatic lung carcinoma
    (C) myocardial infarction
    (D) postcardiotomy pericarditis
    (E) ruptured aortic aneurysm

75. Four months after undergoing coronary artery surgery for left anterior descending and left circumflex CAD, a 69-year-old executive at a Detroit automobile firm complains of chest pain, malaise, and fever. Examination reveals a pericardial effusion with pulsus paradoxus. The ECG shows no evidence of ischemia, and the creatine phosphokinase MB (CPK-MB) isoenzymes and creatine phosphokinase (CPK) levels are normal. Autoimmune pericardial disease (Dressler syndrome) is diagnosed. What is the most useful test for confirming the diagnosis of pericardial effusion?

    (A) stress test
    (B) increased pulmonary artery wedge pressure (PAWP)
    (C) ^{201}Tl scintigraphy
    (D) echocardiography
    (E) increased pulse pressure

76. Three days after a patient underwent hip replacement for a fracture of the neck of the femur, the resident is called to examine the patient and notes hypotension (85/60 mmHg) and a pulse rate of 104 beats per minute (bpm). Fluids are administered, but there is no improvement. The ECG shows peaked T waves and ST elevation. Bedside monitoring reveals a CI of 1.7 L/min/m2 (normal >2.2), stroke work index of 16 g/M2 (normal >30), and a PAWP of 22 mmHg (normal <15). Urgent treatment should involve which of the following?

    (A) rapid hypertonic saline solution administration
    (B) adrenaline
    (C) inotropic agents and, if necessary, intra-aortic balloon counterpulsation
    (D) indomethacin
    (E) atropine

77. A 58-year-old neurologist is admitted to the emergency department with persistent hypotension and shock following an acute MI. He is placed on an intra-aortic balloon pump (IABP). Which following statement is true about IABP?

   (A) The balloon is inflated during systole.

   (B) The balloon is inflated during diastole and systole.

   (C) The pump must be removed after 10 minutes.

   (D) The balloon usually is inserted via the femoral artery.

   (E) Use of an IABP worsens diastolic coronary blood flow.

78. While lying on the examining table before colonoscopy, a 68-year-old electrician notes palpitations. The colonoscopy was scheduled as a routine procedure following removal of a benign polyp 1 year earlier. He had rheumatic fever in infancy. His atrial rate on ECG is 450 bpm, and his ventricular rate is 160 bpm. His pulse rate is 88 bpm. The left atrium is enlarged. Similar findings were noted 1 year ago, but he declined to take any medication. Treatment should entail which of the following?

   (A) continue with colonoscopy

   (B) continue with colonoscopy after administration of parenteral antibiotics

   (C) immediate administration of antibiotics and follow-up colonoscopy at a later date

   (D) immediate administration of anticoagulation and digoxin and follow-up colonoscopy at a later date

   (E) immediate electrocardioversion with a current of 300–400 J

79. During routine clinical examination of a 23-year-old seeking consultation to remove a mole on her left cheek, she develops tachycardia with a pulse rate of 186 bpm. Her pulse is regular. She is otherwise asymptomatic. An ECG reveals supraventricular tachycardia. What should the treatment be?

   (A) alternate pressure on the right and left carotid sinus

   (B) bilateral simultaneous pressure over right and left carotid sinus

   (C) deep eyeball pressure

   (D) morphine sulfate, 4–8 mg IV, given cautiously

   (E) electrical cardioversion

80. After experiencing progressive chest pain for 2 months, a surgical-supply store owner undergoes a CT scan that reveals a space-occupying lesion of the wall of the left atrium, which was confirmed to be a myxoma. There is no evidence of disease elsewhere. What would the next line of treatment be?

   (A) excision of a myxoma performed with a bypass procedure

   (B) excision of a myxoma performed without a bypass procedure

   (C) insertion of a pacemaker

   (D) chemotherapy

   (E) radiotherapy

81. Examination of a 49-year-old male schoolteacher who presents with a swelling in the neck. Palpation reveals a bounding pulse. Which test would be most likely to establish a possible cause of the underlying condition?

   (A) funduscopic eye examination

   (B) liver–spleen scan

   (C) thyroid function studies

   (D) x-ray of the chest and cervical spine

   (E) carotid sinus pressure

82. Following a car accident, a 52-year-old lawyer complains of pain in the left abdomen and back. After arrival of the EMS team, her pulse rate is 84 bpm but of small volume. She states that she has some cardiac condition but is uncertain of its nature. Which is the most likely cause of the small pulse volume?

   (A) aortic stenosis

   (B) syphilis

   (C) hyperthyroidism

   (D) carcinoid syndrome

   (E) aortic incompetence

83. Stenosis of which of the following vessels is associated with the highest patency rates following angioplasty or stenting?

   (A) medial circumflex artery
   (B) iliac artery
   (C) superficial femoral artery
   (D) popliteal artery
   (E) tibial arteries

DIRECTIONS (Questions 84 through 99): Each set of matching questions in this section consists of a list of lettered options followed by several numbered items. For each numbered item, select the appropriate lettered option(s). Each lettered option may be selected once, more than once, or not at all. EACH ITEM WILL STATE THE NUMBER OF OPTIONS TO SELECT. CHOOSE EXACTLY THIS NUMBER.

Question 84

   (A) history of angina and prior MI
   (B) left ventricular ejection fraction of over 50%
   (C) aortic stenosis
   (D) signs of left ventricular failure
   (E) lowered jugular venous distension
   (F) minimal decrease in hematocrit
   (G) presence of groin hernia
   (H) decreased bowel motility

84. An 83-year-old retired navy general shows improvement in claudication following aortoiliac bypass surgery. What is the factor that would cause the greatest concern over the possibility of developing cardiac complications? SELECT ONE.

Questions 85 through 90

   (A) a double aortic arch
   (B) tetralogy of Fallot
   (C) patent ductus arteriosus (PDA)
   (D) coarctation of the aorta
   (E) tricuspid atresia
   (F) umbilical caput medusa
   (G) neurofibromatosis (von Recklinghausen's disease)
   (H) noncyanotic ASD
   (I) spider nevi
   (J) femoral AV fistula
   (K) AV malformation of the vertebral system
   (L) "beading" (notching) of the ribs

85. Cerebrovascular accident occurs most often in which? SELECT TWO.

86. Dyspnea and dysphagia occur with what? SELECT ONE.

87. Differential pressure in right arm and right leg indicates what? SELECT ONE.

88. A child was born with congenital heart disease. The mother had rubella during pregnancy. The child has what? SELECT ONE.

89. Notching of ribs occurs in what? SELECT ONE.

90. Hypoplasia of the right ventricle occurs in what? SELECT ONE.

Questions 91 and 92

A 62-year-old black physician complains of headache, nocturia, and dysuria of 3 weeks' duration. Rectal examination reveals a palpable mass in the prostate, and a biopsy confirms the presence of prostatic carcinoma. He is advised to undergo prostatectomy. His blood pressure is 160/105 mmHg.

   (A) verapamil
   (B) propanalol (inderal)
   (C) deep eyeball pressure
   (D) hydrochlorthiazide diuretic
   (E) calcium phosphate
   (F) digoxin
   (G) cardiac catheterization
   (H) repeat blood pressure assessment in the supine position
   (I) antihistamine

91. The next step in management is which? SELECT ONE.

92. The patient's blood pressure remains elevated when assessment is repeated on several occasions. Investigations fail to reveal an underlying cause of hypertension. Before surgery, he should receive what? SELECT ONE.

Questions 93 and 94

While undergoing a physical examination for life insurance purposes, a 46-year-old executive is noted to have a harsh systolic murmur in the left third and fourth parasternal area. Further evaluation, including echocardiography, reveals pulmonary stenosis.

(A) right ventricular/pulmonary artery gradient of 20 mmHg
(B) right ventricular/pulmonary artery gradient of 65 mmHg
(C) left ventricular hypertrophy
(D) right ventricular hypoplasia
(E) absence of symptoms
(F) hyperbaric oxygen
(G) surgical correction
(H) outflow tract (tunnel) to divert blood from the aorta to the right ventricle
(I) percutaneous balloon valvuloplasty

93. The indication for surgery in pulmonary stenosis is what? SELECT ONE.

94. The appropriate treatment for significant pulmonary stenosis involves which? SELECT TWO.

Question 95

A 23-year-old assistant computer analyst is seen because of lower abdominal pain secondary to an ovarian cyst. Her blood pressure is 180/100 mmHg and remains elevated when she is in bed.

(A) ^{201}Tl scintigraphy
(B) vanillylmandelic acid
(C) analysis of renin and serum potassium levels
(D) 5-hydroxyindoleacetic acid (5-HIAA)
(E) serum lipase
(F) renal arterial angiography
(G) CT scan of the pelvis
(H) renal vein catheterization

95. Which tests are most likely to help exclude a secondary cause of hypertension? SELECT FOUR.

Question 96

On the day of admission for elective cataract surgery, an 84-year-old retired bus driver is noted to have a blood pressure of 255/120 mmHg.

(A) undergo cataract surgery after oral diuretic therapy
(B) undergo cataract surgery without general anesthesia
(C) be given a discharge order and referred to the cardiology clinic
(D) undergo electrocardioversion
(E) be given sodium nitroprusside intravenously
(F) undergo a CT scan of the head
(G) undergo central venous pressure monitoring
(H) undergo arterial blood gas (ABG) measurement

96. Blood pressure assessment is repeated on two occasions, and the same measurements are obtained. What should he do? SELECT ONE.

Questions 97 through 99

    (A) cruciate anastomosis

    (B) long saphenous vein

    (C) caput medusae

    (D) posterior tibial

    (E) iliac veins

    (F) varicocele

    (G) esophageal varices

    (H) anal fissure

97. On the 8th day after undergoing insertion of a prosthesis for a subcapital fracture of the femur, an 81-year-old man develops a massive pulmonary embolus. The most likely site of origin of the embolus is from where? SELECT ONE.

98. A 63-year-old woman complains of pain in the right leg and lower thigh. On examination, there is tenderness on the medial aspect of the leg and induration due to superficial thrombophlebitis. The affected tissue involved is what? SELECT ONE.

99. Portal hypertension causes what? SELECT TWO.

Answers and Explanations

1. **(B)** All the listed conditions may result in isolated digital ischemia. In this age group, atheroembolism is the most likely diagnosis in a man. The atheroma is derived from an occult aortic aneurysm or a proximal ulcerative atherosclerotic lesion. This plaque or ulcer can be any part of the vascular tree proximal to the ischemic toe. Cardiac embolisms also are common in this age group but are a less likely cause in the absence of previous MI, arrhythmia, or valvular disease.

2. **(E)** This patient suffers from thromboangiitis obliterans (Buerger's disease), a disease found most frequently in white men between 20 and 40 years of age. It is a form of panvasculitis involving the artery, vein, and nerve. Heavy tobacco smoking is strongly associated with this disease. Early in the course of the disease, there is involvement of the superficial veins, producing recurrent migratory superficial phlebitis. The distribution of arterial involvement is usually segmental, involving the peripheral arteries. In the lower extremities, the disease occurs generally beyond the popliteal arteries and distal to the forearm in the upper extremities. As long as ulceration or gangrene is confined to a digit, amputation should be postponed as long as possible unless rest pain or infection cannot be otherwise controlled. Bypass surgery is rarely indicated, and long-term anticoagulation has not been of much benefit. The most important aspect of treatment is cessation of smoking, which can halt progression of the disease.

3. **(B)** Atherosclerosis, the etiology of most abdominal aortic aneurysms, is part of a generalized process. Clinical evidence of significant CAD may be present in up to 30% of patients with an abdominal aortic aneurysm. Operative mortality for elective aneurysm operations is most often related to acute MI. It is, therefore, essential that such patients undergo a thorough preoperative cardiovascular evaluation.

4. **(B)** Although aortography, CT, and MRI can all establish the diagnosis of abdominal aortic aneurysm, ultrasound remains the best screening test. It is the preferred method for making the initial diagnosis, because it is reliable, inexpensive, and noninvasive. Aortography is used infrequently because of the small but definite risk it entails and because diagnosis can be made by other means. Once the aneurysm meets the criteria for repair, then a CT scan is done preoperatively to establish the true size and to delineate the aneurysm more accurately. Plain films of the abdomen are inaccurate in establishing the diagnosis.

5. **(A)** Operative treatment is indicated if the diameter of the stenosis is greater than 60%, even if the patient is asymptomatic. The value of prophylactic carotid endarterectomy for hemodynamically significant carotid stenosis is that it decreases the incidence of subsequent cerebral ischemic events if performed with morbidity and mortality rates under 4% (Figure 6–4). Several studies including asymptomatic carotid artery surgery (ACAS) have shown that surgical treatment is superior to medical management if the stenosis is 60% or greater. The ACAS trial has shown the benefits of surgical treatment over medical management if the stenosis, is greater than 60%. However, there are no data to support the use

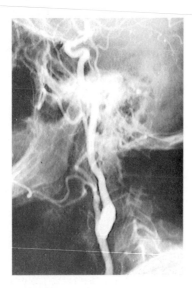

Figure 6–4. Postoperative carotid arteriogram showing restoration of normal luminal size following endarterectomy. (Reproduced, with permission, from Way, LW: Current Surgical Diagnosis & Treatment, 10th ed., Appleton & Lange, 1994.)

of carotid endarterectomy in asymptomatic patients with stenosis of less than 60%. If ischemic events eventually develop, stroke can be the presenting symptom.

6. **(C)** This patient is experiencing recurrent left hemispheric Transient ischemic attack TIA with a hemodynamically significant stenosis of the left carotid artery. This is clearly an indication for surgery because operative management is superior to aspirin in symptomatic carotid bifurcation disease with stenosis greater than 70%. Oral anticoagulants may decrease the incidence of TIAs but not of completed strokes, and they are associated with a considerable risk of hemorrhage. Carotid endarterectomy and not carotid artery bypass, is the surgical procedure of choice. Surgical treatment must be performed before and not after major neurologic deficits are produced from cerebral infarction.

7. **(D)** Popliteal artery entrapment syndrome consists of intermittent claudication caused by an abnormal relation of that artery to the muscles, usually the medial head of the gastrocnemius muscle. As a consequence of developmental abnormalities, the popliteal artery may be com-

pressed by the medial head of the gastrocnemius muscle, resulting in ischemia of the leg at an unusually early age. On examination, the pulses may be diminished or absent, but they may also be normal and be made to disappear on dorsiflexion of the foot. Angiography is essential to establish the diagnosis.

8. **(C)** Phlegmasia cerulae (blue) dolens, indicates that major venous obstruction has occurred. The standard treatment for postoperative thrombosis includes bed rest and anticoagulation. Venous thrombectomy may be indicated when impending gangrene is noted. Vena caval filters are inserted in patients with established pulmonary emboli, but they may be considered as a prophylactic measure when iliofemoral thrombosis is massive. They are also inserted as an adjunct to venous thrombectomy along with creation of an arteriovenous fistula to prevent the venous system from rethrombosing. Thrombolysis of major venous thrombi requires placement of a multihole pigtail catheter inside the thrombus and administration of tPA, including systemic heparinization and is therefore contraindicated postoperatively.

9. **(D)** A through clinical evaluation followed by a venous duplex examination are the two most important steps in managing varicose vein of the lower extremity. An asymptomatic patient without complications of phlebitis, ulceration or hemorrhage should be treated with compression stocking. Duplex evaluation will help map the valvular incompetence of the superficial and deep system including the perforators that guide the extent of the initial surgical intervention, and also investigate if these are primary or secondary varicosities. Sclerotherapy is an alternative to surgery but in the presence of saphanofemoral, saphanopopliteal, or perforator reflux is associated with a high incidence of recurrence and complications.

10. **(C)** A traumatic AV fistula results from a penetrating injury to adjacent artery and vein, permitting blood flow from the injured artery into the vein. The iatrogenic injury in this case occurred during cardiac catheterization. Femoral

artery thrombosis results in signs of limb ischemia. A bruit is usually not heard with venous insufficiency. Traumatic pseudoaneurysm presents as an enlarging pulsating mass. Once the diagnosis of AV fistula is made, an angiogram is performed, and surgical repair (division of the fistula and reconstruction of the artery and preferably of the injured vein as well) is carried out.

11. **(C)** Effort thrombosis, also called Paget–von Schroetter syndrome, is the development of thrombosis of the axillary–subclavian vein as a result of injury or compression. It occurs primarily in young athletes and is disabling. When these patients are seen early, thrombolytic therapy is the first step in management and is followed by a venogram to detect correctable lesions. If effort thrombosis is associated with thoracic outlet syndrome, then thrombolytic therapy should be followed by cervical rib resection. If the condition is chronic, thrombolytic therapy might not be successful; these patients usually respond to limb elevation and anticoagulation.

12. **(B)** Stump prognosis can be judged by transcutaneous oxygen monitoring. Doppler is not fully reliable to select the level of transection, because it cannot calculate the quantity of vascular flow. Transcutaneous oxygen ($PO_2 > 40$ mmHg) offers a fairly accurate prediction of a favorable result; although, Doppler fails to confirm a patent pulse at the level of transection. On the other hand, a duplex evaluation with blood flow of more than 50 cm/s is also a fairly accurate predictor for stump prognosis. The level of transection is 13–15 cm below the level of the medial condyle of the tibia.

13. **(A)** If claudication is the only symptom, elective vascular reconstruction is considered only if claudication is disabling and interferes with day-to-day activity. Because the risk of gangrene occurring in a patient who has only claudication is small, this alone does not constitute a clear-cut indication for operation. Vigorous exercise programs have resulted in marked improvement in claudicants. Revascularization surgery is usually reserved for rest pain or tissue loss (nonhealing ulcer, gangrene). Addition of a phosphodiastraze inhibitor, cilostazol (pletal), or pentoxiphyline (trental) can help increase the claudication distance. It should also be kept in mind that an angiogram is not indicated for claudication. An initial evaluation with noninvasive vascular studies is the investigation of choice. Angiogram is only requested if the decision is made to intervene surgically.

14. **(D)** Splenic artery aneurysms are rare and are most frequently caused by medial necrosis. Small asymptomatic aneurysms caused by atherosclerosis are more commonly incidental findings at autopsy. Larger (>3 cm) aneurysms predominate in women and characteristically may rupture during late pregnancy. Rupture may be preceded by an initial warning bleed into the retroperitoneum, with massive bleeding following after 1 or 2 days.

15. **(E)** Patients with a diabetic foot may have localized arterial occlusion involving the popliteal artery and its branches, usually sparing the femoral artery. Although patients have gangrene of the toes, there may be a palpable pulse in the foot. In the presence of localized disease, trophic ulcers and even gangrene of the toes may respond to local foot care, and major vascular reconstruction or amputations are not required. The trophic ulcers have punched sides. Patients may not realize the gravity of localized gangrene with spreading cellulitis, which develops because of the neurotropic nature of the lesions with the absence of pain sensation.

16. **(C)** Lymphangiosarcoma is a rare complication of long-standing lymphedema, most frequently described in a patient who has previously undergone radical mastectomy (Stewart–Treves syndrome). It usually presents as blue, red, or purple nodules with satellite lesions. Early metastases, mainly to the lung, may develop if it is not recognized early and widely excised. Lymphedema is a complication of radical mastectomy and presents as diffuse swelling and nonpitting edema of the limb. Lymphangitis and hyperkeratosis are complications of lymphedema.

17. **(B)** The most accurate method of confirming the diagnosis of venous thrombosis is the injection of contrast material to visualize the venous system (venography). However, this method is invasive and time-consuming and must be done in the radiology suite. Venous duplex ultrasound is noninvasive, can be done bedside, and has a sensitivity and specificity of 96 and 100%, respectively. The other methods listed are used less often in certain selected patients.

18. **(B)** The mainstay of treatment of chronic venous insufficiency and its complication, venous stasis ulceration, is conservative management. Elastic stocking support, frequent elevation of the legs, and avoidance of prolonged sitting and standing is used for venous insufficiency in the absence of ulceration. If venous stasis ulcers develop, then paste boots (e.g., Unna's boots) are used along with appropriate bed rest and foot elevation until the ulcer heals. Patients whose ulcers fail to heal after such conservative management may need perforator vein ligation. Skin grafting should be considered for chronic stasis ulcers that are large, and perforator incompetance has been treated. Venous reconstruction procedures, including valvuloplasty, can be useful for a selected group of patients, especially those with venous claudication to less than half a block, that have been treated with all the procedures above, including stripping and ligation. Unlike previous opinions, superficial venous stripping and ligation is not always contraindicated in the presence of chronic venous insufficiency and even previous history of deep vein thrombosis.

19. **(E)** The Trendelenburg test is a two-part test used to access the competency of the superficial and perforating veins. The legs are elevated to evacuate the veins, and pressure is applied to the saphenofemoral junction either by hand or tourniquet. The four possible results are: (a) negative/negative response if there is gradual filling of veins from below and continued slow filling after release of pressure, indicating absence of incompetent superficial and perforating veins; (b) negative/positive response if there is gradual filling of veins from below while there is rapid retrograde filling after release of pressure, indicating incompetent superficial veins only; (c) positive/negative response if there is rapid initial filling of the veins from below while only continued slow filling after the release of pressure, indicating incompetent perforators only; and (d) positive/positive response if there is rapid filling of the saphenous vein before and after release of pressure, indicating incompetent superficial and perforating veins.

20. **(D)** The main treatment of DVT is adequate anticoagulation. However, if pulmonary embolism develops during anticoagulant therapy or if there is contraindication to anticoagulation, the insertion of an IVC filter is indicated either to prevent occurrence of or to offer prophylaxis against recurrence of pulmonary embolism (Figure 6–5). Observation alone leaves the patient unprotected against pulmonary embolism, and operative thrombectomy is reserved for limb salvage in the presence of impending venous gangrene. Obviously, if anticoagulation is contraindicated (as in the patient presented), thrombolytic therapy cannot be used.

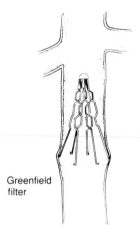

Greenfield filter

Figure 6–5. Surgical prevention of pulmonary embolism. Large emboli can be trapped by partial interruption of the inferior vena cava (Greenfield filter). (Reproduced, with permission, from Way, LW: Current Surgical Diagnosis & Treatment, 10th ed., Appleton & Lange, 1994.)

21. (A) The relatively benign course of intermittent claudication has been well established. The risk of gangrene developing within 5 years in an extremity with claudication as the only symptom is only about 5%. The patient must be encouraged to stop smoking, to exercise, and be placed on a diet that lowers cholesterol.

22. (D) The occurrence of bowel movements during the first 24–72 hours after repair of an abdominal aortic aneurysm (especially if the hemoccult test is positive), should raise suspicion for ischemic colitis. It may develop as a result of interruption of flow to the inferior mesenteric artery with inadequate collateral circulation from either the superior mesenteric artery or the iliac arteries. Aortoduodenal fistula is a late complication of aneurysm repair. Pseudomembranous enterocolitis occurs late in the postoperative course.

23. (D) Popliteal aneurysms are usually arteriosclerotic and are bilateral in at least 50% of cases. Any popliteal aneurysm twice the size of the normal artery is an indication for surgical repair. Although often asymptomatic and small, they should be treated surgically because of their propensity to produce limb-threatening ischemia related to thrombosis or embolism. Spontaneous rupture and/or nerve compression are rare complications of a popliteal aneurysm. The ideal repair consists of ligation of the aneurysm, including its branches and a bypass to the open distal vessels.

24. (B) The presence of acute vascular collapse with history of abdominal or flank pain and associated pulsating abdominal mass is characteristic of a ruptured abdominal aneurysm. Operation should be performed as quickly as possible, because the first priority is to control the hemorrhage. No time should be lost in obtaining diagnostic studies, because these patients often crash in the radiology suite. These patients should not be resuscitated aggressively, because an increase in systolic pressure will only cause more intra-abdominal hemorrhage.

25. (E) The clinical picture presented is that of a subclavian artery stenosis resulting in subclavian steal syndrome, represented by vertebrobasilar symptoms and extremity ischemia. The symptoms are due to a decrease of posterior circulation (vertebral artery) blood flow. Claudication occurs more commonly than ischemic findings. Most patients have no triggering events, and the symptoms are not readily reproducible. Carotid subclavian bypass restores the circulation beyond the stenotic area and corrects the steal syndrome. Ligation of the vertebral artery will correct the steal syndrome but will not improve the circulation of the arm. Anticoagulation has no role in the treatment of this entity. Other treatment options include subclavian artery transposition, axilloaxillary bypass, and subclavian artery angioplasty. Coarctation of the aorta results in pulse and pressure difference between the upper and lower extremities.

26. (D) Spontaneous thrombophlebitis in this age group is unlikely. Plantaris or gastrocnemius tear may occur during physical exertion involving running or walking, causing a sharp pain in this region. After resolution of a hematoma in this region, it may be difficult to exclude cellulitis if there is any question that the integrity of the skin has been damaged. In superficial thrombophlebitis, there is tenderness along the distribution of the long or short saphenous veins. A tear of the medial lemniscus of the knee joint is detected by tenderness over the medical aspect of the knee joint during flexion and internal rotation of the knee joint (McMurray sign).

27. (A) Patients with atrial fibrillation are more likely to develop emboli to different sites throughout the body. Nonocclusive ischemic disease is characterized by spasm of the major mesenteric arterial vessels, with a characteristic beading effect. Early recognition may result in improvement with direct intra-arterial infusion of papaverine (which causes vasodilation), thus avoiding operative intervention.

28. (E) Clinical findings of peritoneal irritation and leukocytosis in patients with suspected visceral ischemia indicate necrosis of ischemic bowel. Immediate arteriography is required to establish the diagnosis and initiate treatment to restore circulation before massive bowel infarction, acidosis, and possible perforation occur. The most likely diagnosis is a mesenteric embolus arising from the heart, especially in the presence of atrial fibrillation. The catheter should be left in place to allow papaverine infusion to an area of borderline ischemic bowel.

29. **(C)** Among all causes of renovascular hypertension, FMD responds best to angioplasty. Intermediate results of PTA for FMD are similar to those of bypass. PTA has lower morbidity, causes less discomfort, and is less expensive. Recurrence can be treated by repeated PTA.

30. **(C)** The heart is the origin of about 90% of lower extremity emboli. The causes are usually mitral stenosis, atrial fibrillation, or MI. A rare source of left atrial emboli is a left atrial myxoma. The remaining 10% arise from ulcerated plaques in the aorta or peripheral arteries. Paradoxical emboli arising from the venous system may reach the arterial circulation through a patent foramen ovale.

31. **(D)** Arterial emboli usually lodge proximal to bifurcations, the most common site being the common femoral artery.

32. **(A)** Once the diagnosis is made clinically, heparin is administered intravenously to prevent the development of thrombi distal to the embolus. Then embolectomy can be done in most instances under local anesthesia. Arteriography to confirm what is already clinically apparent only delays the needed surgical procedure. If there is a doubt, duplex evaluation will help confirm the diagnosis. Lumbar sympathectomy blocks are of dubious value. In patients who have known occlusive disease, absent pulses in the contralateral extremity, absence of clinical features of hyperacute ischemia would be best managed by an angiogram and thrombolytic infusion.

33. **(A)** Patients with combined segmental occlusive disease require correction of proximal hemodynamically significant disease before distal (infrainguinal) bypass. Only about 20% of patients undergoing aortofemoral reconstruction in the presence of superficial femoral artery occlusion will subsequently require femoropopliteal bypass. Combined procedures should be reserved for patients with severe life-threatening ischemia. Lumbar sympathectomy and vasodilator therapy are ineffective in treating severe arterial occlusive disease.

34. **(C)** Most patients are unaware of their abdominal aneurysm until it is incidentally discovered by their physician. The importance of careful deep palpation of the abdomen cannot be overemphasized. On occasion, these aneurysms may expand, causing abdominal or back pain, and may even leak or rupture, mimicking other acute intra-abdominal conditions. Signs and symptoms of acute ischemia in the lower extremities are rare and usually follow thrombosis or embolization from an abdominal aneurysm.

35. **(B)** Leriche syndrome consists of the manifestations of aortoiliac occlusive disease and includes thigh and buttock claudication, atrophy of the leg muscles, diminished femoral pulses, and impotence in men.

36. **(B)** The Nicoladoni–Branham sign can be elicited in some patients with an AV fistula. Occlusion of the fistula or the artery proximal to the fistula may result in slowing of the heart rate. By this compression, the peripheral resistance is increased, venous return is decreased, and the pulse rate falls.

37. **(B)** Peripheral nerve endings are the tissues most sensitive to anoxia in the extremity. Therefore, paralysis and paresthesia are most important when evaluating an extremity with acute arterial occlusion. The second most sensitive tissue is the muscle. This is why an extremity with paralysis and paresthesia will develop gangrene if circulation is not restored. Gangrene is less likely to occur if signs of ischemia are present, but motor and sensory functions are intact.

38. **(E)** The use of an extra-anatomic bypass (axillobifemoral) is indicated in the presence of "hostile" abdomen (infection, dense and severe adhesions, tumors) or if the patient is too sick to undergo an abdominal operation. If a pre-

viously placed graft is contaminated (infection, aortoenteric fistula), the graft must be removed, and the enteric defect must be closed. Although some surgeons advocate removing the infected graft and replacing it in situ with a new graft, the safest approach remains the extra-anatomic route to restore circulation to the lower extremities (axillobifemoral bypass).

39. **(C)** Compartment syndrome can occur following repair of vascular injuries, especially if ischemia time is more than 6 hours or if there have been substantial periods of shock. Other instances include the combination of arterial and venous injury and the presence of concomitant soft-tissue crush injury or bone fracture. Compartment swelling and tenderness, pain disproportionate to the physical findings, paresthesia, and weakness are all clinical signs of compartment syndrome and require urgent surgical decompression. A palpable pulse does not rule out the presence of a compartment syndrome, because compartment pressures are high, even before loss of a palpable pulse

40. **(C)** Rapid warming of the injured tissue is the most important aspect of treatment. The frozen tissue should be placed in warm water, with a temperature in the range of 40°–44°C. Dry heat or hot water carries the risk of thermal injury because of decreased sensation in the injured part. Opening of blisters and debridement of devitalized tissue are contraindicated. Demarcation of gangrenous areas should be carefully observed, often for several weeks, before amputation is performed. The extremity should be elevated, tetanus prophylaxis should be administered as indicated, and antibiotics should be given in the presence of open wounds.

41. **(A)** Carotid body tumors are usually 3–4 mm in size and are located at the carotid bifurcation. They arise from nests of chemoreceptor cells of neuroectodermal origin (carotid body). In normal individuals, the carotid body responds to a fall in P_{O_2} and pH and to a rise in P_{CO_2} and temperature to cause an increase in cardiac contraction, heart rate, and respiratory rate. Carotid body tumors are uncommon, slow growing, and highly vascular. Although large tumors may cause compression of the vagus or hypoglossal nerves, most tumors present as a palpable painless mass at the carotid bifurcation. The treatment is definitely excision whenever possible.

42. **(D)** PTA is technically successful in approximately 90% of iliac lesions with good patency rates. It is more successful for single short stenoses rather than multiple long stenosis or occlusions. The advantages of PTA is that it is less invasive than surgery, has a lower initial cost, has a shorter hospital stay and lower morbidity, enables an earlier return to full activity, and the procedure can be repeated without an increase in morbidity or a decrease in clinical result. It is particularly useful for patients who are high operative risks. The ideal procedure would be and angioplasty and stent placement.

43. **(D)** Aortography and renal ultrasound can detect the presence of renal artery stenosis, but they do not determine the functional significance of the lesion. IVP is not a sensitive enough test to detect the presence of renal artery stenosis. A renal scan can show decrease flow (uptake) or decreased function of the affected kidney, but it, too, lacks sensitivity. The assessment of renal vein renin levels is a good diagnostic test to determine the physiologic significance of renal artery stenosis. It indicates whether the stenosis is significant enough to decrease the glomerular filtration rate and cause the release of renin. In addition, the opposite kidney should have suppression of renin secretion.

44. **(D)** Normal radiographic findings in the presence of severe knee trauma should raise suspicion for posterior dislocation of the knee, which is often associated with popliteal artery thrombosis. A careful vascular examination should, therefore, be made in such a situation. The presence of pain, pallor, and pulselessness (three of the five *p*'s) is indicative of severe ischemia. This patient should undergo urgent exploration for vascular repair. The other options are unlikely to cause the signs and symptoms presented.

45. **(B)** Amaurosis fugax, one type of TIA, is a manifestation of carotid bifurcation atherosclerotic disease. It is manifested by unilateral blindness, being described by the patient as a window shade across the eye, lasting for minutes or hours. It is caused by microemboli from a carotid lesion lodging in the retinal artery, the first intracerebral branch of the internal carotid artery.

46. **(C)** Patients with sudden severe ischemia are prone to "ischemia–reperfusion" syndrome. With revascularization, there is sudden release of the accumulated products of ischemia into the circulation; namely, potassium, lactic acid, myoglobin, and cellular enzymes. Hyperkalemia, metabolic acidosis, and myoglobinuria (red urine, clear plasma) are the key features of the syndrome. Renal tubular acidosis results in myoglobin deposition in the renal tubules. Anticipation and early recognition require the induction of diuresis with mannitol, alkalinization of the urine to avoid precipitation of myoglobin in the renal tubules, and correction of hyperkalemia.

47. **(D)** Despite receiving optimal treatment for DVT, approximately 50% of the patients will develop the post-thrombotic syndrome. The recanalization of the deep veins will result in deformity and subsequently incompetence of the affected venous valves. Although patients with DVT can develop infections secondary to edema, these are usually located about the ankle and resolve with adequate treatment. Patients adequately treated for DVT are not at increased risk of developing pulmonary embolus. Neither the arterial circulation nor the superficial venous system are affected by the development of DVT. Young patients with illiofemoral thrombosis are best managed by thrombolytic infusion, which has been shown to preserve valvular function and decrease the incidence of postphlebitic syndrome.

48. **(A)** The causes of graft failure can be divided into early and late. Although early failure of vein grafts is usually attributed to either technical error or inadequate outflow tract, late failure is usually related to progressive proxi-

mal or distal atherosclerotic disease. Other less common causes of late graft failures include local stenotic areas from trauma or endothelial damage, valve stenosis from fibrosis, and venous aneurysms and subsequent thrombosis. Intimal hyperplasia is a rare cause of late failure.

49. **(C)** Occlusion or stenosis of the subclavian artery proximal to the origin of the vertebral artery results in the "subclavian steal" syndrome. In response to decreased pressure in the distal subclavian artery, especially in instances in which increased perfusion is needed, there is reversal of flow in the vertebral artery. The clinical picture is that of vertebrobasilar symptoms in association with upper extremity exercise. Although this phenomenon is sometimes seen on duplex scanning or angiography, evolution into a clinical syndrome is relatively rare. The other mentioned options do not result in retrograde flow in the vertebral artery.

50. **(C)** Lymphedema is classified by etiology: primary versus secondary. Primary lymphedema is divided into congenital, praecox, and tarda, depending on the age of onset. The diagnosis of Milroy's disease is reserved for patients with familial lymphedema in which clinical factors are present at birth or noticed soon thereafter. Lymphedema is classified as praecox if the age of onset is between 1 and 35 years. Meigs' disease is the familial form of primary lymphedema praecox. If the onset of primary lymphedema is after 35 years of age, it is called lymphedema tarda. Secondary lymphedema usually results from a disease process that causes obstruction of the lymphatic system.

51. **(B)** Increase in pulmonary vascular resistance causes an increased cardiac output. Small shunts (with a pulmonary-to-systemic flow ratio >1.5) do not require surgery but must be treated with prophylactic antibiotics. Larger shunts should be repaired, because the mortality rate exceeds 50% when severe pulmonary pressure (>85 mmHg) occurs. Closure of the VSD in the presence of cyanosis with established reversal of the direction of flow

(right to left) would be detrimental, carrying a very high mortality.

52. **(B)** VSD is the most common cardiac congenital abnormality and results from failure of fusion of the uppermost part of the interventricular septum with the aortic septum. Membranous septal defects account for 90% of VSDs. There is usually a left-to-right shunt and cyanosis does not occur until pulmonary hypertension is severe enough to reverse flow across the VSD. Surgery is indicated in large shunts only when symptoms occur and pulmonary hypertension is evident. Forty percent will close spontaneously in childhood.

53. **(D)** Increase in pulmonary resistance would require more urgent intervention. Because nearly half the cases of VSD in childhood will close spontaneously, elective surgery is deferred to late childhood. Banding procedures are used less frequently today because of the high mortality rate. If symptoms increase in severity, and pulmonary pressure is high more urgent intervention is indicated. If the pulmonary systolic pressure is over 85 mmHg and the left-to-right shunt is small, surgical mortality exceeds 50%.

54. **(B)** Management of compromised respiratory status in the premature infant with PDA includes fluid restriction, adequate oxygenation, attempted closure by medication with indomethacin, and surgical ligation (undertaken when indomethacin is contraindicated). Good results can be anticipated in the absence of other serious complications.

55. **(A)** In full-term infants born with persistent PDA, the anomaly must be closed or excised between 6 months and 3 years of age to avoid cardiac complications, including endocarditis. In PDA, persistence of the communication between the pulmonary trunk and aorta increases pulmonary blood flow, left atrial flow, left ventricular flow, and ascending aorta flow. PDA accounts for 15% of all congenital cardiac abnormalities. Cyanosis does not occur initially, because oxygenated blood is shunted from the aorta to the pulmonary trunk. The murmur is continuous (sounds like machinery) and has harsh features. Its intensity is maximum over the left second intercostal space but radiates to the chest wall and the neck.

56. **(E)** Cardiac catheterization is the definitive test for confirming the diagnosis of ASD. It quantifies the size of the shunt and confirms the increase in oxygen saturation between the right ventricle and the superior vena cava. Beading of the ribs is seen in coarctation, and a decreased carotid pulse is found in aortic stenosis. An elevated sedimentation rate occurs in the presence of infection such as bacterial endocarditis.

57. **(A)** Ostium primum defect occurs low in the septum and may be associated with bicuspid and tricuspid abnormalities. Ostium secundum defect (midseptum) is the most common ASD, present in 80% of cases. In this type, however, symptoms are rarely found in children or adolescents. In contrast, ostium primum defect, which is less common, may result in symptoms in children.

58. **(E)** During inspiration, increased venous return occurs. The increased flow in the right heart increases the murmur of tricuspid valve disease. A time relationship to the carotid or jugular pulse would not help distinguish between a systolic and a diastolic murmur from either site. Tricuspid stenosis is usually secondary to rheumatic fever; tricuspid regurgitation has many causes, including right ventricular overload secondary to left heart failure, inferior MI, endocarditis in drug users, and carcinoid syndrome. In tricuspid regurgitation, the jugular v wave (regurgitant systolic) is prominent, the y descent is rapid, and the x descent is absent or decreased.

59. **(E)** There is decreased vascularity of the lungs seen on chest x-ray. Tetralogy of Fallot includes VSD, right ventricular outflow obstruction, dextroposition of the aorta, and right ventricular hypertrophy. Tetralogy of Fallot accounts for over one-half the cases of congenital cyanotic heart disease.

60. (D) Hepatic enlargement is encountered early in heart failure in children. Prostaglandin E_1 is prescribed to open the ductus arteriosus to increase pulmonary blood flow, and atrial septotomy is performed to improve atrial mixing and decompress the left atrium. In aortic stenosis, the pulses are reduced. In coarctation without PDA, the femoral pulse is absent.

61. (B) Dilation of the left atrium is the obvious complication following long-standing mitral stenosis. Echocardiography is the simplest and most precise method of showing enlargement of the left atrium. Frequently, there is a latency period of 15–20 years before symptoms become evident. Important complications of mitral stenosis include exertional dyspnea caused by an increase in left atrial pressure and backup of blood, with possible pulmonary edema, decreased cardiac output, atrial fibrillation, emboli (15%), and pressure in the intermediate third of the esophagus as seen on an esophogram after barium swallow. The pulse in mitral or aortic stenosis is reduced.

62. (D) Elevation of total cholesterol/high-density lipoprotein is a useful predictor of CAD. Other known main risk factors include genetic predisposition, high cholesterol level, arterial hypertension, and cigarette smoking. Obesity, diabetes mellitus, and personality type are of probable importance as independent risk factors The presence of elevated high-density lipoprotein is a favorable factor.

63. (C) Changes in the nature of angina should alert the physician to the possible progression of the underlying cardiac status. The pain may become more severe and more frequent, may last longer, and may occur with a lesser degree of exertion. Nocturnal pain should likewise signal concern. In the face of unstable angina, 30% of patients are likely to develop myocardial infarction within a 3-month period.

64. (C) In about one quarter of patients with angina pectoris, the ECG findings will be normal. Exercise electrocardiography will reveal ST segment depression and possibly precipitate symptoms if angina pectoris is present.

There is a risk of myocardial death in patients tested, and patients with symptoms after minimal exertion and/or unstable angina are at particular risk with this procedure. If hypotension, ventricular arrhythmia, and supraventricular arrhythmia occur or if the ECG shows a fall in segment ST of over 3 mm, the test should be discontinued. In these cases, ^{201}Tl scintigraphy would be used to detect cardiac ischemia or infarction. Echocardiography during supine exercise may be a helpful test in selected circumstances.

65. (C) ^{99m}Tc pyrophosphate scintigraphy showing a "hot spot." Following injection of ^{99m}Tc pyrophosphate, scintigraphy may show a hot spot in the infarcted area. The hot spot is developed as the radiotracer forms a complex with calcium in necrotic tissue. The test should be requested within the first 18 hours following the onset of acute MI. It is not sensitive enough to detect small infarctions. Following ^{201}Tl scintigraphy, a "cold spot" occurs because of hypoperfusion. The test is performed where exercise or dipyridamole (Persantine) injection can be given. Serum glutamic oxaloacetic transaminase (SGOT) levels are elevated in liver disease. The HIDA scan is used to exclude gallbladder disease. Cardiac enzyme levels and ECG findings are useful to establish a diagnosis of MI.

66. (A) Thrombolytic therapy intravenously with streptokinase, urokinase, or tissue plasminogen activator (tPA) is indicated in most patients with MI presenting early for treatment. This therapy, however, is effective only if initiated within 6 hours after the onset of pain in patients with acute MI. These drugs are fibrinogenolytic, and aspirin and heparin are frequently included in the anticoagulant protocol. Reperfusion rates of 60% can be anticipated; reocclusion rates of 15% usually occur. Vitamin K is not indicated, because it would increase the coagulability of blood. If a diuretic, such as hydrochlorothiazide, 25–50 mg/d is indicated to treat milder hypertension, hypokalemia must be avoided.

67. **(D)** Studies have shown that in men over the age of 50, taking 1 tablet of aspirin (325 mg) on alternate days reduces the incidence of subsequent CAD complications. Nitroglycerin is prescribed if angina pectoris develops, and digoxin would be indicated if CHF is evident. Progression of atherosclerosis should be minimized by appropriate diet and exercise. The intake of excess of cholesterol and saturated fats in the diet causes changes in the vascular endothelium and smooth muscle proliferation, with subintimal fat and fibrous tissue accumulation leading to occlusion of the coronary arteries, their branches, and other arteries.

68. **(B)** Sudden cardiac death is defined as an unexpected death occurring within 1 hour after the beginning of symptoms in a patient who was previously hemodynamically stable. In asymptomatic patients presenting initially with cardiac disease, 20% will die within the first hour of symptoms. Electrolyte imbalance, hypoxia, and conduction system defect are additional factors that increase the risk of sudden death syndrome. Split first heart sound accentuated on inspiration occurs in normal individuals. In CHF, the CVP changes more than 1 cm when pressure is applied below the right costal margin to the liver (hepatojugular reflex) for a 30-second period.

69. **(C)** Mortality figures for elective coronary artery bypass grafting (CABG), for all cases in many centers is less than 1–2%. Patients with impaired ventricular function and failure are poor operative risks. Over 75% of patients undergoing CABG survive more than 5 years. The age limit for CABG has gradually increased, and other risk factors afflicting the patient must be taken into consideration. The functional capabilities of a patient with heart disease can be correlated with prognosis.

New York Classification of Functional Changes in Heart Disease

Class	Limitation of Physical Activity
I	None
II	Slight
III	Marked
IV	Complete (even at rest)

70. **(E)** Endovascular repair of AAA is associated with a higher rate of secondary procedures. Approximately 7–49% of all EAAA repairs require return to the operating room. The most common cause of endoleaks is type II. EAAA is still undergoing evaluation at multiple centers. Interpreting data is difficult, because there are many prosthetic devices undergoing evaluation, and they are constantly undergoing modification, and data are collated using different devices from different centers. Long-term results are still pending. High-risk patients who meet the basic criteria of a aortic diameter of less than 29 mm(device restriction), neck angulation of less than 45 degrees, and infrarenal neck of 1.5cm should be offered EAAA repair. EAAA repair has the same incidence of cardiac morbidity as open repair, and laparoscopic repair is still undergoing evaluation with very few patients to compare against conventional repair.

71. **(A)** EAAA repair has the same rate of morbidity and mortality as open repair. Short duration of hospital stay, acceptable cost effectiveness, and reduced post-operative pain are the main advantages seen during the early phase of studies related to this device study. Procedure time after the initial learning curve is the same as open repair. EAAA repair is associated with a higher complication rate, with endoleaks and graft failure being the most common.

72. **(C)** Type II endoleaks are the Achilles' heel of EAAA repair, most of them are known to thrombose spontaneously; a close follow-up to monitor the leak is advocated. They are caused by persistent retrograde flow from the lumbar or collateral vessels from the aneurysm. Treatment options after an expectant waiting period of 6–12 weeks include endovascular coil embolization, instillation of thrombin in the endoleak region, or laproscopic clipping to persistent lumbar or collateral vessals. Type I leaks are more serious and should be treated when identified.

Endoleak (EL) Classification

Endoleak Type	Synonyms	Description
Type I	Perigraft EL or graft-related EL	Inadequate seal at proximal or distal graft attachment site
Type II	Retrograde El or nongraft-related EL	Persistent retrograde collateral blood flow into aneurysm sac from patent lumbar or collateral vessels
Type III	Fabric tear or modular disconnection	Leakage through a defect in the graft fabric or between segments of a modular graft
Type IV	Graft porosity	Minor blush of contrast on completion angiography emanating from blood diffusion across pores of a highly porous graft

73. **(A)** Mixed venous oxygen represents the amount of oxygen extracted from the tissues. If venous oxygen is greatly reduced, it means that perfusion was less than adequate, and metabolic acidosis may occur. The other parameters listed are still important measurements that may be indicated during surgery.

74. **(D)** Postmyocardial infarction or postcardiotomy pericarditis (Dressler syndrome) may occur in a few patients weeks or months after incision of the pericardium. It is considered an autoimmune event and may recur after successful treatment, which includes use of nonsteroidal anti-inflammatory drugs (NSAIDs) and corticosteroids. Pericarditis may also appear 2–5 days after MI and is caused by transmural myocardial necrosis.

75. **(D)** Several months after suffering MI or undergoing open-heart surgery, patients may develop an autoimmune syndrome (Dressler) that also results in pericardial effusion. Tamponade (intrapericardiac pressure >15 mmHg), however, is rare. *Pulsus paradoxus* results from further impairment of venous filling, and systolic pressure decreases of more than 10 mmHg during inspiration. The echocardiogram is most helpful, because it accurately distinguishes between cardiac failure and pericardial effusion.

76. **(C)** The patient described has cardiogenic shock due to postoperative MI. The mortality rate for patients who develop MI is increased to more than 60% if hypotensive cardiogenic shock also supervenes. Pathology studies of patients dying after such episodes reveal that more than 40% of the heart will have infarcted. Inotropic drugs such as dobutamine are used. If a rapid response is not obtained, intra-aortic balloon tamponade is provided to unload the left ventricle during systole and increase diastolic coronary arterial flow. Hypertonic solutions in graded amounts would be given only if hypovolemia is evident. Atropine and adrenaline would be contraindicated.

77. **(D)** The balloon usually is inserted via the femoral artery. The balloon is inflated during diastole and deflated during systole. It is important that the balloon be adequately deflated during systole to avoid damage to the left ventricle. The pump can be used for a few days if required.

78. **(D)** The major complications occurring in atrial fibrillation are cardiac failure, coronary ischemia, and emboli. Emboli may lead to stroke. Urgent cardioversion is required in patients with auricular fibrillation if heart failure, hypotension, or angina are also present. Immediate cardioversion is indicated in ventricular tachycardia or ventricular fibrillation. If treatment with lidocaine is ineffective, electrocardioversion with 100–200 J for ventricular tachycardia or 300–400 J for ventricular fibrillation is urgently indicated.

79. **(A)** Alternate pressure over the carotid sinus for 20 seconds will end an attack of paroxysmal tachycardia in nearly one-half of cases. The procedure is contraindicated in patients who have had a cerebral TIA or those who have a carotid bruit. Bilateral simultaneous pressure on the carotid sinus carries an additional risk of stroke and must be avoided. The common carotid

artery usually divides at the level of the upper border of the thyroid cartilage or hyoid bone (C3). The carotid sinus may be located either on the proximal internal carotid artery or distal common carotid bifurcation. Eyeball pressure may be effective but carries the risk of retina detachment. If initial measures are unsuccessful, the arrhythmia is treated with intravenous administration of verapamil or a similar drug. Electrocardioversion is indicated in severe cases, particularly if there are adverse symptoms caused by the tachycardia.

80. **(A)** Myxomas constitute more than 50% of all primary cardiac tumors. They are usually polypoid and attached to the septum. Sarcomas constitute 20–25% of primary cardiac tumors. Cardiac metastases are seen in patients with metastatic disease.

81. **(C)** The pulse is bounding when the pulse pressure is magnified because of a wide difference between the systolic and diastolic pressure. It may be due to aortic incompetence, PDA, or noncardiac causes that result in increase in cardiac output and decreased peripheral resistance (e.g., hyperthyroidism, peripheral AV fistula, or anemia).

82. **(A)** A small pulse occurs when the cardiac output is decreased and/or the peripheral resistance is increased. The pulse is reduced in aortic stenosis, heart failure, pulmonary hypertension, pulmonary incompetence, mitral stenosis, and pericardial effusion. The typical cardiac lesion in syphilis is aortic incompetence, which results in a forceful bounding pulse with a wide pulse pressure. Other noncardiac conditions that result in an *increased* pulse pressure include hyperthyroidism, carcinoid syndrome, and aortic incompetence.

83. **(B)** Angioplasty and stenting of the iliac vessels has a patency rate of 75% at 5 years, PTA and stenting of all other vessels has a much lower patency than bypass procedures. The FDA has only approved illiac artery stenting.

84. **(D)** The single most serious prognostic sign for adverse changes after vascular surgery is the presence of CHF. Every effort must be made to correct pulmonary congestion and improve left ventricular function before undertaking elective procedures. MI occurring within 3 months before operation carries a high mortality rate that will be reduced by delaying surgery for 3–6 months when possible.

85. **(B, K)** Cerebrovascular accident is the most important cause of death during the first year of life in patients with tetralogy of Fallot. Over 65% of patients with the tetralogy have cyanosis before 1 year of age. These patients have more severe polycythemia and are particularly liable to develop cyanotic spells of unconsciousness, cerebral thrombosis, hemiplegia, and death. Brain abscess may develop subsequent to infarction and bacteria's entering the systemic circulation via a right-to-left shunt.

86. **(A)** A double aortic arch implies that there are two arches of the aorta; one passes posterior to the esophagus and the other anterior to the trachea. The right side is more common than the left side, and usually one of the arches is smaller than the other. Respiratory difficulty with a labored type of respiration (often precipitated by feeding) usually occurs within the first few months of life. Dysphagia occurs less frequently. Treatment is required only if symptoms are troublesome.

87. **(D)** Coarctation of the aorta is a relatively common anomaly and accounts for approximately 15% of all congenital anomalies. The most common site of coarctation is immediately distal (within 3–4 cm) to the origin of the left subclavian artery. Normally, pressure in the lower extremity is higher than that in the upper extremity, but in coarctation of the aorta, the femoral pulses are absent or markedly reduced. MRI (cine) of chest shows coarctation (Figure 6–6).

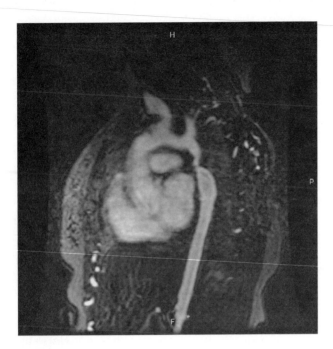

Figure 6–6. MRI (cine) shows coarctation of the aorta distal to the left subclavian artery origin.

88. **(C)** In the fetus, the sixth left aortic arch diverts blood in the pulmonary artery away from the undeveloped lungs. After birth, the channel closes and becomes the ligamentum arteriosum. In rubella, a PDA may be associated with mental retardation and cataracts. Most cases of PDA occur without a clear-cut cause.

89. **(D)** In the presence of coarctation of the aorta, left ventricular enlargement, hypertrophy, and failure to develop occur. As the child grows, collaterals develop between the subclavian artery and the aorta via the intercostal and internal thoracic vessels. In children older than 8 years of age, the intercostal arteries cause typical notching on the inferior margin of the ribs.

90. **(E)** Tricuspid atresia accounts for 5% of cyanotic heart disease. Blood to the lungs is maintained by a PDA.

91. **(H)** Repeat blood pressure assessment in the supine position. Hypertension can be defined as a diastolic pressure above 90 mmHg or systolic pressure above 160 mmHg. Anxiety in an office setting may provide a false high reading of blood pressure. The pressure usually decreases when the individual remains seated and still for a short while. Essential hypertension implies that there is no clear associated cause to explain the hypertension. Ten to 15% of white adults and 20–30% of black adults in the United States suffer from hypertension.

92. **(D)** Diuretics and angiotensinogen-converting enzyme (ACE) inhibitors are more likely to be effective in elderly black men presenting with hypertension. ACE inhibitors inhibit the renin–angiotensin–aldosterone system, sympathetic nervous system activity, and bradykinin degradation and cause an increase in prostaglandin (vasodilator) synthesis. P-Blockers (e.g., propanalol) and calcium channel blockers (e.g., verapamil, nifedipine) are the first line of drugs chosen for young white men presenting with hypertension.

93. **(B)** The presence of mild stenosis (valve gradient/right ventricular pulmonary artery <30 mmHg) in asymptomatic patients does not require surgical correction; such patients can anticipate a normal life expectancy. Moderate to severe stenosis (right ventricular/pulmonary artery gradient of 50–80 mmHg) requires surgical correction.

94. **(G, I)** Percutaneous balloon valvuloplasty is now used in many centers as an initial approach to correct pulmonary stenosis. Right ventricular hypertrophy accounts for the parasternal heave noted on examination. Left ventricular hypertrophy does not occur consequent to pulmonary stenosis. Pulmonary stenosis was once considered rare but now accounts for 10% of cases of congenital heart disease.

95. **(B, C, F, H)** Secondary hypertension accounts for less than 5% of cases involving presentation with asymptomatic hypertension. Vanillylmandelic acid levels would be elevated in pheochromocytoma. Other causes of secondary hypertension include estrogen use, renal disease, renal vascular disease, primary hyperaldosteronism, Cushing's syndrome, and pheochromocytoma. In hyperaldosteronism, there are low renin and potassium levels, and renal vein catheterization may help elucidate the more difficult cases. Renal angiography may reveal renal artery stenosis as a cause of secondary hypertension. 5-HIAA would be elevated in patients with carcinoid syndrome, but the blood pressure is usually lowered.

96. **(E)** Sodium nitroprusside, 0.5–10 μg/kg/min IV, is given to patients (such as the one here) presenting as an urgent hypertensive emergency (e.g., symptomatic hypertension with systolic blood pressure >200 mmHg, or asymptomatic with systolic pressure >240 mmHg). Sodium nitroprusside sodium lowers blood pressure by causing arteriolar and venous dilation. Untreated hypertension may lead to cardiovascular, cerebrovascular, and renal disease. Other complications of hypertension include pulmonary edema, aortic dissection, progressive atherosclerosis, accelerated (malignant) hypertension, and, in pregnant patients, eclampsia.

97. **(E)** Although thrombi are most likely to form in the deep calf veins, emboli to the lungs are more likely to arise from the iliac or larger veins.

98. **(B)** The long saphenous vein arises over the medial malleolus, passes upward superficial to the medial ligament of the knee joint, and enters the femoral vein just below the inguinal ligament. In general, thrombosis in this superficial venous plexus does not lead to pulmonary emboli.

99. **(C, G)** Caput medusae refers to dilated veins around the umbilicus secondary to portal hypertension with backflow from the liver along the round ligament.

CHAPTER 7

Hernia and Breast
Questions

Andrew Ashikari and Max Goldberg

DIRECTIONS (Questions 1 through 49): Each of the numbered items or incomplete statements in this section is followed by answers or by completions of the statement. Select the ONE lettered answer or completion that is BEST in each case.

1. A six-month-old boy presents with an inguinal hernia, first noticed 2 weeks after birth. What is the best treatment choice?

   (A) observation
   (B) laparotomy
   (C) surgical repair when the child is fully grown
   (D) surgical repair of the affected side
   (E) surgical repair of the affected side and exploration of the nonaffected side to search for and repair a sac that was not previously detected by clinical means

2. A 64-year-old man undergoes elective repair of a hernia. At operation, a direct inguinal hernia is found. What is a typical feature of a direct inguinal hernia?

   (A) frequent occurrence in females
   (B) more common in children
   (C) often strangulates
   (D) presents through the posterior wall of the inguinal canal and medial to the deep inguinal ring (Hesselbach's triangle)
   (E) is usually congenital

3. A 70-year-old cigarette smoker presents with a right inguinal mass that has enlarged and has caused discomfort in recent months. He complains of recent difficulty with micturition and nocturia. The swelling, which does not extend to the scrotum, reduces when resting. What is the likely diagnosis?

   (A) direct inguinal hernia
   (B) strangulated indirect inguinal hernia
   (C) hydrocele
   (D) aneurysm of the femoral artery
   (E) cyst of the cord

4. A 62-year-old milliner undergoes emergency surgery for repair of a strangulated indirect inguinal hernia. Which is true in a female patient?

   (A) The sac is formed by the round ligament.
   (B) Correct surgical treatment excludes removal of the sac.
   (C) The sac may extend into the labia majora.
   (D) Risk of strangulation of an inguinal hernia is more likely than that of a femoral hernia.
   (E) An indirect inguinal hernia passes through the internal ring and then through the femoral ring.

5. A 62-year-old Chicago executive goes to the Shouldice Clinic in Canada to have an elective repair of his left inguinal hernia. What does the typical feature of this repair include?

   (A) four-layer approximation of the muscular–aponeurotic arch and transversalis fascia above to the inguinal ligament and transversalis fascia below
   (B) closure of femoral ring
   (C) insertion of mesh
   (D) suture of external oblique to femoral sheath
   (E) fascia lata graft

6. A 28-year-old professional football player has sudden pain and swelling in the right groin when attempting to intercept a pass. He is admitted to the local emergency department. On examination, there is a tender swelling in the right groin. The scrotum and penis show no abnormality. What is the next step in management?

(A) needle aspiration to exclude hematoma
(B) forceful manual reduction
(C) laparotomy within 20 minutes
(D) preoperative preparation and exploration of the groin with hernia repair
(E) morphine and re-evaluation within 12 hours

7. At surgery for a right inguinal hernia, a 72-year-old man is found to have a hernia sac that is not independent of the bowel wall. The cecum forms part of the wall of the sac (Figure 7–1). Such a hernia is properly referred to as which of the following?

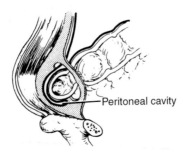

Figure 7–1. Hernia has entered internal inguinal ring. Note that one fourth of the hernia is not related to the peritoneal sac. (Reproduced, with permission, from Way, LW: Current Surgical Diagnosis & Treatment, 10th ed., Appleton & Lange, 1994.)

(A) incarcerated
(B) irreducible
(C) sliding
(D) Richter's
(E) interstitial

8. A 62-year-old construction worker presents with a swelling in the left groin and scrotum of 6 years' duration. It had always been reducible. Twelve hours before hospital admission, the swelling becomes irreducible and painful. After undergoing fluid replacement, he undergoes surgical repair of the hernia, which was noted to be a

Richter's hernia. Which of the following is true of Richter's hernia?

(A) It occurs exclusively in men over the age of 55 years.
(B) It is medial to the linea semilunaris.
(C) It may allow normal passage of stool.
(D) It is treated electively after manual reduction is attempted.
(E) It always contains a Meckel's diverticulum.

9. In Figure 7–2, the patient is being examined to determine if he has an indirect inguinal hernia. The test findings would be positive if, after the patient is directed to cough, the cough impulse is felt where?

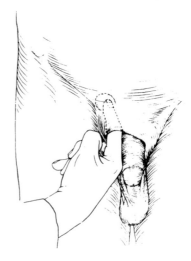

Figure 7–2. Insertion of finger through upper scrotum into external inguinal canal. (Reproduced, with permission, from Way, LW: Current Surgical Diagnosis & Treatment, 10th ed., Appleton & Lange, 1994.)

(A) the examiner's fingertip
(B) the flexor surface of the examiner's finger
(C) the dorsal surface of the examiner's finger
(D) the opposite side of the examiner's finger
(E) not felt

10. A 50-year-old podiatrist complains of severe pain in his ipsilateral testis immediately following hernia repair. The testis is markedly swollen and tender on examination. What is the most likely cause?

(A) acute epididymo-orchitis
(B) mumps

(C) scrotal abscess

(D) compression of the testicular blood supply from too tight a closure of the internal ring during surgery

(E) testicular torsion

11. Which of the following structures would be encountered in a routine repair of a right indirect inguinal hernia?

(A) pudendal nerve

(B) cavernous nerve

(C) Cowper's (bulbourethral) gland

(D) pampiniform plexus

(E) seminal vesicle

Questions 12 and 13

A 70-year-old woman presents with a tender irreducible mass immediately below and lateral to the pubic tubercle. Plain abdominal x-ray shows intestinal obstruction.

12. What is the likeliest diagnosis?

(A) small-bowel carcinoma

(B) large-bowel carcinoma

(C) adhesions

(D) strangulated inguinal hernia

(E) strangulated femoral hernia

13. Treatment with a nasogastric tube and intravenous fluids is initiated. What is the next step in treatment?

(A) sedation to relax the patient and allow spontaneous reduction of the mass

(B) sedation and surgery scheduled for the next elective surgical appointment

(C) sedation and manual taxis (reduction)

(D) emergency surgery on the left groin

(E) emergency laparotomy for intestinal obstruction and hernia repair from the peritoneal cavity

14. In repair of a femoral hernia, the surgeon must take particular care to avoid injury to what?

(A) medial boundary (Gimbernat's ligament)

(B) anterior boundary

(C) lateral boundary

(D) posterior boundary

(E) femoral nerve

15. A male neonate is born with an omphalocele (shown in Figure 7–3). This entity can be distinguished from gastroschisis, because in an omphalocele, the protrusion is what?

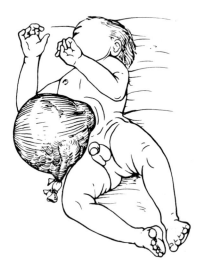

Figure 7–3. Omphalocele. (Reproduced, with permission, from Lindner, HH: Clinical Anatomy, Appleton & Lange, 1989.)

(A) not covered by a sac

(B) a defect in the abdominal musculature

(C) associated with an umbilicus attached to the abdominal wall musculature

(D) associated with partial or complete malrotation of the bowel

16. A 68-year-old obese obstetrician, on chronic steroid medication for rheumatoid arthritis, presents with a large, reducible abdominal hernia, protruding through an old midline incision. Her incision scar is attributed to an operation performed for colon cancer 6 months ago. What is true of incisional hernia?

(A) It occurs mainly in thin individuals.

(B) It is infrequent in patients on steroids.

(C) It should not be repaired, because recurrence is inevitable.

(D) Surgical repair is always urgent.

(E) With a wide neck, it infrequently results in strangulation.

17. A 4-year-old white boy presents with a swelling in the umbilical region. The swelling reduces spontaneously. What is true of hernia at this site?

(A) It occurs more frequently in white than in black children.

(B) It does not require repair, because it does not tend to strangulate.

(C) It should be repaired by mesh.

(D) It is often repaired by the Mayo "pants-in-vest" method, closing the defect in the linea alba.

(E) It is best repaired laparoscopically.

18. A 50-year-old man presents with a complaint of a 1-cm moderately painful, tender mass situated one-third of the way between the xiphisternum and the umbilicus (Figure 7–4). What is the most likely diagnosis?

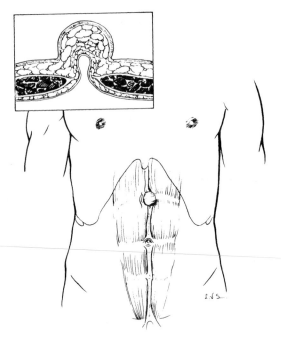

Figure 7–4. Epigastric lesion. (Reproduced, with permission, from Way, LW: Current Surgical Diagnosis & Treatment, 10th ed., Appleton & Lange, 1994.)

(A) fibrosarcoma of the abdominal wall

(B) omphalocele

(C) spigelian hernia

(D) fat necrosis

(E) epigastric hernia

19. What is true of Spigelian hernia?

(A) It occurs exclusively in males.

(B) It involves part of the circumference of the bowel wall.

(C) It is best repaired by the classical Bassini technique of inguinal ligament repair.

(D) It occurs at the lateral edge of the linea semilunaris.

(E) It always contains the vermiform appendix.

20. A 55-year-old woman who has recently been dieting and lost 10 lbs in weight presents with acute small-intestinal obstruction and severe pain that radiates down the inside of her thigh to the knee. Vaginal examination reveals a soft swelling, and an ultrasound of the abdomen and pelvis shows no abdominal finding. What is the likely diagnosis?

(A) strangulated obturator hernia

(B) small-bowel lymphoma with obstruction

(C) ovarian cancer

(D) osteoarthritis of the hip

(E) strangulated femoral hernia

21. A 40-year-old male undergoes a right inguinal hernia repair under local anesthesia. After discharge from hospital, he complains of severe pain in the inguinal scrotal region. The pain is moderate, persistent, and made worse with physical activity. In evaluating the need for further treatment, which is the nerve most likely injured?

(A) femoral

(B) pudendal

(C) ilioinguinal

(D) lateral femoral cutaneous

(E) obturator

22. A 52-year-old male undergoes laparoscopic preperitoneal repair of a left indirect inguinal hernia. Following surgery, he complains of pain. The most likely complication that could account for his symptoms is operative injury to which of the following?

(A) femoral nerve

(B) ureter

(C) iliac artery

(D) seminal vesicle

(E) lateral femoral cutaneous nerve

23. A 62-year-old pharmacist underwent radical mastectomy 7 years earlier. She now complains of back pains radiating to the right lower costal margin. An x-ray reveals an osteolytic lesion of the body and transverse process of T8 and T9 vertebrae. Her chest x-ray findings are unremarkable. Breast carcinoma may spread to the vertebrae before the lungs. Why?

(A) Bone is an excellent tissue for the growth of cancer cells.

(B) The breast lymph nodules drain into the spine.

(C) Deep intercostal veins communicate with the vertebral venous plexus.

(D) The intercostal artery anastomoses with the vertebral artery.

(E) The axillary nodes communicate with the vertebral lymphatic system.

24. A 35-year-old professional dancer presents with a well-defined, tense, smooth mass in the upper outer quadrant of the left breast. She states that the mass becomes larger just before onset of her periods. Aspiration yields a clear yellow fluid and the mass disappears. The most likely diagnosis is:

(A) fibroadenoma in a cyst

(B) fibrocystic disease of the breast

(C) carcinoma in a cyst

(D) lipoma

(E) galactocele

25. An 18-year-old clerk who works at a boutique presents with a well-circumscribed 2-cm mass in her right breast. The mass is painless and has a rubbery consistency and discrete borders. It appears to move freely through the breast tissue. What is the likeliest diagnosis?

(A) carcinoma

(B) cyst

(C) fibroadenoma

(D) cystosarcoma phylloides

(E) intramammary lymph node

26. Galactorrhea, a milky discharge from the nipple in nonpregnant women, is most likely to be associated with which of the following?

(A) fibroadenoma

(B) pituitary adenoma

(C) pineal tumor

(D) hyperparathyroidism

(E) breast abscess

27. Following delivery of her second baby, a 38-year-old statistician develops a breast abscess. She should be treated with which of the following?

(A) antibiotic therapy for gram-negative infection

(B) antibiotic therapy and should express milk from the infected breast

(C) needle aspiration of abscess

(D) mastectomy, because an underlying carcinoma is usually present

(E) incision and drainage

28. A 28-year-old ice-skating star presents several weeks after having sustained an injury to her left breast. She has a painful mass in the upper outer quadrant. Skin retraction is noticed, and a hard mass, 3–4 cm in diameter, can easily be palpated. What is the most likely diagnosis?

(A) infiltrating carcinoma

(B) breast abscess

(C) hematoma

(D) fat necrosis

(E) sclerosing adenosis

29. A 36-year-old woman who recently immigrated from Russia complains of a 3-month history of bloody discharge from the nipple. At examination, a small nodule is found, deep to the areola. Careful palpation of the nipple–areolar complex results in blood appearing at the three o'clock position. Mammogram findings are normal. What is the likeliest diagnosis?

(A) breast cyst
(B) intraductal papilloma
(C) intraductal carcinoma
(D) carcinoma in situ
(E) fat necrosis

30. A 40-year-old lawyer comes into your office after seeing some information on the Internet about breast cancer. She is interested in determining her risk factors. She should be informed that the incidence of breast cancer is increased in which patients?

(A) Those whose paternal cousin had breast cancer.
(B) Those who delivered children as teenagers.
(C) Those who breast-fed their children.
(D) Those who test positive for the BRCA-1 gene.
(E) Those who have undergone previous hysterectomy and bilateral oophorectomy.

31. During a routine screening offered to employees of the county, a 62-year-old science teacher is informed by letter that changes are evident on her mammogram, and she should consult her physician. She can be reassured that the findings that indicate a benign condition are which of the following?

(A) discrete, stellate mass
(B) fine, clustered calcifications
(C) coarse calcifications
(D) solid, clearly defined mass with irregular edges
(E) discrete, nonpalpable mass that has enlarged when compared with a mass shown on a mammogram taken 1 year previously

Questions 32 and 33

A 43-year-old waitress inquires about the implications of positive estrogen receptors in the carcinoma that is excised from her left breast.

32. She should be informed of what?

(A) They are more often positive in patients under 50 years of age.
(B) If the receptors are positive, antiestrogen therapy is not indicated.
(C) If the receptors are positive, the outlook is more unfavorable.
(D) Estrogen and progesterone receptor status should be determined in all cases of breast carcinoma.
(E) Estrogen receptors are usually negative when progesterone receptors are positive.

33. Estrogen receptors are positive in breast cancers in what percentage of cases?

(A) 2.5%
(B) 8%
(C) 25%
(D) 55%
(E) 95%

34. A 52-year-old office administrator undergoes a left modified mastectomy for a 2-cm mass. She has recently become engaged and is anxious about her future outlook and decision to go through with her marriage. She should be informed that the factor that will most likely provide the greatest impact on her prognosis is which of the following?

(A) the size of the primary tumor
(B) the histological type of the carcinoma
(C) the number of axillary nodes positive for metastases
(D) hormonal receptor status of the primary tumor
(E) positive findings on tests for the presence of the BRCAI gene

35. A 46-year-old woman presents with a mammogram that shows a 1-cm cluster of fine microcalcification in the right breast. Following mammographic wire localization, the lesion is excised and the pathology reported as ductal carcinoma in situ (DCIS) with comedo features. Resected margins are free. What advice should be given to the patient?

    (A) If untreated, about 30% of such lesions become invasive over a 10-year period.
    (B) Comedo DCIS seems to be less aggressive than noncomedo DCIS.
    (C) Bilateral mastectomy and radiotherapy are the preferred treatments.
    (D) Axillary node dissection is always indicated.
    (E) Total mastectomy carries a high (50%) risk of carcinoma recurrence.

36. A 43-year-old premenopausal housewife has a biopsy at another hospital, and the pathology shows focal lobular carcinoma in situ (LCIS) in the area of calcification. With regard to the LCIS, you should tell the patient which of the following?

    (A) She needs a simple mastectomy.
    (B) She must be placed on tamoxifen and chemotherapy.
    (C) This is a premalignant lesion, and she requires additional lumpectomy and radiotherapy.
    (D) She is at increased risk of breast cancer, and she should just be observed closely.
    (E) LCIS often presents with a mass.

37. A partially blind 65-year-old mother of five children complains of pain the right shoulder. On examination a slight change in color of the areola of the left breast is noted as an incidental finding. An eczematous rash of the left areola persist for 3 weeks. Biopsy of the areola reveals Paget's disease, and x-ray shows osteoarthritis of the right shoulder. In Paget's disease of the nipple which of the following is true?

    (A) Carcinoma of the breast is rarely found.
    (B) Surgical therapy often fails to cure Paget's disease.

    (C) The diagnosis should be made by nipple biopsy when suspected.
    (D) The underlying carcinoma when present is very large.
    (E) Paget's disease of the bone is commonly encountered.

38. A 39-year-old patient presents to your office with a left 3.5 cm breast tumor, which on core needle biopsy, is shown to be an invasive ductal cancer. On left axillary examination, she has a hard nonfixed lymph node. A biopsy of a left supraclavicular node is positive for malignancy and her staging is classified as which of the following?

    (A) IIIB
    (B) IV
    (C) IIB
    (D) IIIC
    (E) IIA

39. A 45-year-old woman presents with a hard, palpable mass in the central area of her left breast. Mammography shows a normal right breast. On the left side, mammogram shows a stellate 2-cm mass in the central area and a clustered area of fine of microcalcifications in the upper outer quadrant. Stereotactic biopsies are performed. The palpable lesion is an infiltrating ductal carcinoma, and the area of microcalcification is reported to be DCIS. The best surgical treatment is which of the following?

    (A) lumpectomy with sentinel node dissection and radiation therapy
    (B) lumpectomies of both areas plus axillary node dissection and radiotherapy
    (C) simple mastectomy plus radiotherapy
    (D) modified radical mastectomy and radiotherapy
    (E) modified radical mastectomy

40. A 75-year-old woman presents to the emergency department with a fracture of the left hip. An x-ray reveals osteolytic changes in the proximal femur. There is no previous history to suggest underlying cancer. The most likely primary site is which of the following?

(A) pancreas

(B) jejunum

(C) stomach

(D) breast

(E) colon

41. After undergoing modified radical mastectomy for cancer of the right breast, a 52-year-old female teacher becomes aware that the medial end of the scapula becomes prominent, and this change is more prominent in protraction movements at the shoulder. She also complains of some weakness in complete abduction of the same shoulder. What nerve was cut?

(A) long thoracic

(B) dorsal scapular

(C) median

(D) ulnar

(E) intercostobrachial

42. Tamoxifen is an antineoplastic drug that has which following characteristics?

(A) antimetabolite properties

(B) corticosteroid properties

(C) competes with estrogen at the binding site of breast tissue

(D) is useful in patients whose breast carcinoma is estrogen receptor-negative

(E) causes hypocalcemia

43. Five years of tamoxifen treatment should be recommended to all the following patients with breast cancer, EXCEPT those patients with which of the following?

(A) still have their uterus

(B) are premenopausal and whose tumor is ER−/PR−

(C) are premenopausal

(D) have a tumor that is ER+/PR−

(E) have DCIS carcinoma

44. A 43-year-old female requests breast augmentation surgery. She has no family history of breast cancer and her clinical examination fails to reveal any evidence of pathology. What should she be informed about the procedure?

(A) In the United States only gel-filled and not saline-filled implants are performed.

(B) Breast implants increase the incidence of malignancy of the breast.

(C) The occurrence of subsequent breast cancer occurs at a later stage than those without implants.

(D) Saline implants have a more natural appearance than gel-filled implants.

(E) Implants in the submuscular plane allow better mammographic findings than those placed in the subglandular position.

45. A 56-year-old radiotherapy technician has had a breast lump for 2 years. Initially, the lesion is considered to represent gynecomastia. Part of the swelling becomes hard, and a biopsy confirms the presence of carcinoma. Of all breast cancers, the rate of occurrence in males is which of the following?

(A) less than 1%

(B) 4%

(C) 7%

(D) 10%

(E) over 10%

46. A 25-year-old nonalcoholic man has had noticeable right gynecomastia since age 20. He is most uncomfortable and reluctant to swim or exercise at a gym for fear of being an object of derision. He should be advised to have which of the following?

(A) right mastectomy

(B) observation

(C) needle biopsy of the breast

(D) endocrine workup and right subcutaneous mastectomy

(E) testosterone therapy by transdermal patch

47. A 36-year-old operating room technician presents with a substantial breast enlargement. She had presumed that this was normal, but on examination, a large, firm tumor is palpated by the attending physician. There is early erosion on the skin. A favorable outlook can be anticipated if the lesion is which of the following?

(A) sarcoma

(B) cystosarcoma phylloides

(C) colloid carcinoma

(D) infiltrating carcinoma

(E) inflammatory carcinoma

48. A premenopausal 44-year-old woman undergoes a quadrantectomy and node dissection for a 2-cm infiltrating carcinoma of the left breast. The margins are clear, and five out of 15 axillary lymph nodes is involved. Estrogen and progesterone receptors are positive. Recommended adjuvant therapy should include which of the following?

(A) radiotherapy only

(B) estrogen therapy alone

(C) modified radical mastectomy

(D) chemotherapy alone

(E) chemotherapy, radiotherapy, and tamoxifen

49. A 55-year-old postmenopausal woman undergoes a left axillary lymph node biopsy, which turns out to be an adenocarcinoma. Breast examination fails to show any abnormality. Bilateral mammography, bilateral ultrasound, and other metastatic work-ups are negative. The tumor is ER+/PR+. The following statements are true EXCEPT for which of the following?

(A) Recurrence and survival results for this patient are worse than those identified with tumor in the breast.

(B) This is most likely a lesion from the larynx or pharynx.

(C) This is a common site for papillary carcinoma of the thyroid to metastasize.

(D) The treatment should be a left axillary dissection followed by radiation therapy and chemotherapy.

(E) A primary breast cancer is only found in 10–20% of mastectomy specimens.

DIRECTIONS: (Questions 50 through 57): The set of matching questions in this section consists of a list of lettered options followed by several numbered items. For each numbered item, select the appropriate lettered option(s). Each lettered option may be selected once, more than once, or not at all. EACH ITEM WILL STATE THE NUMBER OF OPTIONS TO SELECT. CHOOSE EXACTLY THIS NUMBER.

Questions 50 and 51

(A) femoral vein

(B) iliac crest

(C) inguinal ligament

(D) pectineal (Cooper's) ligament

(E) quadrate lumborum muscle

(F) Gimbernat's (lacunar) muscle

(G) internal oblique muscle

(H) symphysis pubis

(I) latissimus dorsi

(J) external oblique muscle

(K) 12th rib

50. What forms the boundaries of a femoral hernia? SELECT ONLY FOUR.

51. What forms the boundaries of Petit lumbar hernia? SELECT ONLY THREE.

Questions 52 through 54

(A) foramen of Bochdalek

(B) Littré's hernia

(C) Richter's hernia

(D) sliding hernia

(E) Spigelian hernia

(F) foramen of Morgagni

(G) obturator hernia

(H) epigastria hernia

52. A male neonate is born 4 weeks prematurely with respiratory distress. Loops of small intestine are seen in the left chest. What is the most likely hernia? SELECT ONLY ONE.

53. A 64-year-old male presents with intermittent retrosternal pain. Barium gastrointestinal series shows that a barium-filled loop of bowel enters the thorax during the Trendelenburg maneuver.

The lateral chest x-ray locates the bowel loop to the anterior mediastinum. The hernia, which is reducible, is what? SELECT ONLY ONE.

54. A 26-year-old female presents with abdominal distention of 2 days' duration. She had had a bowel movement and passed flatus immediately before hospital admission. Examination showed abdominal distention, and on auscultation increased bowel sounds were heard. There was no evidence of a groin hernia. Vaginal examination revealed a left-sided swelling. Laparotomy was performed, and part of the circumference of the bowel showed ischemic changes; the remaining circumferences of the same bowel were entirely normal. The findings include what? SELECT ONLY TWO.

Questions 55 through 57

(A) tubular
(B) medullary
(C) colloid
(D) infiltrating ductal carcinoma
(E) infiltrating lobular carcinoma
(F) adenoidcystic
(G) inflammatory carcinoma
(H) DCIS
(I) LCIS
(J) carcinoma en cuirasse
(K) Mondor's disease

55. Which of the above invasive histology has a more favorable prognosis compared with other invasive cancers on a stage-by-stage comparison? SELECT ONLY THREE.

56. Which of the above favorable histologys tends to occur in younger women and be hormone receptor negative? SELECT ONLY ONE.

57. Microscopic examination on this malignancy shows large, vacuolated cells. SELECT ONLY ONE.

Answers and Explanations

1. **(E)** Inguinal hernias in infancy are almost always congenital and indirect and are often bilateral. Bilateral exploration is recommended, except when the surgery is performed for incarceration.

2. **(D)** Direct inguinal hernia is more common in men. It seldom strangulates and is usually acquired in adult life. It protrudes through the transversalis fascia, where it is posterior to the inguinal canal. It tends to occur more often in smokers, those with chronic bronchitics, and others with conditions that lead to a chronic increase in intra-abdominal pressure. At operation, a direct hernia protrudes through the posterior wall of the inguinal canal, medial to the inferior epigastric vessels and the internal ring.

3. **(A)** Direct hernias are more common in older patients. There is an increased incidence in patients with a chronic cough and prostatic obstruction. They are rarely encountered in children and women. This type of hernia does not extend to the scrotum and rarely undergoes strangulation.

4. **(C)** An indirect sac represents failure of the processus vaginalis to obliterate. The sac often contains small bowel, and strangulation is a substantial risk. Although indirect inguinal hernia in females occurs at least as frequently as femoral hernia, strangulation is more likely to occur in patients presenting with femoral rather than inguinal hernias.

5. **(A)** The Canadian method popularized the four-layer repair of transversalis fascia and aponeurotic structures to the inguinal ligament. This operation is frequently performed under local anesthesia, and the patient is discharged on the same day that surgery is performed.

6. **(D)** Unexplained recent onset of swelling in the groin that is not reducible should be considered to be a strangulated inguinal or femoral hernia until proved otherwise. Needle aspiration may cause fecal perforation and forceful manual reduction may result in the return of gangrenous bowel to the peritoneal cavity.

7. **(C)** The term *sliding* refers to the peritoneum that slides along with the hernia in its passage along the cord (Figure 7–5). The viscus forms part of the wall of the sac. The peritoneum should not be removed from the bowel wall, because devascularization may occur.

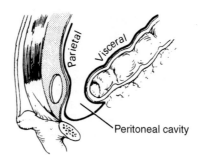

Figure 7–5. Note cecum and ascending colon sliding on fascia of posterior abdominal wall. (Reproduced, with permission, from Way, LW: Current Surgical Diagnosis & Treatment, 10th ed., Appleton & Lange, 1994.)

8. **(C)** In Richter's hernia, part of the wall of the bowel is caught in the hernia sac in a patient with strangulation. Thus, gangrene may occur in the presence of a normal bowel movement.

The full circumference of the bowel wall must always be defined before reducing the hernia at operation. The presence of a Meckel's diverticulum (Littré's hernia) inside a hernia sac is extremely rare.

9. **(A)** In an indirect inguinal hernia, a cough impulse will be transmitted in a direction followed by the cord and thus to the external ring to reach the examiner's fingertip. In a direct inguinal hernia, the impulse is medial to the inferior epigastric vessels (Hesselbach's triangle), and the cough impulse will be found more on the flexor aspect of the examiner's finger (Figure 7-6).

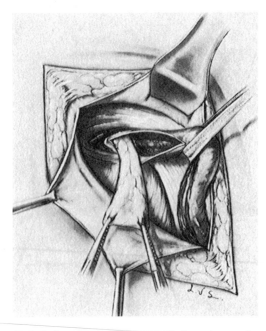

Figure 7–6. Indirect inguinal hernia. Inguinal canal opened and spermatic cord retracted upward and medially. The internal spermatic fascia is incised to reveal the sac of an indirect inguinal hernia directed downward and inferiorly toward the external ring. (Reproduced, with permission, from Way, LW: Current Surgical Diagnosis & Treatment, 10th ed., Appleton & Lange, 1994.)

10. **(D)** During hernia repair, excessive closure of the internal and external ring should be avoided to prevent compression of the cord. The repair should admit the tip of one finger at both rings.

11. **(D)** The pampiniform plexus constitutes the venous return from the testis and is found in the spermatic cord (within the internal spermatic fascia layer) together with the testicular artery, lymphatics, and the vas deferens. The seminal vesicles are located posterior to the prostate. Cowpers glands surround the membranous urethra, and their drainage ducts perforate the perineal membrane to enter the penile urethra.

12. **(E)** Strangulated femoral hernia is located below and lateral to the pubic tubercle and is more common in females. Inguinal hernias occur in similar frequency in females, but compared to femoral hernias, they are less likely to undergo strangulation.

13. **(D)** This patient has a strangulated femoral hernia. Emergency surgery after appropriate resuscitation is the correct treatment. Gangrene of strangulated bowel may be present. No attempt at manual reduction should be made, because gangrenous bowel may be returned to the peritoneal cavity.

14. **(C)** The femoral vein is immediately lateral to the femoral canal and may be accidentally lacerated or constricted with a suture. The femoral canal contains Cloquet's gland and major lymphatics that drain the lower abdominal wall, perineum, and lower extremity in their passage to the para-aortic lymph nodes.

15. **(D)** In omphalocele (see Figure 7–7), the swelling is covered by a membrane formed by the peritoneum, Wharton's jelly, and amnion. The membrane is transparent, and underlying intestine can be seen. The other features listed are characteristic of gastroschisis. In gastroschisis, the protrusion is not covered by a membrane and the other features listed apply.

16. **(E)** Incisional hernias are more frequent in patients who are obese or malnourished, are on steroids, or have had a severe wound infection after surgery or a faulty surgical closure occurs. If the hernia has a wide neck and is asymptomatic, repair is not urgent.

17. **(D)** Failure to repair the hernia may result in strangulation. If the diameter of the umbilical hernia is above 1.5–2 cm, the defect is most unlikely to close spontaneously. If the swelling is under 1 cm, only 5% will still be evident at 5 years of age.

A
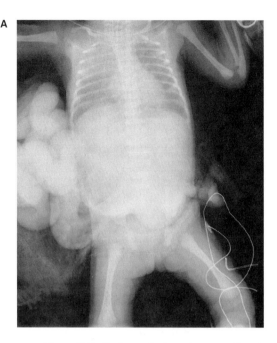

B
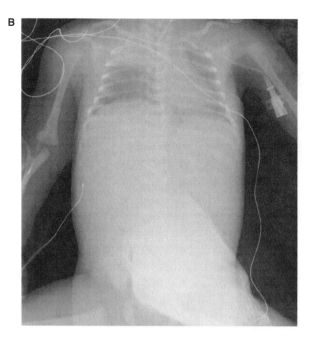

Figure 7–7. Radiograph shows large swelling due to gastroschisis. **A,** Multiple loops of bowel lying on the right side and outside of the abdomen. **B,** Bowel loops wrapped in synthetic bag to reduce bowel sequentially.

18. **(E)** Epigastric hernia is a defect in the linea alba between the umbilicus and the xiphisternum. It usually contains preperitoneal fat rather than omentum or bowel. It may cause pain and is commonly encountered in older patients. Sometimes it is located on either side of the midline. Spigelian hernia occurs lateral to the linea semilunaris.

19. **(D)** Spigelian hernia occurs at the semilunar line, which extends along the lateral border of each rectus abdominis muscle. The posterior rectus sheath is deficient at the level of the arcuate line (semicircular line) about one-third of the distance between the umbilicus and the pubic symphysis; this is the most common site for Spigelian hernia to occur through the linea semilunaris. It occurs in both sexes. The Bassini technique refers to inguinal hernias only. A hernia that involves part of the bowel wall is known as a Richter's hernia. The appendix may or may not form part of the contents of the sac.

20. **(A)** Strangulation of a bowel loop may occur at the obturator fossa, especially after weight loss. Compression of the obturator nerve accounts for referred pain on the medial aspect of the thigh just above the knee region.

21. **(C)** Compression on the ilioinguinal nerve after inguinal hernia repair is the common cause of severe pain radiating into the inguinal scrotal region. Both the ilioinguinal nerve and the genital branch of the genitofemoral nerve require careful identification to avoid injury during groin surgery. The other nerves listed are somatic nerves within the inguinal region but are not likely to be injured during groin surgery. See Answer 22 for possible injury to the lateral femoral cutaneous nerve during a mesh repair of an inguinal hernia.

22. **(E)** The lateral femoral cutaneous nerve is visible in the laparoscopic preperitoneal approach to the inguinal canal. A mesh is stapled into position during the repair, and the nerve can be easily injured. Following such injury, severe burning pain and parasthesia along the lateral aspect of the thigh may occur. Injury to this nerve is unlikely if staples are not inserted lateral to the internal inguinal ring. Compression of this nerve (independent of surgery) may cause myalgia paresthetica when the nerve is compressed as it traverses the lateral aspect of the inguinal ligament.

23. **(C)** The vertebral plexus receives tributaries from the deep intercostal veins and also from the

pelvic plexus. This provides a route for the dissemination of cancer cells. There are connections between the pelvis and abnormal veins of the posterior abdominal wall that account for the similar mechanism for the spread of cancer.

24. **(B)** Breast cysts are often well demarcated and tend to get larger premenstrually. Needle aspiration yields a non-blood-stained fluid, and cytology is required to exclude malignant cells.

25. **(C)** Fibroadenomas are most often found in teenage girls. They are firm in consistency, clearly defined, and very mobile. The typical feature on palpation is that they appear to move freely through the breast tissue ("breast mouse").

26. **(B)** Galactorrhea is fairly common up to old age. The discharge may vary in color from brown to milky. Hormonal causes are associated with elevated prolactin levels or with pituitary or thyroid disorders. Tranquilizers have also been implicated. Simple abscesses do not cause galactorrhea.

27. **(E)** Incision and drainage remains the standard treatment of choice for a breast abscess. Breast abscesses are most common during lactation. The usual organism is *Staphylococcus aureus*, but streptococci may also cause them. When they are untreated, extensive damage may result. They are rarely associated with underlying breast carcinoma.

28. **(D)** Fat necrosis is a rare condition that follows injury. Diagnosis may be difficult, and mammography and excision may be necessary to rule out carcinoma. Sclerosing adenosis is a variant of fibrocystic disease and may present with a hard mass. In a hematoma, evidence of resolving ecchymosis may be present.

29. **(B)** Intraductal papilloma is the most common cause of bloody discharge from the nipple. The lesion is treated by excision and is benign in most cases. Cancer is present in 5% of cases. Preoperative ductography is advised to locate the lesion precisely.

30. **(D)** The incidence of breast cancer has been shown to be increased in carriers of both the BRCA-1 and BRCA-2 genes. Risks vary but can be as high as a 60% lifetime risk in families where a known genetic mutation occurs. Breast cancer incidence has not been shown to be increased in families with distant paternal relatives affected by this malignancy. Having children at a younger age (below 30 years) is a protective factor against subsequent development of breast cancer.

31. **(C)** Coarse calcifications are usually benign. Fine, clustered calcifications are often malignant and require biopsy. Solid tumors of the breast, especially those that have increased in size or have changed in appearance, are suspicious for carcinoma and require biopsy.

32. **(D)** Estrogen and progesterone receptor status should be determined in all cases of breast carcinoma. Positive estrogen and progesterone receptors are indicative of an improved outlook and likelihood of response with antiestrogen medication. Positive progesterone receptors do not predict negative estrogen receptor status.

33. **(D)** The overall estrogen receptor positive rate is 55%, but the figure is higher in postmenopausal women. Receptor's positive status increases with age.

34. **(C)** The number of positive axillary nodes remains one of the best prognostic indicators in breast carcinoma. In one study from California, of over 1,500 axillary node dissections, 36% contained evidence of metastatic disease, and the 12-year median survival was 54%. In patients who were node negative, the survival over a corresponding period was 85%.

35. **(A)** DCIS is a noninvasive lesion. Comedo DCIS is more aggressive than noncomedo DCIS. Axillary disease is uncommon in DCIS, and lymph node staging is generally not required. Unless extensive or multifocal, breast-conserving therapy can be performed as long as negative margins can be obtained. Radiation therapy after breast-conserving surgery is indicated.

36. **(D)** She is at increased risk of breast cancer and she should be observed closely. LCIS is usually an incidental finding. Although multifocal throughout both breasts, it is thought not

to be precancerous itself but rather an indicator of cancer risk. Therefore, wide resection is not indicated. Careful examinations every 6 months and yearly mammograms are done to detect invasive carcinoma at the earliest time. Lifetime risk is about 30%.

37. **(C)** The diagnosis should be made by nipple biopsy when suspected. Paget's disease represents a ductal carcinoma that has grown along the ducts into the nipple/areola region. The lesion often presents with an eczematous rash, which does not resolve and can be easily diagnosed with a small incisional nipple biopsy. Typical swollen vacuolated Paget's cells are found on histological examination. Many cases involve small carcinomas, which are missed on clinical examination and mammogram. Surgical therapy is often curative. This is unrelated to Paget's disease of the bone.

38. **(B)** Ipsilateral supraclavicular lymph node disease is stage IIIC in breast cancer. The new classification of AJCC will include ipsilateral supraclavicular nodes as IIIC and not IV. These patients are not benefited by surgery primarily and typically require appropriate metastatic work-up and chemotherapy.

39. **(E)** A modified radical mastectomy is indicated because of the multifocal nature of this cancer. Breast conservation therapy is generally not advisable because of the invasive nature of the cancer, and node dissection is performed for staging. Currently, a sentinel node procedure is not indicated in patients with multifocal disease.

40. **(D)** Breast, thyroid, lung, kidney, and prostate cancers commonly metastasize to the bone. Alimentary tract cancers seldom spread to bone. Prostatic metastases are usually sclerotic on x-ray.

41. **(A)** Axillary dissection during a modified radical mastectomy requires exposing the long thoracic and thoracodorsal nerves (Figure 7–8). Injury to

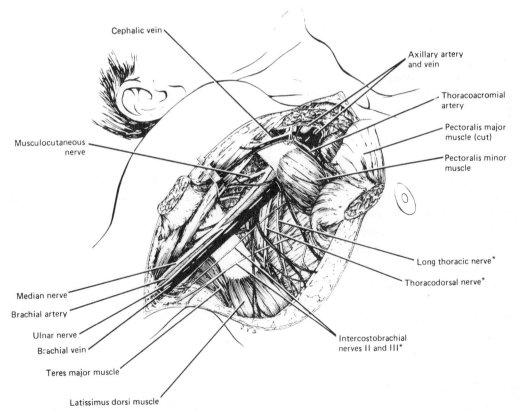

Figure 7–8. Structures that may be exposed in radical breast surgery. *Note position of the long thoracic, thoracodorsal, and intercostobrachial nerves. (Reproduced, with permission, from Lindner, HH: Clinical Anatomy, Appleton & Lange, 1989.)

the long thoracic nerve that supplies the serratus anterior muscle causes "winging of the scapula." The thoracodorsal nerve innervates the latissimus dorsi muscle. The intercostobrachial nerve supplies sensory innervation to the skin in the axilla and proximal upper extremity.

42. **(C)** Tamoxifen competitively blocks estrogen binding sites and thus reduces estrogen stimulation of breast tissue. Tamoxifen has been shown to benefit patients with a history of breast cancer as well as those who are at high risk of developing breast cancer. The FDA in June 2002 issued a cautionary note on the use of tamoxifen in those without proven breast cancer because of the increased incidence in a small percentage of patients of the development of highly aggressive uterine sarcoma.

43. **(B)** A large meta-analysis of patients treated with invasive breast cancer showed a benefit in all groups except premenopausal women who have receptor status ER–/PR–ve.

44. **(E)** There is no evidence that long-term insertion of breast implants leads to an increased incidence of breast cancer or detection of the cancer at an inappropriate late stage. Although the use of silicone gel implants is confined by the FDA guidelines to select circumstances (e.g., breast reconstruction following mastectomy), retrospective studies to date have failed to demonstrate a significant increase in the incidence of collagen disease in patients who have had a silicone breast implant.

45. **(A)** Cancer of the breast in males constitutes less than 1% of total cases. It tends to present at a more advanced stage in men than in women, because it is often overlooked. It may easily be confused with the more commonly occurring condition of gynecomastia. Careful clinical and radiological follow-up studies are indicated.

46. **(D)** In general, persistent gynecomastia should be evaluated to rule out endocrine abnormalities. In most cases, none are found. Subcutaneous mastectomy is indicated if the patient is self-conscious.

47. **(B)** Cystosarcoma phylloides is a tumor that is very slow growing and has a good prognosis if treated by mastectomy. It is characterized by large polygonal cells with abundant cytoplasm and lymphoid infiltration.

48. **(E)** Current NIH Consensus Conference advises chemotherapy for all invasive cancers >1 cm as well as for node-positive breast cancers. Radiotherapy is required whenever breast-conserving surgery is undertaken and tamoxifen for all ER+ tumors.

49. **(D)** Occult primary breast cancer is a rare but well-known entity. Stage for stage these patients have a similar prognosis as other patients with node-positive breast cancer. The primary tumor is often found in the breast. Either modified radical mastectomy and chemotherapy or just axillary dissection and chemotherapy are accepted treatment choices.

50. **(A, C, D, F)** The femoral canal is bordered medially by Gimbernat's (lacunar) ligament, laterally by the femoral vein, anteriorly, by the inguinal ligament, and posteriorly by the pectineal (Cooper's) ligament. A femoral hernia presents through the femoral ring. The sudden appearance of a reducible hernia in this region requires urgent surgical consultation. Delay in recognizing a femoral hernia may result in the involved loop of bowel undergoing gangrene and infarction.

51. **(B, I, J)** A Petit's hernia is a lumbar hernia, which occurs as a weakness in muscles situated in the flank. The hernia is bordered by the iliac crest inferiorly, the external oblique muscle anteriorly, and the latissimus dorsi muscle posteriorly.

52. **(A)** The foramen of Bochdalek is a posterolateral defect in the diaphragm and occurs most commonly on the left side. Intestinal loops of bowel enter the left thorax to cause severe respiratory compromise.

53. **(F)** The foramen of Morgagni is a diaphragmatic hernia that occurs more commonly in adults and is also called an *anterior diaphragmatic hernia*. It

occurs at the junction of the xiphoid and the costal fibers of the diaphragm. A *Littré's hernia* is a rare Richter's hernia, which includes Meckel's diverticulum.

54. **(C, G)** A Richter's hernia implies that only part of the circumference of the loop of bowel is caught up in the hernia sac. The involved segment may undergo strangulation and gangrene. The importance of recognizing this variation is that the diagnosis of obstruction may be overlooked as intestinal contents and air may pass through the partially occluded intestinal loop. In an obturator hernia in females, pain may radiate to the knee (obturator nerve) and vaginal examination may detect the hernia.

55. **(B, C, F)** In their pure forms (present without any other more aggressive histologic pattern),

they can be treated without chemotherapy in node negative-patients, even when the diameter of the tumor reaches 3 cm.

56. **(B)** The medullary subtype has a tendency to occur in younger women and is often hormone receptor negative.

57. **(L)** Paget's disease is characterized by these large vacuolated intradermoid cells usually arising from a ductal carcinoma that has grown along the duct to the nipple. Mondor's disease is a benign superficial thrombophlebitis of the breast. Inflammatory breast carcinoma is a very aggressive form of breast cancer characterized by dermal tumor spread. Carcinoma en cuirasse is a diffuse infiltration of the skin or subcutaneous tissue of the chest wall causing a "woody" induration and spread of the cancer.

CHAPTER 8

Male and Female Genitourinary Systems
Questions

Scott I. Zeitlin, Haroon Durrani, and Simon Wapnick

DIRECTIONS (Questions 1 through 63): Each of the numbered items or incomplete statements in this section is followed by answers or by completions of the statement. Select the ONE lettered answer or completion that is BEST in each case.

Questions 1 and 2

A 62-year-old African American male attorney presents to a prostate-screening clinic during National Awareness Week. On careful questioning, he has noted slight urgency, frequency nocturia, and a decrease in the force of micturition

1. He is referred to have blood tests to include which of the following?

    (A) carcinoembryonic antigen (CEA)
    (B) prostatic acid phosphatase
    (C) alkaline phosphatase
    (D) prostate-specific antigen (PSA)
    (E) lactic dehydrogenase (LDH)

2. General examination by his urologist is normal. Rectal examination reveals hemorrhoids and a left-sided irregular mass in the prostate. Following normal blood tests, he should have which of the following?

    (A) computed tomography (CT) scan of the pelvis
    (B) magnetic resonance image (MRI) of the prostate
    (C) colonoscopy and biopsy of the prostate under general anesthetic
    (D) biopsy of the nodule
    (E) bone scan

3. During her eighth month of pregnancy, a 29-year-old woman is noted to have polyhydramnios. Further testing shows anencephalus. Polyhydramnios in this patient is caused by which of the following?

    (A) impairment of the fetus's swallowing mechanism
    (B) tumor of the fetus's brain
    (C) a secretory peptide from the placenta
    (D) excess antidiuretic hormone (ADH) from the fetus
    (E) renal agenesis

4. A 62-year-old police officer develops minimal urinary symptoms. His PSA level is elevated and continues to increase during a 6-month period of observation. Because of positive biopsy findings, he undergoes a radical prostatectomy (Figure 8–1). The pathology report reveals an unfavorable high-grade tumor (Gleason score: 9), and several lymph nodes are shown on microscopy to be involved. Where is the most likely site for prostatic cancer metastasis to occur?

    (A) liver
    (B) kidney
    (C) lung
    (D) bone
    (E) brain

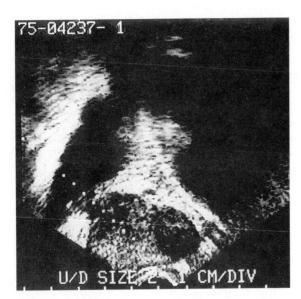

Figure 8–1. Transrectal ultrasound of the prostate. Sagittal plane showing large hypoechoic prostate cancer at arrows. (Reproduced, with permission, from Way, LW: Current Surgical Diagnosis & Treatment, 10th ed., Appleton & Lange, 1994.)

5. A 69-year-old man is examined for severe pain in the iliac crest. Metastatic disease from prostatic cancer is confirmed. What is the treatment offered initially to most patients with metastatic prostatic cancer?

(A) cortisone and pituitary ablation
(B) radical prostatectomy
(C) luteinizing releasing hormone (LRH) agonist (leuprolide)
(D) local irradiation and testosterone
(E) hyperthermia

6. Which of the following statements is true of testicular cancer?

(A) It is the most common solid tumor in men over 50 years of age.
(B) It is not associated with a higher incidence of infertility.
(C) It presents as a painless mass in the scrotum in more than 70% of patients.
(D) It accounts for 10% of malignant tumors in men.
(E) It rarely metastasizes.

7. What is a benign ovarian fibroma with associated ascites and hydrothorax called?

(A) Brenner tumor
(B) dysgerminoma
(C) Wolffian duct remnant
(D) Krukenberg tumor
(E) Meig's syndrome

8. During a workup for infertility, a 34-year-old man is noted to have a solid tumor in the anterior aspect of his right testis. What is the most likely diagnosis?

(A) torsion of the testis
(B) cyst of the epididymis
(C) lipoma of the cord
(D) cancer of the testis
(E) epididymo-orchitis

9. Improved survival after lymphadenectomy for testicular tumors occurs after which of the following?

(A) seminoma
(B) embryonal cell carcinoma
(C) Leydig cell tumor
(D) Sertoli cell tumor
(E) lymphoma

10. A 41-year-old man requests information concerning vasectomy for sterilization. In this procedure, which of the following statements is true?

(A) The incidence of sexual dysfunction is not influenced in those with with dependent personalities.
(B) The success rate in re-establishing continuity of the vas deferens is greater than 80% at 10 years.
(C) The failure rate occurs in 1/400 patients.
(D) Recanalization of the vas deferens does not occur.
(E) The procedure is difficult and requires laparotomy.

11. A 6-month-old boy was born with hypospadias. This condition is due to failure in the development of which of the following?

(A) urogenital fold
(B) Müllerian system

(C) genital tubercle

(D) urachus

(E) vitelline duct

12. A 16-year-old boy climbs a tree and sustains a straddle injury to the penile urethra. In such injuries (Figure 8–2), urine extravasates to involve which of the following?

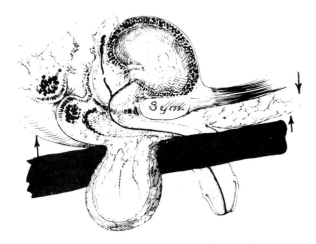

Figure 8–2. Injury to the bulbous urethra due to an injury to the perineum, resulting in crushing of the urethra against the inferior edge of the pubic symphysis. (Reproduced, with permission, Tanagho, EA and McAninch, JW: Smith's General Urology, 13th ed., Appleton & Lange, 1992.)

(A) femoral triangle

(B) prostate

(C) perianal region

(D) anterior abdominal wall

(E) posterior abdominal wall

13. In children, what is the most frequent site of tumor formation in the genital tract?

(A) vulva

(B) vagina

(C) cervix

(D) uterus

(E) ovary

14. What is the highly malignant vaginal lesion that occurs in young girls?

(A) clear cell adenocarcinoma

(B) sarcoma botryoides

(C) mesonephroma

(D) carcinosarcoma

(E) squamous carcinoma

15. A 64-year-old woman notes an ulcer on her left labia majora. Biopsy reveals carcinoma. What is the treatment?

(A) wide local excision

(B) radiotherapy

(C) preoperative radiotherapy followed by wide local excision

(D) wide excision and unilateral groin dissection

(E) radical vulvectomy and bilateral groin dissection

16. What is the most common solid malignant renal tumor in children?

(A) a Wilm's tumor

(B) neuroblastoma

(C) lymphoma

(D) renal cell carcinoma

(E) rhabdomyosarcoma

17. In repair of a third-degree perineal laceration, which structure shown in Figure 8–3 is *least* likely to be divided?

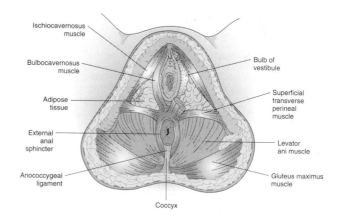

Figure 8–3. Skin and subcutaneous tissues removed to reveal structures in perineum. (Reproduced, with permission, from DeCherney, AH and Pernoll, ML: Current Obstetric & Gynecologic Diagnosis & Treatment, 8th ed., Appleton & Lange, 1994.)

(A) bulbocavernosus muscle

(B) vaginal mucosa

(C) superficial transverse perineal muscle

(D) external anal sphincter

(E) ischiocavernosus muscle

18. A 24-year-old man had been treated for gonorrhea 2 months previously. He develops an ulcerative lesion in the glans of the penis that is noted to be condylomata lata. The etiology of condylomata lata is which of the following?

   (A) a mixture of organisms
   (B) *Haemophilus ducreyi*
   (C) *Herpesvirus hominis,* type 2
   (D) *Treponema pallidum*
   (E) *Neisseria gonorrhoeae*

19. A 23-year-old woman has a cesarean section in which a Pfannenstiel incision (Figure 8–4) is used. In the Pfannenstiel incision, which of the following is true?

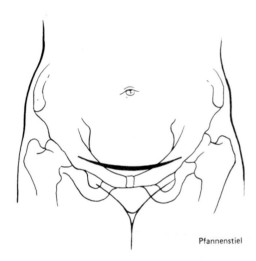

Figure 8–4. Pfannenstiel incision. (Reproduced, with permission, from Lindner, HH: Clinical Anatomy, Appleton & Lange, 1989.)

   (A) The recti and fascia are separated transversely.
   (B) The recti and fascia are separated vertically.
   (C) Fascia lata graft is used.
   (D) A prosthetic graft is used.
   (E) The upper abdomen can readily be explored.

20. What is the most common cause of failure of radiotherapy for stage II cervical carcinoma?

   (A) liver metastasis
   (B) bone metastasis
   (C) para-aortic node metastasis
   (D) resistance of the central tumor
   (E) undifferentiated tumor histology

21. Twelve years after menopause, a 60-year-old woman undergoes laparotomy for an ovarian carcinoma. The ovarian tumor that is most likely to respond to radiotherapy is which of the following?

   (A) Krukenberg tumor
   (B) dysgerminoma
   (C) arrhenoblastoma
   (D) granulosa cell tumor
   (E) Brenner tumor

22. A 24-year-old woman has been unsuccessful becoming pregnant. She is admitted with abdominal pain; her blood pressure is 90/60 mmHg, her pulse rate is 102 beats per minute (bpm), and her hematocrit is 28. Features of ectopic pregnancy include which of the following?

   (A) pain referred to the supraclavicular region
   (B) pulsus paradoxus
   (C) tenderness below the right subcostal margin (Murphy's sign)
   (D) elevated blood pressure on assuming an erect position
   (E) ecchymosis around the umbilicus

23. After undergoing a partial cystectomy for carcinoma of the rectum, an 84-year-old woman develops a genitourinary fistula. The repair will have a higher chance of success if which of the following occurs?

   (A) Repair is performed within 7–14 days of symptom onset.
   (B) Scar tissue is not excised.
   (C) The bladder wall is closed under tension.
   (D) It is performed more than 6 months after the causative operation.

24. After pelvic irradiation for cancer in a 49-year-old man, which is true of supravesicular urinary diversion?

(A) It should not include a conduit from the ileum, transverse colon, or sigmoid colon.

(B) It has an increased rate of complications if irradiated bowel is used.

(C) It is not associated with a high rate of postoperative pyelonephritis.

(D) It is complicated by the development of urinary fistulas in more than 40% of patients.

(E) none of the above

25. After being treated for ovarian carcinoma, a 65-year-old woman develops complications attributed to cisplatin (*cis*-diamminedichloroplatinum). What is a common side effect of cisplatin?

(A) multiple lipoma

(B) ankylosing spondylitis

(C) peripheral neuropathy

(D) pulmonary fibrosis

(E) megaloblastic anemia

26. A 33-year-old woman is seen for evaluation of infertility. She complains of dyspareunia. On vaginal examination, tender nodularity along the uterosacral ligaments is noted. What is the diagnosis?

(A) adenomyosis

(B) diethylstilbestrol (DES)-related disease

(C) subserosal fibroids

(D) endometriosis

(E) adrenogenital syndrome

27. Following a radical nephrectomy, a 60-year-old, diabetic male develops necrotizing fasciitis. After treating the infection, the plastic surgeon places an omental graft, which is based on blood supply from the which of the following?

(A) omental branch of the abdominal aorta

(B) middle colic artery

(C) gastroepiploic artery

(D) middle sacral artery

(E) epigastric artery

28. After sustaining an injury, a 32-year-old motorcyclist is noted to have signs of abdominal tenderness and guarding. Which of the following organs is most commonly involved in blunt visceral injuries?

(A) spleen

(B) intestine

(C) liver

(D) bladder

(E) pancreas

29. In pelvic fracture, which of the following statements is true?

(A) An isolated fracture never occurs.

(B) Pain is relieved on walking.

(C) Open lavage is a useful indication for the need to perform laparotomy.

(D) Fracture of the coccyx requires surgical excision in most patients.

(E) Dislocation of the sacroiliac joint is usually associated with a fracture of the pubic ramus or separation of the symphysis.

30. A 62-year-old woman with cardiac disease undergoes a pudendal nerve block to remove a tumor from the vulva. Fibers forming the pudendal nerve originate from which of the following?

(A) L2–L4

(B) L3–L5

(C) L4, L5, S1

(D) S1–S3

(E) S2–S4

31. A 42-year-old man has recurrent cystitis. Cystoscopic examination and biopsy confirm the presence of locally invasive muscle (T_2) carcinoma of the bladder. What is the next step in management?

(A) repeat cystoscopic resection

(B) cystoscopic fulguration

(C) partial cystectomy

(D) radical cystoprostatectomy

(E) radiotherapy

32. During a tubosalpingectomy, a ureter is accidentally cut. To minimize injury to the ureter, the surgeon should recognize what about this structure?

    (A) It enters the pelvis at the level of the aortic bifurcation.
    (B) It passes posterior to the iliac vessels.
    (C) It passes above the uterine artery.
    (D) It enters the pelvis 4 cm medial to the bifurcation of the common iliac artery.
    (E) It enters the pelvis immediately distal to the common iliac artery bifurcation.

33. A 56-year-old woman is admitted to the emergency department complaining of upper abdominal pain. An ultrasound of the abdomen reveals a thin-walled gallbladder filled with fluid and a solid left renal mass. What should be the next test ordered?

    (A) HIDA scan
    (B) intravenous pyelogram (IVP)
    (C) CT scan of the abdomen
    (D) oral cholecystogram
    (E) upper gastrointestinal (GI) series

Questions 34 and 35

A mentally retarded child and with cerebral palsy is admitted for repair of a left indirect inguinal hernia. Clinical palpation reveals a large left retroperitoneal abdominal mass.

34. What is the most common presentation for a patient with a Wilm's tumor?

    (A) unilateral flank mass
    (B) back pain
    (C) hematuria
    (D) urinary tract infection (UTI)
    (E) weight loss

35. Before radiologic investigation, which is the best method to distinguish a Wilm's tumor from a neuroblastoma?

    (A) physical examination of the abdomen
    (B) shifting dullness
    (C) catecholamine levels

    (D) auscultation for bowel sounds
    (E) cortisol administration

36. A kidney graft between identical twins is likely to survive for which period of time?

    (A) 1–6 weeks
    (B) 7–52 weeks
    (C) 1–10 years
    (D) 11–25 years
    (E) more than 25 years

37. A 32-year-old woman with chronic renal failure undergoes successful renal transplantation. Tests carried out after the operation indicate the presence of cytomegalovirus (CMV). What is true of this condition?

    (A) It cannot be measured by immunofluorescent assay.
    (B) It is detected in most patients after surgery.
    (C) It should not cause additional problems with regard to tissue rejection.
    (D) It results in infection that usually is fatal.

38. A 4-year-old girl has a yellow, blood-tinged, foul-smelling, vaginal discharge. On examination, the external genitalia are red, and a malodorous, blood-tinged discharge is noted. The most likely cause of these findings is:

    (A) *Chlamydia trachomatis*
    (B) gonorrhea
    (C) treponema
    (D) foreign body
    (E) vaginal cancer

39. A 46-year-old man is on a waiting list to secure a renal transplant. The genetic locus of transplant antigens in humans is known as which?

    (A) rhesus (Rh)
    (B) IgA and IgM
    (C) human leukocyte antigen (HLA)
    (D) ABO
    (E) hepatitis B surface antigen (HBsAg)

40. A 64-year-old man underwent transplantation that was complicated by graft-versus-host reaction. He had undergone a transplantation of which of the following?

    (A) kidney
    (B) skin
    (C) bone marrow
    (D) cornea
    (E) liver

41. In evaluating the role of the autonomic nervous system related to urinary incontinence that developed in a 67-year-old man after prostatectomy, it is determined that the sympathetic nerves are injured. What is the natural hormone in the catecholamine pathway?

    (A) norepinephrine
    (B) dopamine
    (C) vasoactive intestinal peptide (VIP)
    (D) isoproterenol
    (E) acetylcholine

42. During evaluation of the cause of varicocele in a 36-year-old man, attention is directed to the method of drainage of the left testicular vein, which usually enters which of the following?

    (A) left adrenal vein
    (B) left renal vein
    (C) left inferior mesenteric vein
    (D) inferior vena cava (IVC)
    (E) left inferior epigastric vein

43. A 42-year-old man presents with cancer of the left testis. To exclude lymphatic metastasis, which is the site that should be initially examined?

    (A) vertical chain of inguinal glands
    (B) horizontal chain of inguinal glands
    (C) retrorectal glands
    (D) para-aortic glands
    (E) obturator nodes

44. As a result of a traffic accident, a 42-year-old female has a pelvic fracture, confirmed on x-ray of the pelvis. What does she require?

    (A) surgical repair under local anesthesia
    (B) open lavage and, if positive, immediate laparotomy
    (C) immobilization of the pelvis in a plaster cast
    (D) analgesics and observation
    (E) skeletal traction

45. A 62-year-old woman with metastatic cancer has mild chronic renal disease. Renal excretion of antineoplastic drugs is least likely to be affected by which of the following?

    (A) nonsteroidal anti-inflammatory drugs (NSAIDs)
    (B) probenecid
    (C) aspirin
    (D) alkalinizing urine
    (E) aminoglycosides

46. A 62-year-old farmer had received chemotherapy for cancer of the head and neck. He has developed classical multidrug resistance (MDR) to which of the following?

    (A) alkylating agents
    (B) antimetabolites
    (C) bleomycin
    (D) vinca alkaloid
    (E) cyclosporine

Questions 47 and 48

A 32-year-old female has chronic pyelonephritis with chronic renal failure. She is scheduled to have a renal transplantation. The donor kidney will be obtained from her brother-in-law, and a limited renal incision and laparoscopic nephrectomy is planned. The donor kidney operation (left side) will be performed in a separate operating room under general anesthesia.

47. Where will the donor kidney be placed?

    (A) in the groin
    (B) left iliac fossa
    (C) at site of bifurcation of aorta
    (D) into the portal system
    (E) inferior vena cava

48. With reference to the donor kidney, which statement is true?

    (A) The left side is preferred, because the left renal artery is larger than that on the right.
    (B) The left renal vein passes posterior to the aorta.
    (C) Renal arteries are end arteries.
    (D) Anomalous arteries are a contraindication for elective use in transplantation.
    (E) Renal fascia separates segments of kidney.

49. A 64-year-old male is admitted to the emergency department following a car accident. His pulse is 94, blood pressure 95/60, and HCT 30%. Severe hematuria is evident. Following resuscitation, his blood pressure is elevated to 120/80. A CT scan reveals extensive contusion confined to the left kidney and perirenal fat. His blood pressure declines to 80/40, and urgent laparotomy is performed where?

    (A) through the left flank
    (B) through a midline abdominal incision and peritoneal covering the posterior abdominal wall
    (C) through an incision confined to the peritoneal cavity
    (D) through a thoracoabdominal incision
    (E) extraperitoneal groin incision

50. A 42-year-old male presents with a solid swelling in the left testis of 2 months duration. Biopsy reveals this to be a Leydig cell tumor. The function of the Leydig cell is to produce what?

    (A) follicle-stimulating hormone (FSH)
    (B) inhibin
    (C) testosterone
    (D) luteizing hormone
    (E) progesterone

51. A 63-year-old male has had declining ability to achieve an erection over the past 18 months. He received a prescription of sildenafil (Viagra), which works via which route?

    (A) cGMP mechanism
    (B) inhibiting type 5 phosphodiesterase

    (C) nitric oxide (NO)-induced mechanism
    (D) all of the above
    (E) none of the above

52. A 65-year-old male patient complains of loss of libido and is found to have a low free and total testosterone level. Treatment is commenced with testosterone supplemental therapy. What follows testosterone administration?

    (A) PSA levels are increased.
    (B) Testosterone levels are decreased.
    (C) Decrease in size of benign prostatic tissue lesions occurs.
    (D) Decrease in size of prostatic cancer occurs.
    (E) Anemia occurs.

53. A 45-year-old male CIA employee presents with a 3-week history of a tumor in the scrotum. The patient has a known history of diabetes controlled by diet. There is minimal discomfort. On examination, the lesion is located posteriorly and does not transilluminate to light. Both testes are clinically normal. What is the most likely diagnosis?

    (A) spermatocele
    (B) teratoma
    (C) adenomatoid lesion of the epididymis
    (D) varicocele
    (E) torsion of a testicular appendiceal cyst

54. A 63-year-old man undergoes a peripheral vascular procedure under general anesthesia. A decrease in urine formation and excretion are noted. Decreased urine flow under general anesthesia occurs because of which of the following?

    (A) vasopressin
    (B) aldosterone suppression
    (C) depression of glucocorticoid
    (D) depression of thyroid function
    (E) specific effect of anesthesia on renal tubules

55. A 32-year-old athletic long distance runner complains of severe pain in the left loin. There is no radiation of the pain to the groin. Examination reveals mild tenderness in the left flank. Investigations confirm the presence of renal

calculi. The stone is most likely which of the following?

(A) cystine
(B) ammonium magnesium phosphate (Struvite)
(C) calcium oxalate
(D) uric acid
(E) calcium phosphate

56. If the stone is shown to consist of struvite (ammonium magnesium phosphate) it would be which of the following?

(A) always translucent
(B) show increased solubility by alkalinization of urine
(C) seen only in sterile urine
(D) confined to animals
(E) all of above.

57. Following nonsurgical management of the stone, the patient is readmitted with severe colicky pain radiating to the left groin. There is minimal tenderness in the left abdomen. An x-ray shows a stone in the ureter at the level of the 5th lumbar vertebra. Surgical intervention should be considered for which reason?

(A) for all ureteric stones
(B) if analgesics are required
(C) if urinary tract infection is present
(D) for uric acid stones
(E) if impaired renal function occurs

Questions 58 and 59

A 42-year-old female seeks advice concerning dyspareunia, dysuria, and urinary incontinence. Symptoms were mild for the past 3 years but have become more troublesome in the past 6 months. She has had five full-term deliveries. Symptoms are worse with coughing and sneezing.

58. Which of the following statements is true concerning this condition?

(A) It occurs in 5% of woman over the age of 50.
(B) It is most likely due to interstitial cystitis.

(C) It causes urgency incontinence if due to a urinary fistula.
(D) It is suggestive of a urethral diverticulum if a suburethral mass is present.
(E) Kegel pelvic muscle exercises would aggravate this condition.

59. Treatment for urinary incontinence involves which of the following?

(A) should exclude Kegel pelvic muscle exercises
(B) Kegel's pelvic muscle exercises, involving exclusively the thigh and abdominal wall muscles
(C) is by routine hysterectomy
(D) includes cholinergic drugs
(E) is by transabdominal or transvaginal surgical repair

60. A 32-year-old female had been unable to become pregnant for 6 years. Three weeks previously, she missed her period. She was admitted to hospital with left-side lower abdominal pain and nausea. Her β subunit HCG and pelvic ultrasound confirms an ectopic pregnancy. Treatment includes which of the following?

(A) immediate laparotomy and salpingectomy
(B) if unruptured, the fallopian tube should be spared
(C) avoid incidental appendectomy
(D) if stable, avoid surgery
(E) transfer embryo to uterus

61. Which statement is true in gestational trophoblastic disease?

(A) It always leads to malignancy.
(B) It is more common in multiple pregnancy.
(C) Gestational trophoblastic disease has complete moles that are diploid and have a 20% risk of malignancy.
(D) Gestational trophoblastic disease has partial moles that are triploid and always undergo neoplasia.
(E) Gestational trophoblastic disease with hydatiform mole is then treated by hysterectomy.

62. Which statement is true in gestational tropho-blastic neoplasia?

    (A) It follows abortion or pregnancy in 25% of cases.
    (B) It is high risk if HCG titer is above 4,000 mIU/mL.
    (C) It is low risk if present for more than 4 months.
    (D) If low risk, it is treated with multiple chemotherapeutic agents.

63. In evaluating the menstrual cycle, which is true?

    (A) Estrogen secretion predominates during week prior to menstruation.
    (B) Ovulation follows a surge in LH.
    (C) Progesterone predominates the first week after menstruation.
    (D) FSH is released at midcycle.

DIRECTIONS (Questions 64 through 74): Each set of matching questions in this section consists of a list of lettered options followed by several numbered items. For each numbered item, select the appropriate lettered option(s). Each lettered option may be selected once, more than once, or not at all. EACH ITEM WILL STATE THE NUMBER OF OPTIONS TO SELECT. CHOOSE EXACTLY THIS NUMBER.

Questions 64 through 66

    (A) ulcerative colitis
    (B) hidradenitis
    (C) rheumatoid arthritis
    (D) hemolytic anemia
    (E) cancer of the thyroid
    (F) Crohn's disease
    (G) Behçet's syndrome
    (H) glomus tumor
    (I) renal agenesis
    (J) granuloma inguinale

64. A 44-year-old woman complains of pain in the perineum. On vaginal examination, she is noted to have a 2-cm ulcer on the posterior wall of the vagina. The most likely cause of vulvar ulcer with associated perineal fistula and/or a weeping pustular lesion is which? SELECT TWO.

65. Sexually transmitted diseases are caused by which? SELECT ONE.

66. What is characterized by genital and oral ulcers? SELECT ONE.

Question 67

    (A) invades the rectum
    (B) invades the uterus
    (C) invades superficial muscle (T_1)
    (D) is superficial
    (E) is associated with schistosomiasis (*Bilharzia*)
    (F) is associated with peritoneal metastasis
    (G) invades adjacent intestine
    (H) is associated with liver metastasis

67. Fulguration is the treatment of choice when a bladder does which? SELECT ONE.

Question 68

    (A) perineum
    (B) retroperitoneum
    (C) internal ring
    (D) inguinal canal
    (E) pubis
    (F) liver
    (G) spleen
    (H) diaphragm

68. A 12-year-old boy presents for repair of an ectopic testis situated where? SELECT TWO.

Questions 69 and 70

    (A) expanding retroperitoneal hematoma
    (B) confined retroperitoneal hematoma
    (C) renal parenchymal injury not entering calyceal system
    (D) renal parenchyma injury involving calyceal system
    (E) absent kidney vessels on angiography
    (F) associated splenic injury with fall in HCT to 30%
    (G) penetrating neck injury
    (H) avulsion of left renal vessels following falls on the buttock with contracoux injury to renal pelvis

69. Urgent exploration of the kidney follows blunt trauma resulting in which? SELECT FOUR.

70. Bleeding affects tissue around adrenal gland and kidney in which cases? SELECT TWO.

Question 71

(A) sebaceous cyst on the skin of the scrotum
(B) cyst of the epididymis
(C) hydrocele
(D) direct inguinal hernia
(E) femoral hernia
(F) Richter's hernia
(G) torsion of testis
(H) Fournier's gangrene of the scrotum

71. A 46-year-old man has a swelling in the scrotum. It shows clear transillumination anterior to the testis when a light is applied to the scrotum in a dark room. What is the most likely diagnosis? SELECT ONE.

Question 72

(A) vasoconstriction of the leg
(B) impotence
(C) infertility
(D) peptic ulcer
(E) failure of ejaculation
(F) loss of sensation in the scrotum
(G) absent bulbocavernous reflex
(H) rectal incontinence

72. A 25-year-old man undergoes orchiectomy and is advised to undergo retroperitoneal lymphad-enectomy. Which complications are most likely to occur? SELECT TWO.

Question 73

(A) thalidomide
(B) oral DES
(C) oral contraceptive tablets
(D) German measles
(E) alcohol consumption
(F) cortisone
(G) cocaine abuse
(H) pneumococcal vaccine

73. At the age of 20, a patient has vaginal bleeding that is confirmed to be from a clear-cell adeno-carcinoma of the vagina. Her mother most likely was exposed to what? SELECT ONE.

Question 74

(A) mucinous cystadenocarcinoma
(B) serous cystadenocarcinoma
(C) corpus luteum cyst
(D) dermoid cyst
(E) benign serous cyst
(F) pseudocyst
(G) endometriosis cyst
(H) Hydatid cyst

74. On pelvic examination, a 42-year-old woman is noted to have a questionable pelvic mass. Ultrasound examination reveals a small left-sided ovarian cyst. Which is the most common cyst in the ovary in a premenopausal patient? SELECT ONE.

Answers and Explanations

1. **(D)** All men over the age of 50 years should undergo annual PSA level measurement and a digital rectal examination to exclude early prostatic cancer. Marginal elevation of PSA levels may indicate benign disease, but transrectal prostatic biopsy under ultrasound guidance is indicated. Patients with abnormal PSA levels require careful follow-up monitoring, even if the initial biopsy results are negative.

2. **(D)** The upper two-thirds of the anal canal and rectal wall are supplied by the autonomic nervous system. Thus, a prostatic biopsy performed without anesthesia through the rectal wall in this region is usually relatively well tolerated by the patient.

3. **(A)** This abnormality is relatively common and occurs in 1/1,000 pregnancies, four times more commonly in whites than blacks and four times more commonly in females than males. The abnormality can be identified on an x-ray, because the vault of the skull is absent. Anencephalus is due to failure of the cephalic part of the neural tube to close off.

4. **(D)** Bone metastasis is a characteristic feature of prostatic cancer. The lesions are typically osteoblastic on x-ray, and the serum acid phosphatase level becomes elevated.

5. **(C)** LRH agonist is given by injection. This method of androgen deprivation has the advantage that orchidectomy is not required. The PSA level typically falls dramatically. Ninety-five percent of testosterone is produced by the Leydig cells of the testis and the remainder by conversion of other hormones in the peripheral blood.

6. **(C)** Testicular tumors account for 1–2% of all malignant tumors in men.

7. **(E)** Meig's syndrome with pleural effusion responds to removal of the ovarian fibroma. Brenner tumor is a fibroepithelial tumor of the ovary with low malignant potential. Dysgerminomas contain germ cells and infiltration with lymphocytes. Krukenberg tumor is metastasis of a primary alimentary tract adenocarcinoma to the ovary.

8. **(D)** Testicular tumors account for 1–2% of all malignant tumors in men. In the 15–35 age group, they are the most common nonhematogenous malignant tumors. In 15–30% of these tumors, there is associated pain in the involved testicle.

9. **(B)** Embryonal cell carcinoma should be treated by retroperitoneal lymph node dissection, if tumor spread is confined to the peritoneal cavity—30% of patients will have lymph node metastases at the time of diagnosis. Seminoma and embryonal cell carcinomas account for about 70% of all testicular tumors. Nearly all patients with testicular tumors are young, and most are under 40 years of age. Testicular tumors occur more frequently in undescended testicles.

10. **(C)** The failure rate occurs in 1/400 patient. Recanalization of the vas deferens may occur spontaneously more than 1 year after the procedure.

11. **(A)** Embryologically, the genital tubercle develops into the penis. The edge of the cloacal membrane forms the urogenital fold and by a process

of invagination forms the urethral groove and finally the penile urethra. The severity of hypospadias depends on the location of the anomalous opening onto the penile urethra. The mildest degree is where the opening is on the glans and the most severe form at the penile–scrotal junction.

12. **(D)** Fascia of Camper and Scarpa's fascia are the two layers of superficial fascia. The deeper membranous (Scarpa's) layer fuses with the fascia lata but is continuous over the penis and the scrotum as Colles's fascia to fuse with the urogenital membrane. Urine will, therefore, only escape upward over the anterior abdominal wall (Figure 8–5).

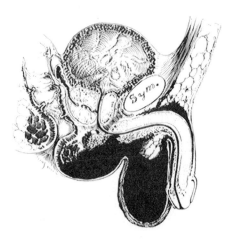

Figure 8–5. Injury to the bulbous urethra due to an injury to the perineum resulting in crushing of the urethra against the inferior edge of the pubic symphysis. Extravasation of blood and urine enclosed within Colle's fascia. (Reproduced, with permission, from Tanagho, EA and McAninch, JW: Smith's General Urology, 13th ed., Appleton & Lange, 1992.)

13. **(E)** In children, the most common site of tumor formation in the genital tract is the ovary. Uterine, vulval, vaginal, and cervical tumors are extremely rare in children. Previously, there was a concern for adolescent females whose mothers had received DES during pregnancy to develop vaginal cancer; however, this drug is no longer used during pregnancy. Sarcoma botryoides is a very rare tumor of the cervix in girls.

14. **(B)** Sarcoma botryoides usually occurs as a grapelike polypoid mass in the vagina of young

girls. Clear-cell adenocarcinoma occurs at an older age, in the second decade of life. It is associated with the administration of DES to patients' mothers during pregnancy. Squamous carcinoma is the most common tumor of the vagina in postmenopausal patients. However, malignant tumors of the vagina are rare in children.

15. **(E)** Radical vulvectomy and bilateral groin dissection has improved survival in patients with carcinoma of the vulva. The deep and superficial nodes are removed. If the lymph nodes are not involved, the cure rate exceeds 70%. The overall survival figure is 50%. Radiotherapy has not offered additional benefit.

16. **(A)** Wilms's tumors represent 5% of childhood cancers and have an equal male/female ratio. Neuroblastomas arise from the adrenal gland, sympathetic chain, or paraganglia (Figure 8–6).

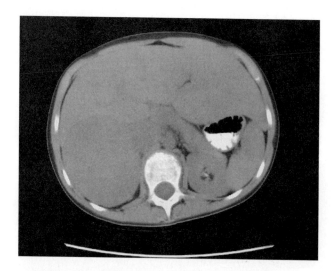

Figure 8–6. Note that the retroperitoneal neuroblastoma tumor arises outside the kidney area. Neuroblastoma is an extrarenal tumor.

17. **(E)** Third-degree lacerations of the perineum do not involve the ischiocavernosus muscle. The ischiocavernosus muscle originates at the ischial tuberosity and inserts at the base of the clitoris.

18. **(D)** Condylomata lata are a manifestation of secondary syphilis. The treatment for condylomata lata is penicillin. They are distinguished from condylomata acuminata in that the latter are

velvety and filiform in appearance. Condylomata acuminata result from human papillomavirus (HPV) infection.

19. **(B)** In the Pfannenstiel incision, the rectus muscles and the peritoneum are separated in a vertical fashion after the skin is incised transversely.

20. **(C)** In stage II disease, the incidence of nodal involvement is 25–40%. Most tumors are not radioresistant, and distant metastases (i.e., a more advanced stage) are a late complication of more advanced stages of the disease.

21. **(B)** Dysgerminoma (like seminoma in men) is very radiosensitive. The Krukenberg tumor is a metastatic tumor to the ovary and is not treated by radiation. The other tumors are best treated by surgery. The Brenner tumor is most often a benign tumor. Arrhenoblastoma and granulosa cell tumors are hormone-producing tumors.

22. **(A)** Free bleeding in the peritoneal cavity results in pain referred to the right supraclavicular region due to diaphragmatic irritation. Patients who present with abdominal pain and (usually) a history of a missed period should undergo a pregnancy test after hospital admission.

23. **(D)** Repair of a genitourinary fistula is recommended after enough time has passed to allow a reduction in the inflammatory reaction and even spontaneous closure of a small fistula (and inserting a Forley catheter into the bladder to drain the urine). When the fistula is repaired, it is wise to excise the tract, perform a meticulous repair, and avoid placing tension on approximated edges of the anastomosis. An omental interposition will facilitate healing.

24. **(B)** After irradiation, supravesicular urinary diversion may be performed by creating a conduit from the ileum, transverse colon, or sigmoid colon. This is associated with a high rate of postoperative pyelonephritis. In cases of urinary diversion, urinary fistula formation does occur, but at a much lower rate than 40%.

25. **(C)** Peripheral neuropathy, ototoxicity, and nephrotoxicity may be encountered following cisplatinum treatment. Nephrotoxicity can be minimized by hydrating the patient well during treatment.

26. **(D)** Tender uterosacral ligaments usually are a sign of endometriosis. Although the other conditions listed may be associated with some form of pelvic pain, they do not produce tender uterosacral ligaments.

27. **(C)** The greater omentum is supplied by the right and left gastroepiploic arteries. There is no omental branch from the aorta. The middle sacral artery is a pelvic artery that does not supply the omentum, and the epigastric arteries supply the anterior abdominal wall.

28. **(A)** In blunt trauma, the spleen is most commonly involved, with kidneys, intestine, and liver next in frequency. If the spleen is involved, attempts should be made to conserve this organ when possible.

29. **(E)** Dislocation of the sacroiliac joint is usually associated with a fracture of the pubic ramus or separation of the symphysis. In elderly patients with osteoporosis, a fall may lead to a fracture of the pubic ramus, coccyx, or sacrum. In all patients involved in automobile accidents, the pelvis should be examined for local tenderness, and appropriate x-rays should be ordered when a fracture is suspected. Open lavage in fracture of the pelvis does not differentiate between a simple pelvic fracture and one associated with visceral injury. Fracture of the coccyx is treated by avoiding local pressure when sitting. In a few patients, the persistence of pain may require excision of the coccyx.

30. **(E)** The pudendal nerve is formed from the fibers of S2–S4. In males, this nerve supplies the scrotum and penis. In females, the clitoris, distal vagina, and more than 80% (posterior part) of the vulva is innervated by the pudendal nerve. Pudendal nerve block with local anesthetic infiltration may be offered to patients during vaginal delivery and/or repair of an episiotomy.

31. **(D)** The main type of carcinoma in this country is transitional. Cystoscopic removal of the tumor

is indicated for small, superficial tumors. The standard of care for muscle invasive bladder cancer is radical cystectomy with pelvic lymph node dissection.

32. **(E)** It is very important to be familiar with the ureter's course in the pelvis in order to be able to minimize injury to this structure during pelvic and colon operations. The ureter enters the pelvis immediately distal to the bifurcation of the common iliac artery. It then passes (posterior to the ovary) toward the bladder, where it travels *inferior to* the uterine artery—about 12 mm lateral to the cervix and upper vagina.

33. **(C)** The ultrasound findings of the gallbladder are normal. A CT scan is required to determine the nature and further course of management of renal cancer if this is confirmed. Pre- and post-contrast CTs will indicate if the tumor enhances and is thus more likely to be malignant.

34. **(D)** Imaging of the genitourinary system, usually by CT scan, is essential before surgery. Clinically, a tumor that protrudes posteriorly is more likely to be an adrenal rather than a kidney tumor. In neuroblastoma, the tumor tends to secrete dopamine (epinephrine precursors) so that urinary vanillylmandelic acid (VMA) levels, rather than catecholamine levels, are elevated.

35. **(A)** Clinically, a tumor that protrudes posteriorly is more likely to be an adrenal rather than a kidney tumor. In a large renal Wilms's tumor, the splenic flexure (resonant to percussion) passes inferior to the solid kidney tumor. In an adrenal mass, the splenic flexure is separated by the intervening (normal tumor). In neuroblastoma, the tumor tends to secrete dopamine (epinephrine precursor) so that urinary vanillylmandelic acid (VMA) levels rather that catecholamine levels are elevated. In the CT scan shown in Figure 8–5, the adrenal mass is separate from that of the right kidney.

36. **(E)** Immunosuppression will not be required after grafting between identical twins (isograft). Kidneys taken from live donors have done better than those taken from cadavers. Grafts taken from siblings can be expected to yield a 75% 5-year functional status.

37. **(C)** CMV infection may cause serious disease in immunosuppressed patients. In general, the CMV titer is elevated before transplantation in the recipient and only occasionally is attributed to transmission from the donor kidney. Although over one-half of patients with kidney grafts have a positive CMV titer, only a small fraction develop serious disease.

38. **(D)** The possibility of sexual assault should be considered in the differential diagnosis of a child presenting with an unexplained vaginal discharge.

39. **(C)** HLA was one of the first studied. The transplant antigen is located on the surface. The strongest transplant antigen is known as the major histocompatibility complex (MHC) and is found in humans on chromosome 6.

40. **(C)** Normal bone marrow cells are destroyed readily by drugs and ionizing irradiation; the red blood cell (RBC) stem cell in particular is sensitive to damage. The marrow is not destroyed by the host if transplanted into an immunosuppressed host. The transplanted bone marrow develops mature stem cells that have immunologic competence that now reject those of the host (graft-versus-host reaction). Diarrhea, dermatitis, weight loss, and infection occur.

41. **(A)** The metabolic pathway of catecholamines is initiated by conversion of tyrosine to dopa, which in turn, forms dopamine. Dopamine forms norepinephrine, which is the precursor of epinephrine. Epinephrine is the main amine secreted during life and is concerned with the "fight or flight" reaction.

42. **(B)** The left testicular vein empties into the left renal vein, and the right testicular vein empties into the IVC. Partial occlusion of the right renal vein is an uncommon cause of varicocele and may signify an associated retroperitoneal malignancy.

43. **(D)** Testicular lesions metastasize to the para-aortic glands at the L2 level. Lymphatic drainage corresponds to the route of the testicular vessels. If the skin of the scrotum is involved, then the inguinal lymph nodes may be involved.

44. **(D)** In all patients in automobile accidents, the pelvis should be examined for local tenderness, and appropriate x-rays should be ordered when a fracture is suspected. Open lavage in fracture of the pelvis does not differentiate between a simple pelvic fracture and one associated with visceral injury.

45. **(A)** NSAIDs may decrease renal blood flow. Probenecid and aspirin inhibit excretion of methotrexate.

46. **(D)** The hallmark of classic MDR is the development of cross-resistance to several drugs after exposure to a single drug such as dactinomycin, anthracycline, vinca alkaloid, or doxorubicin; the mechanism is a glycoprotein transmitter (Pgp) that is a result of the MDR-1 gene. Cyclosporine and verapamil block the effect of Pgp.

47. **(B)** In general, the left external iliac vessels of the recipient are chosen for anastomosis of the renal artery and renal vein of the recipient. The ureter of the donor kidney is anastomosed directly to the bladder.

48. **(C)** In general, there are five segmental arteries supplying each kidney. Segmental arteries are end arteries and, therefore, occlusion of a segmental will lead to infarction of the affected segment. The segmental arteries arise from the main renal artery. In about 70% of normal kidneys, there is a single renal artery arising from the aorta to supply each kidney. In 30%, multiple arteries arise from the aorta. In 10% of cases, there are at least two veins draining into the IVC on the right side. Duplication of venous drainage on the left side occurs much less frequently. The left renal vein passes anterior to the aorta and is of longer length, which offers advantage for the selection of the left kidney as a donor organ. If a kidney is in an abnormal location, vascular anomalies are encountered more frequently.

49. **(B)** After entering the abdominal cavity the inferior mesenteric vein is isolated to the left of the 4th part of the duodenum and Treitz's suspensary ligament. An incision is made between the 4th part of the duodenum and the inferior mesenteric vein lateral to the aorta. This approach exposes the left renal kilum and allows early and accurate exposure and control of the left renal kilum. The approach allows exposure of the left kidney and enables the surgeon to determine if a renal repair or nephrectomy is needed. It also allows exposure to the opposite kidney.

50. **(C)** LH released from the anterior pituitary acts on Leydig cells to synthesize testosterone. Testosterone is a paracrine mediator and with FSH acts on the Sertoli cells to promote spermatogenesis. Testosterone inhibits release of Gn RH from the hypothalamus. It also has a direct effect in preventing release of LH from the anterior pituitary. The Sertoli cells releases inhibin, which inhibits FSH secretion from the anterior pituitary.

51. **(D)** Sidenafil, better known as Viagra, is a type 5 phosphodiesterase inhibitor. It potentiates the effect of cGMP and increases the ability of the cavernosal smooth muscle to relax. Nitric oxide is released from the nerve terminal to cause the release of cGMP.

52. **(A)** PSA levels are increased. Both benign and malignant prostatic tissue are sensitive to testosterone (hormonal) therapy. There is increased prostatic growth with elevation of PSA and possible polycythemia.

53. **(C)** Adenomatoid is the most common tumor of the epidydimus. The epididymis is posterior, and a cyst of the epidydimis transilluminates to light. A hydrocoele also transilluminates, but it is anterior to the testis. A cyst of the testis is a remnant of the proximal part of the paramesonephros (Müller's) duct. In the presence of a normal FSH, testicular biopsy would most likely confirm normal sperm formation. The presence of varicocele is unlikely to result in azospermia.

54. **(A)** The antidiuretic hormone vasopressin (released from the posterior pituitary) is secreted to a large extent when a patient is under anesthesia. Thus, urine formation is suppressed. The metabolic response to anesthesia and surgery tends to be retention of fluids; therefore, one must be careful to avoid administering large amounts of fluid to patients with early or overt heart failure during this period.

55. **(C)** More than 70% of renal calculi are calcium oxalate stones. Nearly half of calcium oxalate stones contain phosphate in addition to oxalate. Calcium containing stones are radio opaque and can be visualized on plain x-rays. Struvite (ammonium magnesium phosphate) and cystine stones may also be radio-opaque.

56. **(B)** Although struvite (ammonium magnesium phosphate) stones show increased solubility in urine which is acidified, urea-splitting organisms release ammonium that causes alkalinization effect. Effective therapy must be directed to eradicate associated infection. Struvite stones are the second most common type of renal calculi (after calcium oxalate stones)

57. **(E)** Surgical intervention by endoscopic percutaneous or open surgical procedure is indicated for stones more than 5 mm in diameter that cause persistent obstruction, intractable pain, impaired renal function, or persistent urinary tract infection. In over 90% of cases, a ureteric stone <4 mm will pass naturally.

58. **(D)** Patients with urethral diverticulum show a triad of dysuria, dyspareunia, and dribbling of urine The commonest form of urinary incontinence, called stress incontinence, is due to multifactorial causes, and frequently there is an anatomic defect of the bladder neck. Urge incontinence is attributed to detrusor bladder instability and may be associated with neurological causes such as Parkinson's disease. The urethral syndrome and intestitial cystitis are sensory bladder disorders usually occurring in younger patients who do not have urinary infection.

59. **(E)** Initial treatment for urinary incontinence revolves around well-planned Kegel pelvic floor muscles and sympathomimetic drugs (to increased urethral pressure). Surgery includes the Marshall Marchetti retropubic urethropexy. Transvaginal correction is equally effective.

60. **(B)** If unruptured the fallopian tube should be spared; laparoscopic surgery is indicated, on the side of the ectopic pregnancy. An incision is made into superior (antimesenteric) border of the fallopian tube and the products of conception removed by gentle traction. Preserving the fallopian tube may improve the chances of future conception. The appendix should be removed to avoid possible confusion of the diagnosis at a subsequent date.

61. **(C)** Complete moles are diploid and have a 20% risk of malignancy. Partial moles are triploid and do not as a rule undergo malignant change. Gestational trophoblastic disease is divided into: (a) hydatiform mole (partial or complete); and (b) gestational trophoblastic neoplasia. Hydatiform moles are from paternal and maternal origin. Hydatiform moles are treated by suction curettage through the cervix.

62. **(A)** In the majority (50%), the condition is consequent to molar pregnancy and 25% occurs following normal pregnancy. Patients considered high risk with gestational neoplasia have a poor prognosis if HCG > 40,000 mIU/mL (before treatment), have cerebral or hepatic metastasis, or present with unsuccessful response to chemotherapy within a 4-month trial period. High-risk (poor prognosis) gestation trophoblastic neoplasia is treated with multiple-agent chemotherapy.

63. **(B)** The proliferative (follicular) phase (estrogen) is between the first days of menstrual bleeding to ovulation. If fertilization does not take place, progesterone release results in the endometrial proliferative phase. FSH stimulates the cycle of follicular proliferation.

64. **(B, F)** Crohn's disease usually causes perineal fistulas, and suppurative hidradenitis can cause weeping pustular lesions. Carcinoma, syphilis, Crohn's disease, hidradenitis, granuloma inguinale, and Behçet syndrome are some of the more common causes of ulcerative lesions of the vulva.

65. **(J)** Granuloma inguinale is a lesion related to a contagious, sexually transmitted disease. Identification of Donovan bodies in tissue prepared with Giemsa stain establishes the diagnosis. Treatment is with tetracycline.

66. **(G)** Behçet syndrome is characterized by oral and genital ulcers, ocular inflammation, disorders of the skin resembling erythema nodosum or multiforme, and disturbances of the central nervous system (CNS). Arthritis and thrombophlebitis are not commonly associated with this condition. The etiology is not well understood, and it may be an autoimmune disease. Cortisone has been used as treatment with variable results.

67. **(D)** Patients with noninvasive bladder cancer can be treated by fulguration transurethrally. This procedure must be followed up by regular cystoscopic examinations.

68. **(A, E)** The perineum, pubis, and the region anterior to the inguinal ligament are the main sites where an ectopic testis is found. Ectopic testis must be distinguished from failure of descent of the testis, in which the testis may be held up in the retroperitoneum, internal ring, or inguinal canal. The other sites listed are not recognized places for an ectopic testis to occur.

69. **(A, D, E, H)** Following blunt trauma, patients who are stable with trauma, confined to renal parenchyma or retroperitoneum require observation.

70. **(A, B)** The kidney is surrounded by the perirenal capsule, which, in turn, is surrounded by the perirenal fat and renal fascia. Any lesion (tumor, infection or hemorrhage) that surrounds the kidney and adrenal glands will enter the pararenal fat (Gerota's fascia) if the renal fascia layer is penetrated. Lesions in the pararenal space are confined (i.e., within) the fascia transversalis (endoabdominal fascia). In approaching a kidney with an expanding extraperitoneal hemorrhage, the surgeon should enter the kidney anteriorly at the hilum if the approach is through Gerota's pararenal fat layer. If this is not observed, excessive loss of blood may occur before control of renal vasculature at the hilum.

71. **(C)** In adults, this is diagnostic, but in children, transillumination is also seen in an indirect inguinal hernia. An epididymal cyst may transilluminate but is posterior to the testis.

72. **(C, E)** Infertility and failure of ejaculation occur because of sympathetic denervation. Infertility is found in many patients with testis cancer. In retroperitoneal dissection (and any surgery in the region of the aortic bifurcation or promontory of the sacrum), the sympathetic branches to the hypogastric plexus must be identified and preserved when possible. In the case discussed here, the patient's ability to have an erection should not be interfered with, because the pelvic splanchnic nerves are remote from the operating site.

73. **(B)** Oral DES was given to patients who were unable to conceive. Fortunately, this complication is unlikely to occur, because DES has been withdrawn as a drug used for this purpose.

74. **(C)** A corpus luteum cyst is functional and usually regresses within one menstrual cycle. If a cyst is larger than 5–6 cm, one should re-evaluate the patient in 4–6 weeks before suggesting laparotomy. Dermoid cysts are benign variations of teratomas. They usually are cured by simple excision, but the opposite ovary may be involved in 10% of cases.

CHAPTER 9

Thorax, Head, and Neck
Questions

Alan Berkower, Jaroslaw Bilaniuk, and Simon Wapnick

DIRECTIONS (Questions 1 through 84): Each of the numbered items or incomplete statements in this section is followed by answers or by completions of the statement. Select the ONE lettered answer or completion that is BEST in each case.

1. Following a vacation in Florida, a 43-year-old man notes shortness of breath. He is a non-smoker. His wife points out that his face has become slightly swollen. On examination, his blood pressure is normal. His pupils are equal and respond to light. Dilated veins are noted around the shoulders, upper chest, and face. An x-ray of the chest reveals an opacity in the superior mediastinum. What is the most likely diagnosis?

   (A) thymoma
   (B) neurogenic tumor
   (C) lymphoma
   (D) teratodermoid tumor
   (E) pheochromocytoma

2. A 64-year-old assistant hair stylist undergoes a vaginal hysterectomy under spinal anesthesia. Bleeding occurs when an attempt is made to separate and exclude the right ureter from the operating field. After a short interval, respiratory arrest occurs and intubation must be instituted. What is the most likely cause of respiratory arrest during during this procedure under spinal anesthesia?

   (A) paralysis of the intercostal muscle
   (B) paralysis of the diaphragm (phrenic nerves)
   (C) centrally induced mechanism secondary to decreased cardiac output

   (D) diffusion of anesthetic to the level of the pons
   (E) diffusion of anesthetic to the level of the medulla

3. In the evaluation of a 64-year-old woman with fluctuating neurological signs of ptosis, eleventh and twelfth cranial nerve palsy, and generalized extremity weakness are noted. Edrophonium (Tensilon) given intravenously results in clinical improvement. A computed tomography (CT) scan shows a lesion in the anterior mediastinum, and a biopsy confirms the presence of a thymoma. She should undergo which of the following?

   (A) high-dose steroid administration
   (B) irradiation of the anterior mediastinum
   (C) calcium administration
   (D) thymectomy
   (E) pneumococcal vaccination

4. A 54-year-old construction worker has smoked two packs of cigarettes daily for the past 25 years. He notes swelling in his upper extremity and face, along with dilated veins in this region. A CT scan and venogram of the neck are performed. What is the most likely cause of the obstruction?

   (A) aortic aneurysm
   (B) metastasis
   (C) bronchogenic carcinoma
   (D) chronic fibrosing mediastinitis
   (E) granulomatous disease

5. During a routine chest x-ray offered by a department store to all its employees, a 42-year-old business manager is found to have a 1.5-cm nodule in the upper lobe of the lung with a central core of calcium. He has no symptoms. The management of this lesion should involve which of the following?

(A) transbronchial biopsy
(B) percutaneous needle biopsy
(C) thoracotomy
(D) periodic x-ray follow-up evaluation
(E) mediastinoscopy

6. A 54-year-old manager of a bank is noted to have a solitary 1.5-cm nodule on a routine chest x-ray. He is asymptomatic. The most suggestive feature of malignancy would be the finding of which of the following?

(A) a lesion in the lingula lobe
(B) central calcification
(C) a laminated calcium pattern
(D) indistinct margins
(E) none of the above

7. An asymptomatic 56-year-old man is found on routine chest x-ray to have a 2-cm nodule-central tumor in the upper lobe of the right lung. The lesion is not calcified. No previous x-rays exist. What is the most appropriate initial step toward making a diagnosis?

(A) fiberoptic bronchoscopy
(B) bone scan
(C) thoracotomy
(D) observation at follow-up examination in 6 months
(E) mediastinoscopy

8. At the age of 46, an accountant has developed hoarseness due to an inoperable cancer of the left upper lung lobe. He has smoked heavily since the age of 14. Which of the following features of cancer of the lung indicates distant spread?

(A) hypercalcemia
(B) Cushing-like syndrome
(C) gynecomastia
(D) syndrome of inappropriate secretion of antidiuretic hormone (SIADH)

(E) brachial plexus lesion (Pancoast syndrome)

9. Surgery is indicated in the initial management of lung cancer in the presence of which of the following?

(A) hypercalcemia
(B) vocal cord paralysis
(C) superior vena cava syndrome
(D) small-cell anaplastic carcinoma
(E) chest wall and anterior abdominal wall metastasis

10. Pneumonectomy for carcinoma of the lung is contraindicated with which of the following?

(A) total atelectasis of the involved lung
(B) P_{CO_2} over 60 mmHg
(C) cardiac index (CI) of 3 L/min
(D) P_{O_2} of 80 mmHg
(E) maximal breathing capacity of 75% of predicted value

11. After undergoing a percutaneous needle biopsy, a 49-year-old electrical engineer is found to have small-cell carcinoma. The chest x-ray shows a lesion in the peripheral part of the right middle lobe. The patient should be advised to undergo which of the following?

(A) right lobectomy
(B) right pneumonectomy
(C) excision of lesion and postoperative radiotherapy
(D) combination chemotherapy
(E) radiotherapy

12. While walking to the train station from college, a sophomore is accosted and stabbed in the chest immediately above the second rib. On admission to the hospital, he is bleeding from the wound and the blade of the knife is protruding from the skin. A chest x-ray reveals that the knife is at the level of the inferior margin of the fourth thoracic vertebra. The patient has a blood pressure of 100/60 mmHg. Which structure is the most likely cause of bleeding?

(A) arch of the aorta
(B) left ventricle

(C) hemizygous vein

(D) vertebral artery

(E) right subclavian artery

13. Four years previously, a 56-year-old fisherman underwent thyroidectomy for cancer of the thyroid gland. He is now noted to have a single 4-cm lesion in the upper lobe of the left lung. There is no other evidence of disease, and he is in excellent health. Endobronchial biopsy confirms that the lesion is malignant but the organ of origin cannot be determined. What should he be given?

(A) radiotherapy

(B) combination chemotherapy

(C) attempted curative lung resection

(D) exploration of the neck for thyroid recurrence

(E) androgen therapy

14. A 72-year-old retired miner complains of progressive dyspnea, chest pain, and a 20-lb weight loss. He is a nonsmoker. Examination reveals clubbing of the fingers. CT scan shows a pleural effusion and nodular, irregular thickening of the right lung and involvement of the celiac lymph nodes. Cytology, repeated on several occasions, is not helpful. Which test will most likely establish the diagnosis?

(A) laparoscopy

(B) bronchoscopy

(C) open pleural biopsy

(D) repeat cytology

(E) gastroscopy

15. A 28-year-old bank employee undergoes investigation for infertility that revealed oligospermia. On further inquiry, it is found that he has suffered from repeated bouts of coughing since childhood and episodes of recurrent pancreatitis. Clubbing of the fingers is evident. Which test is most likely to reveal the cause of his chronic lung disease?

(A) chest x-ray

(B) x-ray of the humerus

(C) sweat chloride elevated to over 80-mEq/L

(D) sweat chloride reduced to less than 50 mEq/L

(E) aspergillus in the sputum

16. A 58-year-old male factory worker scheduled to undergo a left inguinal hernia repair is noted to have a severe chronic cough. Further pulmonary function tests revealed reduction of forced expiratory volume in 1 second (FEV_1) and reduction of FEV_1/FVC (forced vital capacity) ratio associated with emphysema. Before rescheduling surgery, which of the following would improve residual function?

(A) trial of ipratropium bromide bronchodilator therapy

(B) cromolyn

(C) cough suppressants

(D) bilateral carotid body resection

(E) intermittent positive-pressure breathing (IPPB)

17. The chest x-ray of a 62-year-old woman who complains of weakness, dyspnea, and hemoptysis shows multiple nodules in the right lung. She states that the dyspnea is worse in the supine position (platypnea) and improves on sitting up. On examination, the physician notes multiple hemorrhagic telangiectasia in the mouth and in the skin of the upper chest wall. There is a mild increase in the erythrocyte count, and the Po_2 is 90. An angiogram shows multiple pulmonary arteriovenous (AV) fistula in both lungs. What should be the next step in treatment?

(A) needle biopsy of lesion

(B) irradiation

(C) therapeutic embolization

(D) endobronchial biopsy

(E) sympathomimetic inhalation therapy

18. A 32-year-old male janitor complains of a swollen face during the past week. A CT scan reveals an expanding hematoma in the superior mediastinum. Mediatinal tamponade is most likely to manifest as which of the following?

(A) hypertension

(B) increased pulse pressure during inspiration

(C) paresis of the right arm

(D) venous congestion in the upper extremity

(E) hyperhidrosis

19. After returning from vacation, a 67-year-old retired judge is admitted to the emergency department with severe dyspnea. On examination, an inspiratory stridor, ecchymosis in his neck, and swelling of soft tissue and veins in his face and upper extremity veins are evident. The CT scan shows an expanding superior mediastinal hematoma. What is the most common source of mediastinal hemorrhage?

    (A) parotid gland surgery
    (B) trauma
    (C) dissecting thoracic aneurysm
    (D) mediastinal tumor
    (E) hemorrhagic diathesis

20. A 42-year-old man known to have Marfan's syndrome is admitted to the emergency department with severe chest pain radiating to the back. His blood pressure is 190/130 mmHg. An electrocardiogram (ECG) shows no evidence of myocardial infarction (MI). A type I (ascending aorta) dissecting aneurysm is detected on angiography. What should he undergo?

    (A) percutaneous transluminal coronary angioplasty (PTCA)
    (B) nitroprusside and attempted resection of the ascending aorta
    (C) intra-aortic balloon pumping (IABP)
    (D) immediate thoracotomy
    (E) steroid administration

21. In interpreting a follow-up x-ray to exclude metastatic disease in an elderly man with prostatic cancer, the radiologist reports sclerotic metastasis to all floating rib(s). *Floating rib* refers to ribs

    (A) 1
    (B) 2
    (C) 3–7
    (D) 8–10
    (E) 11 and 12

Questions 22 and 23

A 36-year-old man is crossing a bridge when he is suddenly swept by a torrent into the river. After rescue and resuscitation, he is admitted to the intensive care unit (ICU) of the local hospital with adult respiratory distress syndrome (ARDS).

22. Which of the following associated features would suggest a diagnosis of ARDS?

    (A) high lung compliance
    (B) activation of surfactant
    (C) consolidation confined to the lingula
    (D) interstitial edema with normal pulmonary capillary wedge pressure (PCWP)
    (E) hypoxia responding rapidly to oxygen therapy

23. Which is one of the most important principles of treatment of ARDS?

    (A) steroid use
    (B) avoidance of positive end-expiratory pressure (PEEP)
    (C) tracheobronchial toilet
    (D) use of large amount of fluids
    (E) early and vigorous use of PEEP and highest FIO_2

24. On his return from a 3-year visit to India, a United Nations research worker complains of night sweats, cough, weight loss, and tiredness. An x-ray shows an apical radiopaque lesion (Figure 9–1). Several enlarged glands are palpable in the posterior triangle of the neck. The next step toward establishing the diagnosis should involve which of the following?

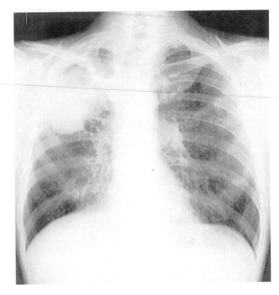

Figure 9–1. Cavity lesion of the right upper lobe. (Reproduced, with permission, from Lindner, HH: Clinical Anatomy, Appleton & Lange, 1989.)

(A) determination of antitrypsin 3 level

(B) Kweim skin test

(C) examination of sputum for cytology

(D) thoracotomy and open-lung biopsy

(E) sputum culture for mycobacterium

25. A student with known human immunodeficiency syndrome (HIV) infection has lost 6 lb in weight and his sedimentation rate is increased to 40. He has no other symptoms. The Mantoux (tuberculin) test results show a change of 7 mm (positive), and x-ray findings reveal a small lesion in the apex of the right lobe of the lung. How should this patient be managed?

(A) hospitalized in a public ward

(B) hospitalized in an isolated hospital room

(C) treated as an outpatient with triple antituberculous drug therapy for 2 weeks

(D) treated as an outpatient with multiple antituberculous drug therapy for 2 months and then appropriate antituberculous drugs for 4 more months

(E) observed and undergo repeat skin test after 8 weeks

26. A 12-year-old girl with leukemia develops a lower respiratory tract infection with hemoptysis that is shown to be due to right-sided bronchiectasis. In addition to treatment for the underlying leukemia, the patient should receive which of the following?

(A) undergo right pneumonectomy

(B) receive selective antibiotics, physiotherapy, and bronchodilator therapy

(C) undergo tracheostomy

(D) have cough-suppressant medication

(E) undergo weekly suction by endotracheal intubation

27. An 18-year-old man develops a severe cough with productive sputum due to *Pseudomonas aeruginosa*. He has had similar episodes in the past, and previous studies revealed bronchiectasis. Which of the following will help elucidate the most likely underlying cause of bronchiectasis?

(A) small-intestinal obstruction successfully treated at birth

(B) low concentration of DNA in the bronchial sputum

(C) mycobacterium culture from sputum

(D) fungus grown from sputum

(E) immunodeficiency studies

28. After suffering an episode of hemoptysis, a 14-year-old boy is found, on chest x-ray, to have a well-circumscribed mass that contains both fluid and air. Surgical excision is carried out, and a localized mass adjacent to the carina is excised. What is the most likely diagnosis?

(A) tuberculosis

(B) bronchogenic carcinoma

(C) bronchogenic cyst

(D) chronic obstructive pulmonary disease (COPD)

(E) AV fistula

29. Following thoracotomy, in a 20-year-old man a lesion is detected in the right lower lung lobe and is found to be nonfunctioning lung tissue that is served by vessels separate from those of the adjacent lung tissue. What is the most likely diagnosis?

(A) mesothelioma

(B) hiatal hernia

(C) glomus tumor

(D) bronchopulmonary sequestration

(E) cystic hygroma

30. A 64-year-old man complains of pain in the lower chest. A CT scan confirms the presence of a tumor of the lung at T10 level to the left of the midline and invading the surrounding left lung base. Because of the structure most likely involved and penetrating the diaphragm at this level, what could be associated?

(A) hoarseness

(B) latissimus dorsi palsy

(C) Budd–Chiari syndrome (hepatic venous outlet obstruction)

(D) dysphagia

(E) tracheobronchial fistula

31. An 8-year-old girl with a prominent chest wall deformity that pushes the sternum inward (i.e., in a posterior direction) is asymptomatic, and she participates fully in athletic activities at school. Surgical correction is recommended. What is the most likely cause of the deformity?

    (A) funnel chest (pectus excavatum)
    (B) pectus carinatum (protrusion at the sternum)
    (C) flail chest
    (D) cystic hygroma
    (E) rickets

32. After suffering a respiratory tract infection, a 64-year-old female biochemist develops chronic lung disease requiring intubation in the ICU for an 8-week period. Tracheal stenosis is noted. What is the most likely cause of tracheal stenosis?

    (A) prolonged intubation
    (B) tuberculosis
    (C) scleroderma
    (D) Riedel struma (fibrous thyroiditis)
    (E) achalasia

33. In evaluating the chest x-ray findings in a 60-year-old man with pleural effusion, which of the following constitutes an abnormal finding of the pleural cavity?

    (A) communication between the right and left pleural cavities
    (B) intersection of the twelfth rib posteriorly
    (C) existence of both a parietal and visceral layer in the upper parts
    (D) existence of different attachments on the right and left sides
    (E) extension of the cavity above the levels of the clavicles

34. Because of his involvement in a motor vehicle accident, a 23-year-old football player has a chest wall injury. The only abnormal findings on clinical and radiologic examination are a fracture of the left fifth to seventh ribs and a small hemothorax. What should treatment include?

    (A) insertion of an intercostal drain to avoid pneumothorax

    (B) thoracotomy to treat a small hemothorax in the left base
    (C) insertion of a metal plate to fix the fracture
    (D) administration of analgesic medication
    (E) administration of cortisone to prevent callus formation

35. In chest surgery, which is true regarding a thoracoabdominal incision?

    (A) It should be used for most abdominal and thoracic procedures.
    (B) It enters the third to fifth intercostal space.
    (C) It causes less postoperative pain.
    (D) It allows division of the costal margin and the diaphragm.
    (E) It causes severe denervation of the anterior abdominal wall.

36. A rope used to elevate a heavy metal object breaks causing the object to fall on a 55-year-old factory worker and producing chest wall injury. Which is true of associated sternal injury?

    (A) It occurs most commonly at the work site.
    (B) It usually involves the body of the sternum.
    (C) It usually is vertical.
    (D) It involves the hemizygous system.
    (E) It causes miosis of the pupil owing to sympathetic injury.

37. After undergoing an emergency operation for dehiscence of a colon suture line, a 62-year-old patient requires endotracheal intubation. Following prolonged intubation, it is noted that she has tracheal stenosis. What is the most appropriate treatment?

    (A) administration of steroids
    (B) resection of segment of tracheal stenosis
    (C) irradiation
    (D) treatment with an intrathoracic under–water drain if a tracheoesophageal fistula is present
    (E) none of the above

38. A 22-year-old student is scheduled to undergo parathyroidectomy for hyperparathyroidism associated with familial multiglandular syndrome. His sister developed peptic ulcer disease secondary to a Zollinger–Ellison (hypergastrinemia) tumor of the pancreas. On examination, a swelling was noted over the posterior aspect of the patient's fifth rib. What is the most likely finding?

   (A) metastasis from a parathyroid carcinoma
   (B) osteitis fibrosa cystica (brown tumor) and subperiosteal resorption of the phalanges
   (C) dermoid cyst
   (D) eosinophilic granuloma
   (E) chondroma

39. After suffering a severe bout of pneumonia, a 46-year-old renal transplantation patient develops a lung abscess. She has been receiving immunosuppression therapy since her last kidney transplantation 3 years ago. What is the most appropriate treatment?

   (A) needle aspiration
   (B) urgent thoracotomy
   (C) antituberculous therapy
   (D) antibiotics and vigorous attempts to obtain bronchial drainage
   (E) insertion of an intercostal pleural drain

40. What is true of branchial cleft cysts?

   (A) They usually appear in the axilla.
   (B) They may become infected after an upper respiratory tract infection (URTI).
   (C) They may be traced to the stomach.
   (D) They arise from endodermal tissue.
   (E) They frequently cause brachial plexus lesions.

41. A 9-year-old boy complains of a swelling on the left side of his neck in the supraclavicular region. The swelling is translucent; a diagnosis of cystic hygroma is established. What is true of cystic hygroma?

   (A) It arises from sweat glands in the neck.
   (B) It is usually an anterior midline structure.
   (C) It may occur in the mediastinum.

   (D) Its lesions are usually easy to enucleate.
   (E) It is premalignant.

42. A 48-year-old woman presents with a 6-month history of intermittent cranial nerve palsy that has become progressively worse in the past 2 weeks. On examination, ptosis and diplopia are evident. Her condition shows a favorable response to the anticholinesterase inhibitory drug prostigmin (neostigmine). What is the most likely diagnosis?

   (A) cerebral palsy
   (B) pineal gland tumor
   (C) adenoma of the pituitary
   (D) myasthenia gravis
   (E) tetany

43. Squamous cell carcinoma of the lip is least likely to develop in which of the following?

   (A) Scandinavian fisherman
   (B) redheaded pornographic actress with a gorgeous year-round tan
   (C) man from Lohatchie, Alabama, who smokes a clay pipe
   (D) brunette secretary who constantly drinks tea
   (E) mentally defective man who smokes 40 cigarettes a day and keeps the butt in his mouth

44. A 43-year-old male tennis champion develops cancer of the lip. What is true of this condition?

   (A) It involves the upper lip in 90% of patients.
   (B) It is more common at the lateral commissure than in the middle.
   (C) It usually occurs beyond the vermilion border.
   (D) It results in cure in about 60% of cases.
   (E) It requires radical neck dissection.

45. A 58-year-old fisherman has been heavily exposed to the sun for more than 30 years. He develops a thickened, scaly lesion extending over two-thirds of the lower lip. There is no ulceration. Histology reveals hyperkeratosis. What should he undergo?

(A) steroid ointment application three times daily

(B) antihistaminic medications

(C) lip stripping and resurfacing with mucosal advancement

(D) radical neck dissection

(E) observation and biopsy of any new ulcers

46. A 24-year-old computer technician notes a progressive increase in the size of his left jaw. After x-rays are taken and a biopsy is done, a diagnosis of ameloblastoma is established. What should be the next step in management?

(A) radiotherapy

(B) laser beam therapy

(C) curettage and bone graft

(D) excision of lesions with 1–2 cm of normal mandible

(E) mandibulectomy with bilateral radical neck dissection

47. Which of the following benign salivary gland lesions occurs exclusively in the parotid gland?

(A) glandular hypertrophy secondary to vitamin A deficiency

(B) cystic dilation

(C) Mikulicz's disease

(D) pleomorphic adenoma

(E) papillary cystadenoma (Warthin's tumor)

48. A 62-year-old man undergoes excision of a cylindroma of the submandibular gland. He is most likely to have an injury to which of the following?

(A) maxillary branch of the trigeminal nerve

(B) lingual nerve

(C) vagus nerve

(D) floor of the maxilla

(E) frontozygomatic branch of the facial nerve

49. A 62-year-old alcoholic presents with an indurated ulcer, 1.5 cm in length, in the right lateral aspect of her tongue (not fixed to the alveolar ridge). There are no clinically abnormal glands palpable in the neck, and a biopsy of the tongue lesion reveals squamous cell carcinoma. What should she undergo?

(A) chemotherapy

(B) local excision of the ulcer

(C) wide excision and right radical neck dissection

(D) antibiotic therapy and should be encouraged to stop smoking

(E) none of the above

50. A 59-year-old woman has discomfort in the posterior part of her tongue. A biopsy confirms that the lesion is a carcinoma. What is true in carcinoma of the posterior third of the tongue?

(A) Lymphoid tissue is absent.

(B) Lymph gland spread is often encountered.

(C) There is an excellent prognosis.

(D) The tissue is well differentiated.

(E) The recurrent laryngeal nerve is infiltrated.

51. Adenocarcinoma is the predominant malignant lesion in which of the following?

(A) hard palate

(B) lip

(C) anterior two-thirds of the tongue

(D) larynx

(E) esophagus

52. The prognosis for squamous carcinoma of the floor of the mouth is adversely affected by which of the following?

(A) poor differentiation of tumor

(B) verrucous carcinoma

(C) presence on right side

(D) superficial tongue involvement

(E) all of the above

53. A 15-year-old immigrant from China presents with a mass in the left supraclavicular region. He is asymptomatic. Findings on endoscopy and biopsy show that this is a metastatic nasopharyngeal tumor. Clinical evidence of complications of this tumor would most likely be indicated by which of the following?

(A) decreased growth hormone levels
(B) bitemporal hemianopsia
(C) lateral rectus palsy
(D) hoarseness
(E) deviation of tongue to the side of lesion

54. A 49-year-old man suffering from depression attempts suicide by jumping out of the window of his third floor apartment. He requires multiple operations during a prolonged, complicated hospital stay. Endotracheal intubation is attempted in the ICU but is unsuccessful because of tracheal stenosis, which is attributed to which of the following?

(A) prolonged nasotracheal intubation
(B) orotracheal intubation
(C) tracheostomy tubes
(D) all of the above
(E) none of the above

55. A 46-year-old Texan develops a lesion in the vestibule of his mouth that, on histological examination is revealed to be verrucous carcinoma of the upper aerodigestive tract. What is true of this lesion?

(A) It is most commonly found on the inside of the cheek.
(B) It is associated with a high metastatic rate.
(C) It is ulcerating in appearance.
(D) It is best treated with radiation.
(E) It is more common in the northeastern part of the United States.

56. A 16-year-old boy complains of difficulty in breathing through his nose. Endoscopy reveals a tumor infiltrating the nasopharynx. Histology reports this as a juvenile nasopharyngeal hemangiofibroma. The boy's anxious mother requests information concerning the lesion. What should she be told?

(A) It is a premalignant lesion.
(B) It usually occurs with laryngeal obstruction.
(C) It is treated with radiotherapy.
(D) It may proceed to destroy surrounding bone.
(E) It is found equally in teenaged girls and boys.

57. A 52-year-old woman has metastatic epidermoid carcinoma on the left side of her neck. Complete head and neck workup fails to identify the primary tumor. What is the recommended treatment?

(A) close follow-up monitoring until the primary tumor is found
(B) exploratory laparotomy
(C) radical neck dissection
(D) full course of radiotherapy to the head and neck
(E) combination chemotherapy using 5-fluorouracil (5-FU), vincristine, hexamethanilamine, and prednisone

58. A 58-year-old woman undergoes excision biopsy of a tumor in the left posterior triangle of her neck. Histology suggests that this is a metastatic cancer. What is the most likely site of the primary tumor?

(A) ovary
(B) adrenal gland
(C) kidney
(D) piriform fossa
(E) stomach

59. Arterial infusions via the external carotid artery with methotrexate and 5-FU for head and neck carcinoma have shown a 50% response rate. Widespread use, however, is limited. Why?

(A) The internal carotid is inadvertently perfused in a large percentage of patients.
(B) Ipsilateral facial slough has occurred in 3% of patients.
(C) Blindness occurs in 30% of patients.
(D) The response is transient, lasting only 2–3 months.
(E) There is a prohibitive incidence of leukemia.

60. The classic complete neck dissection for palpable adenopathy in the posterior triangle of the neck includes removal of which of the following?

(A) the transverse process, C2–C4
(B) the spinal accessory nerve
(C) both thyroid lobes
(D) the trapezius
(E) the vagus

61. A 69-year-old endocrinologist complains of progressive facial weakness and loss of taste sensation on the right side of her tongue. What is the most likely structure affected?

(A) lingual nerve
(B) middle ear
(C) ansa hypoglossi
(D) twelfth cranial nerve
(E) ninth cranial nerve

62. What is true of the thymus gland?

(A) It is located in the posterior mediastinum.
(B) It arises from the first branchial arch.
(C) It controls calcium metabolism.
(D) It can be excised through a low cervical incision.
(E) It results in severe pneumococcal infection when removed in adults.

63. A 29-year-old woman develops difficulty in swallowing. Examination reveals acute pharyngitis. Which organism is most likely to be isolated?

(A) viral
(B) *treponema*
(C) anaerobic
(D) *Staphylococcus aureus*
(E) *Escherichia coli*

64. A 43-year-old man suddenly develops odynophagia. Which organism is most likely to be isolated on throat culture?

(A) mononucleosis
(B) *S. aureus*
(C) normal pharyngeal flora

(D) group A streptococci
(E) diphtheroid

65. A 72-year-old man presents to the emergency department complaining of frequent nosebleeds. What is the most likely site of acute epistaxis?

(A) turbinate
(B) septum
(C) maxillary sinus
(D) ethmoid sinus
(E) sphenoid sinus

66. What is true of carotid body tumors?

(A) They secrete catecholamines.
(B) They are more common at sea level.
(C) They arise from structures that respond to changes in blood volume.
(D) They arise from the structures that respond to changes in P_{O_2}.
(E) They are usually highly malignant.

67. A newborn male is brought to the physician's office with a history of poor feeding and recurrent fever. Examination of the baby's ears demonstrates bilateral otitis media. Which is the most common organism isolated from the middle ear space in a newborn with otitis media?

(A) *E. coli*
(B) *S. aureus*
(C) *Mycobacterium tuberculosis*
(D) *Pseudomonas aeruginosa*
(E) *Bacteroides fragilis*

68. A 32-year-old pregnant female presents with a 1-day history of drooping of the right side of her face. A thorough history and physical examination do not reveal an obvious cause of the condition. What is the most likely cause of the patient's facial nerve weakness?

(A) labyrinthitis
(B) parotid tumor
(C) Lyme disease
(D) herpes zoster
(E) idiopathic

69. A six-year-old girl complains of otalgia, fever, and irritability. Physical examination reveals a stiff, bulging, red tympanic membrane. Previous history of ear infections is denied. Clinical response to amoxicillin is maximized at which following duration?

    (A) 1 day
    (B) 5 days
    (C) 7 days
    (D) 10 days
    (E) 2 weeks

70. After undergoing a minor nasal operation, a 65-year-old man is given a neuroleptic agent. What is the most commonly used neuroleptic?

    (A) droperidol (inapsine)
    (B) ketamine
    (C) fentanyl
    (D) morphine
    (E) thiopental (tentothal) be achieved for as long as 4–5 minutes

71. Following surgical resection of a large thyroid mass, a patient complains of persistent hoarseness and a weak voice. What is the most likely cause of these symptoms?

    (A) traumatic intubation
    (B) prolonged intubation
    (C) injury to the recurrent laryngeal nerve
    (D) injury to the superior laryngeal nerve
    (E) scar tissue extending to the vocal cords

72. A 9-month-old girl is brought to the physician's office for noisy breathing. The child is otherwise healthy, and her gestation and delivery were uncomplicated. On physical examination, mild inspiratory stridor is heard. What is the most likely cause of stridor in an infant?

    (A) bilateral vocal cord paralysis
    (B) laryngomalacia
    (C) tracheal stenosis
    (D) epiglottitis
    (E) Arnold–Chiari malformation

73. A 32-year-old teacher presents at her physician's office complaining of hearing loss in her right ear. Physical examination reveals cerumen completely obstructing the ear canal. Ear wax removal is recommended using which of the following?

    (A) jet irrigation (Water Pik)
    (B) 3% hydrogen peroxide ear drops
    (C) irrigation of the eardrum if perforated
    (D) aqueous irrigation if a bean is present
    (E) aqueous irrigation if an insect is present far in the ear

74. A 4-year-old boy requires prolonged intubation and nasogastric tube placement in an intensive care setting following a closed head injury incurred in a car accident. He develops recurrent fever but is hemodynamically stable. What is the most likely source of sepsis?

    (A) sinusitis
    (B) bacterial tracheitis
    (C) epiglottitis
    (D) small-bowel necrosis
    (E) deep vein thrombosis (DVT)

75. What is the most common site for foreign bodies in the head and neck?

    (A) eye
    (B) ear
    (C) nose
    (D) throat
    (E) esophagus

76. A 25-year-old accountant is seen by her family practitioner for a sore throat. Her physician performs a *Streptococcus A* direct swab test (SADST). What is the specificity of SADST as compared to the standard culture method for the diagnosis of streptococcal pharyngitis?

    (A) 25%
    (B) 45%
    (C) 65%
    (D) 80%
    (E) 85%

77. A 33-year-old female noted a discharge from a sinus in the overlying skin below the right angle of the mandible. She recalls previous episodes of fullness and mild pain in this region over the past several years. What is the most likely cause?

    (A) thyroglossal duct cyst
    (B) branchial cyst
    (C) teratoma
    (D) myeloma
    (E) trauma to the neck

78. An 85-year-old hypertensive man is evaluated in the emergency department for recent onset epistaxis. His blood pressure is 150/80, and a hematocrit is 39%. What is the most likely source of bleeding?

    (A) posterior nasal septum
    (B) anterior nasal septum
    (C) inferior turbinate
    (D) middle turbinate
    (E) floor of nose

79. An elderly man complains of ear pain. During evaluation, the physician asks if the patient has tinnitus. What is tinnitus?

    (A) a subjective sensation of noise in the head
    (B) a complication of chronic metal ingestion
    (C) an audible cardiac murmur
    (D) dizziness with sounds
    (E) nystagmus

80. A 4-year-old girl is diagnosed with bilateral otitis media and is treated for 10 days with an oral broad-spectrum antibiotic. The patient completes the full course of antibiotics and returns for regular follow-up visits. In most children, the appearance of the tympanic membrane returns to normal following a single antibiotic regimen for an episode of otitis media within what period?

    (A) 1 week
    (B) 2 weeks
    (C) 3 weeks
    (D) 1 month
    (E) 3 months

81. During an examination, the dentist notices a lump between the earlobe and mandible in a 6-year-old boy. It feels soft, but it is difficult to distinguish from the rest of the parotid gland. What is the most likely diagnosis?

    (A) lymphoma
    (B) squamous cell carcinoma
    (C) metastatic skin cancer
    (D) benign mixed tumor
    (E) hemangioma

82. During a baseball game, the pitcher is hit in the left eye with a hard-hit line drive. He is rushed to the nearest emergency department where CT scan reveals left orbital rim and floor fractures and fluid in the left maxillary sinus. What are physical findings likely to include?

    (A) enophthalmos
    (B) vertical diplopia
    (C) cheek numbness
    (D) epistaxis
    (E) all of the above

83. A 4-year-old child presents with chronic bilateral nasal discharge and diffuse headaches. Examination reveals a thin, irritable child who is mouth breathing. X-ray evaluation of sinuses most likely reveals opacification of which of the following?

    (A) maxillary
    (B) sphenoid
    (C) ethmoid
    (D) frontal
    (E) all of the above

84. A 2-year-old child undergoes tympanostomy tube placement for treatment of chronic bilateral serous otitis media. Which of the following complications is least likely to occur subsequent to surgery?

    (A) otorrhea
    (B) chronic perforation
    (C) cholesteatoma
    (D) tympanosclerosis
    (E) scarring of the external auditory canal

DIRECTIONS (Questions 85 through 97): Each set of matching questions in this section consists of a list of lettered options followed by several numbered items. For each numbered item, select the appropriate lettered option(s). Each lettered option may be selected once, more than once, or not at all. **EACH ITEM WILL STATE THE NUMBER OF OPTIONS TO SELECT. CHOOSE EXACTLY THIS NUMBER.**

Question 85

  (A) recurrent laryngeal

  (B) internal laryngeal

  (C) external laryngeal

  (D) pharyngeal branch of vagus

  (E) phrenic

  (F) sympathetic

  (G) glossopharyngeal

  (H) ansa hypoglossi

85. After undergoing a left thyroid operation, a 42-year-old opera singer notes no change in speech, but she has difficulty in singing high-pitched notes. Which nerve is most likely to be injured? SELECT ONLY ONE.

Question 86

  (A) scrofula

  (B) carotid body tumor

  (C) ganglioneuroma

  (D) Virchow node

  (E) sternomastoid tumor

  (F) glomus tumor

  (G) cervical rib

  (H) sarcoid

86. A 67-year-old woman has lost weight and complains of night sweats. She had previously undergone treatment for tuberculosis. She has lymph node enlargement in the neck that has broken down to form sinus with overhanging bluish edges. What is the diagnosis? SELECT ONLY ONE.

Question 87

  (A) erysipelas

  (B) eczema

  (C) scarlet fever

  (D) mucor mycosis

  (E) coccydynia

  (F) ameba

  (G) schistosomiasis

  (H) actinomycosis

  (I) tuberculosis

87. A 63-year-old man with insulin-dependent diabetes develops a black crusting lesion in the nose and left maxillary sinus. Biopsy reveals nonseptate hyphae, which confirms the diagnosis of what? SELECT ONLY ONE.

Question 88

  (A) cholesteatoma

  (B) dermoid cyst

  (C) glomus tumor

  (D) neurofibroma

  (E) hemangioma

  (F) epidermoid cyst

  (G) Mikulicz lesion

  (H) sarcoma

88. This develops along lines of embryological fusion in the floor of the mouth. SELECT ONLY ONE.

Question 89

  (A) optic neuroma

  (B) constricted pupil

  (C) cerebellar dysfunction

  (D) hamartomatous polyps in the small intestine

  (E) diverticulitis

  (F) melanosis coli

  (G) cancer of the breast

  (H) melanoma

89. A 32-year-old man presents with abdominal pain. On examination, he is noted to have pigmented spots in the buccal region. He is diagnosed to have Peutz–Jeghers syndrome, which also results in what? SELECT ONLY ONE.

Question 90

(A) lymphoma

(B) squamous cell carcinoma

(C) metastatic skin cancer

(D) benign mixed tumor

(E) hemangioma

(F) neurofibroma

(G) Paget's disease

(H) ranula

90. A businessman notices a lump in front of his ear while shaving one morning. His wife thinks it has been there for several months. What is the most likely cause of a mass in the parotid gland in this patient? SELECT ONLY ONE.

Questions 91 and 92

(A) foramen cecum

(B) foramen ovale

(C) foramen rotundum

(D) foramen spinosum

(E) foramen magnum

(F) foramen jugulare

(G) foramen of Munro

(H) foramen of Magendi

91. A 46-year-old accountant notices that he keeps cutting the right side of his lower face while shaving. On self-examination, he notes a loss of sensation of the skin and lower teeth on that side. At his physician's office, a CT scan is ordered. Which structure should be carefully evaluated for this patient's complaint? SELECT ONLY ONE.

92. A 4-year-old boy is brought to the physician's office by his father for evaluation of small stature. A thyroid scan is ordered and shows no uptake in the neck. Which structure is embryologically related to the thyroid gland and should be carefully evaluated? SELECT ONLY ONE.

Question 93

(A) HPV

(B) Epstein–Barr virus

(C) HIV

(D) varicella zoster virus

(E) herpes type 2 virus

(F) microcytic anemia

(G) autoimmune deficiency

(H) meningioma

93. Mononucleosis in the blood is associated with what? SELECT ONLY ONE.

Question 94

(A) mental status change

(B) anosmia

(C) hypopituitarism

(D) meningitis

(E) neck mass

(F) deafness

(G) bitemporal hemianopsia

(H) neck stiffness

94. A middle-aged woman from China presents at her physician's office with a history of nasopharynx cancer. A medical history is obtained about her illness. What is the most common complaint of patients presenting with nasopharynx cancer? SELECT ONLY ONE.

Question 95

(A) lymphoma

(B) squamous cell carcinoma

(C) metastatic skin cancer

(D) benign mixed tumor

(E) hemangioma

(F) sebaceous cyst

(G) Sjögren syndrome

(H) ectopic thyroid

95. A 63-year-old bartender presents at his physician's office complaining of a painful sore on his tongue. On examination, it is found that he has an ulcerated lesion on his tongue and a mass in the submandibular gland triangle. What is the most likely diagnosis? SELECT ONLY ONE.

Question 96

(A) funnel chest (pectus excavatum)

(B) pectus carinatum (protrusion at the sternum)

(C) flail chest

(D) cystic hygroma

(E) rickets

(F) sebaceous cyst

(G) dermoid cyst

(H) nevi

(I) lipoma

(J) Tay–Sachs disease

96. Midline swelling causing a double chin appearance is what? SELECT ONLY ONE.

Question 97

(A) metastasis from a parathyroid carcinoma

(B) osteitis fibrosa cystica (brown tumor) and subperiosteal resorption of the phalanges

(C) atypical mycobacterium

(D) eosinophilic granuloma

(E) chondroma

(F) dermoid cyst

(G) thyroglossal duct cyst

(H) laryngoc) cele

(I) Warthin's tumor

97. A 5-year-old boy is taken to his pediatrician for a laceration on his right knee. A mass on his neck is noticed; his mother states it has been there for several months and is slowly getting larger. The mass is slightly to the left of midline. Ultrasound findings are shown in Figure 9–2. What is the most likely diagnosis? SELECT ONLY ONE.

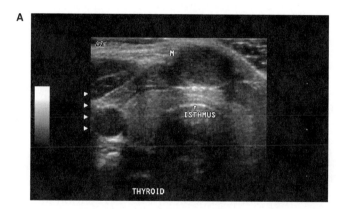
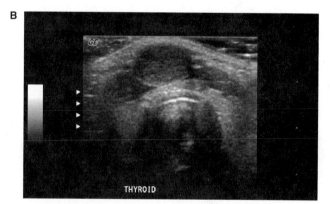

Figure 9–2. A, Ultrasound of neck. Midline hypoechogenic mass anterior and superior to the thyroid gland. **B,** Both poles and isthmus at a higher level.

Answers and Explanations

1. **(B)** The most common cause of primary mediastinal tumor is a neurogenic tumor (20–25%), and 10% are malignant (more likely in children). They usually arise from an intercostal nerve or sympathetic ganglion. Varieties of neurogenic tumors include neurilemmoma (schwannoma), neurofibroma, ganglioneuroma, and neuroblastoma. Next in frequency (of primary mediastinal tumors) are thymoma, congenital cysts, and lymphoma. New diagnostic techniques have resulted in detection of larger numbers of these lesions.

2. **(C)** Spinal anesthesia induces venous vasodilation because of sympathetic blockade. Venous pooling can seriously impair venous return. It is the sympathetic blockade and not somatic nerve blockade that is responsible for the vasomotor and respiratory changes. It is important to ensure that volume depletion is corrected before spinal anesthesia, because venous return and hence cardiac output are diminished. These changes are aggravated by keeping the head up.

3. **(D)** The role of thymectomy in treating patients with myasthenia gravis who have a thymoma is well established. The thymus gland is located in the anterior mediastinum and can be approached by a cervical or mediastinal approach. It arises from the third and fourth branchial arches. Thymectomy is frequently advised for patients with myasthenia gravis who do not have a thymoma; however, there are some authorities who would treat these patients initially with an anticholinesterase drug such as pyridostigmine (Mestinon). Corticosteroid therapy may be indicated when thymectomy has failed, but it must be undertaken cautiously,

because the drug may precipitate severe weakness. Pneumococcal infections (which may occur after splenectomy performed in children) are not a specific complication noted after thymectomy.

4. **(C)** Bronchogenic carcinoma accounts for 70–80% of all cases of superior vena cava (SVC) obstruction; primary mediastinal tumors are the second most common cause. The main bronchial lymphatics are located at the tracheal bifurcation and immediately to the right and left of the trachea. Tuberculosis and mycotic infections are the most likely causes of chronic fibrosing mediastinitis.

5. **(D)** CT is useful, because it delineates the calcification and shows the pattern of the calcification. There is no need for intervention at this stage, because most lesions of this nature are probably benign granulomas.

6. **(D)** By definition, a solitary nodule is one that is 5 cm or less in diameter. In most series, 60% of such lesions are benign, and 40% are malignant. The presence of irregular margins, the absence of calcification, a recent onset of symptoms, or an increase in size of the lesion within a relatively short period (several months) indicate the greater likelihood of malignancy. Thin-section CT scanning may add further information.

7. **(A)** Bronchoscopy is the initial step, particularly if the patient is a smoker and a good risk for surgery. If cancer is confirmed, thoracotomy will probably be undertaken. Patient age is an important consideration in the management of a solitary pulmonary nodule; malignancy occurs in less than 1% of patients under 35 years of age.

Benign lesions, such as bronchopulmonary sequestration, which usually affects the posterior aspect of the inferior lobes of the lung, must be considered. Bronchopulmonary sequestration is usually asymptomatic, unless complications occur.

8. **(E)** In apical lung cancers, the malignant tumor may extend above the thoracic inlet, penetrate the suprapleural membrane, and infiltrate the structures found at the root of the neck. The first thoracic nerve and lower trunk of the brachial plexus are most likely to be involved initially, as T1 passes along the inner border of the first rib to reach the neck. If the sympathetic nerve is involved, pupil constriction and ptosis may be evident (Horner syndrome). The other listed items are all features of the paraneoplastic syndrome associated with lung cancer and do not necessarily indicate extranodal metastasis. Cushing's syndrome in lung cancer occurs more frequently in men and in an older age group and has a more rapid downhill course than typical Cushing's syndrome. SIADH should be suspected if the patient with a lung lesion develops unexplained mental changes and an extremely low serum sodium level. Fluid restriction is required. Urine osmolarity is low.

9. **(A)** Hypercalcemia is attributed to the secretion of parahormone from a localized squamous cell carcinoma (paraneoplastic effect); as such, improvement may be seen after surgical resection. Following extension of the tumor into the chest wall, radiotherapy and subsequent extensive resection carried out in selected cases may occasionally be indicated. Small-cell carcinoma (also known as oat-cell carcinoma) accounts for 20–25% of cases of bronchogenic carcinoma, arises centrally and tends to metastasize widely. The initial treatment is combination chemotherapy followed by radiotherapy in those whose cancer responds.

10. **(B)** Uncorrected hypercarbia is the major contraindication to total pneumonectomy. Surgery is the treatment of choice for non–small-cell carcinoma of the lung. Although 25% of patients with bronchogenic carcinoma may undergo thoracotomy, many of these patients will have un-

resectable lesions. Patients with a FEV_1 less than 2 L, a FVC under 70% of predicted value, and maximal voluntary ventilation (MVV) under 50% are likely to tolerate operation poorly. The normal FEV_1/FVC ratio is 0.7 or less; in severe obstructive dysfunction, it is under 0.45. Total atelectasis of the lung may be associated with obstruction of the main bronchus by the tumor.

11. **(D)** Patients with small-cell carcinoma should not be treated initially by thoracotomy. This cancer responds favorably to combination chemotherapy, but few patients survive for more than 1 year. More than 160,000 cases of bronchogenic carcinoma are diagnosed in the United States per year. It accounts for 33% of all cancer deaths in men and 20% of all cancer deaths in women. The most common cancers of the lung are squamous carcinoma, 30% (tumor tends to be central); adenocarcinoma, 30%, (tumor tends to be peripheral) small-cell carcinoma, 20% (tumor tends to be central); and large-cell carcinoma, 15% (tumor tends to be peripheral).

12. **(A)** The arch of the aorta is above the arbitrary line drawn between the manubriosternal angle (of Louis) and the lower border of the fourth thoracic vertebra level. Therefore, it is located entirely in the superior mediastinum behind the manubrium. The projected line passing behind the manubriosternal junction and the lower border of T4 is a key surgical anatomic landmark of this region. The ascending aorta (anteriorly), descending aorta (posteriorly), and pulmonary trunk are below this level. The left recurrent laryngeal nerve curves around the ligamentum arteriosus, the arch of the azygous vein enters the SVC, and the upper third of the esophagus are separated arbitrarily from the middle third at this level. On a plain film of the chest, the tracheal bifurcation (carina) is a useful marker of this line.

13. **(C)** Although there is a history of previous thyroid cancer, the presence of a solitary nodule on chest x-ray is more likely to represent a primary carcinoma of the lung than a solitary secondary metastasis. In metastasis, the lesions are more often multiple, they frequently appear bilaterally, and they more commonly present in the

lower area of the lungs. A CT scan would be helpful in delineating the pulmonary findings.

14. **(C)** The most likely diagnosis, malignant epithelioma, commonly occurs following chronic (> 20–40 years) exposure to asbestos. We need to consider this diagnosis in those employed in milling and construction, as well as in workers in pipe, textiles, gaskets, and other industries in which asbestos (especially crocidolite form) is used. In 75%, the diffuse (malignant) form occurs; fewer than 25% will survive more than 1 year after the diagnosis is established. In advanced disease, lesions below the diaphragm are frequently encountered.

15. **(C)** Cystic fibrosis is the most common cause of chronic obstructive lung disease (COLD) in children and adolescents. It is an autosomal-recessive disease that affects widespread exocrine glands. COLD is evident in all patients who survive childhood. (See Figure 9–3).

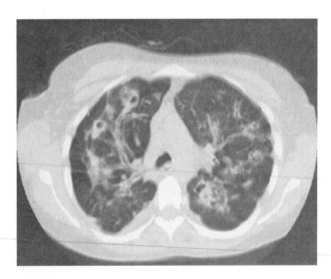

Figure 9–3. X-ray of chest shows typical tree and bud sign attributed to mucus plugs occluding the bronchioles. Bronchioles thickened with cyst formation. Patient with cystic fibrosis.

16. **(A)** Ipratropium bromide bronchodilator therapy will frequently improve pulmonary function in patients with COPD. Two to four inhalations every 4–6 hours are prescribed. COPD is due to emphysema (COPD type A) or chronic bronchitis (COPD type B). In the early stages, small airway dysfunction (abnormal closing volume) is

found. As the disease proceeds, the FEV_1 is reduced, then the FEV_1/FVC ratio (< 0.7).

17. **(C)** The presence of multiple masses on a chest x-ray should alert the physician to the possible diagnosis of pulmonary AV fistula. Needle biopsy and endobronchial biopsy of the lesion should *not* be attempted, because severe hemorrhage may be precipitated. Paradoxical emboli, brain abscess, and hemothorax are recognized complications. If the fistula is localized, resection is undertaken; in multiple lesions, therapeutic embolization is done. In addition to AV malformation, multiple masses on a chest x-ray could be due to metastasis, granulomatous infection, or sarcoid or rheumatoid arthritis.

18. **(D)** In mediastinal tamponade, hypotension, dyspnea, cyanosis, and a decrease in pulse pressure will be evident. During inspiration, the pulse pressure is further impeded to cause obstruction to transmitted ACV waves in the neck; in congestive cardiac failure, the ACV waves recorded in the neck are more prominent. Paresis of the arm is unlikely to occur, because the lower part of the brachial plexus (T1) passes along the inner border of the first rib to reach the neck.

19. **(B)** Mediastinal hemorrhage after trauma may result from blunt or penetrating injuries. Tamponade should be suspected if hypotension, cyanosis, dyspnea, and venous congestion occur.

20. **(B)** Dissecting thoracic aneurysm should be suspected in Marfan's syndrome, pregnancy, bicuspid aortic valves, and coarctation. The onset of pain is sudden and severe and radiates to the back. Pulse discrepancy is frequently seen. The hypertension should be treated initially before any surgery is contemplated. The mortality rate of immediate (within 24 hours) surgical resection of the ascending aorta (type A) is 20%; however, if surgery is delayed, the mortality is 50% at 2 weeks and 90% at 3 months.

21. **(E)** The 11th and 12th ribs are free anteriorly and like other ribs articulate with costal cartilage anteriorly. However, the anterior margins of these ribs are free (float) and do not form part of the costal margins. The pleural reflection

posteriorly intersects the 12th rib. Ribs that articulate with the sternum are called true (ribs 1–6 or 7); the remainder are called false ribs.

22. **(D)** In ARDS, poor alveolar gas exchange and interstitial edema are evident in the presence of normal or lowered PCWP. The changes are caused by damage to capillary and alveolar epithelial cells consequent to the release of pro-inflammatory cytokines, which in turn arise from stimulated lymphocytes and macrophages. Other clinical features suggestive of ARDS are diffuse ("fluffy") pulmonary infiltrates and refractory hypoxemia ($P_AO_2/FIO_2 < 200$).

23. **(C)** ARDS is caused by pulmonary or systemic insult. It is characterized by bilateral pulmonary infiltrates, hypoxemia, noncompliant lungs, and a normal or low PCWP, and steroids have no proved value in the management of ARDS, and their use may be deleterious in the presence of sepsis. PEEP, if required, should be used cautiously with the lowest FIO_2 that maintains the PO_2 above 60 mmHg. Excessive fluid overload should be avoided. Ventilation with lower tidal volumes and decreasing peak airway pressures. Management strategies in ARDS are aimed largely at supportive care, maintaining tissue oxygenation and preventing further lung injury secondary to mechanical ventilation. Smaller tidal volumes are used (5–7 mL/kg) to prevent volutrauma as well as to decrease the peak inspiratory pressures.

24. **(E)** Culture for mycobacterium usually requires 6 weeks before a diagnosis can be made. The clinical and x-ray features are suggestive of tuberculosis. The sedimentation rate is increased in the presence of active disease. The incidence of tuberculosis in the United States has increased in recent years. In many cases of primary infection, resolution occurs without symptoms. The pulmonary focus remains dormant (Ghon) and may become activated, causing caseation of the lung, formation of a thick-walled fibrous cavity, tuberculous bronchitis, bronchiectasis, hemoptysis, and cavitation. Sputum examined for acid-fast bacilli may be inadequate, because saprophytic organisms may be detected. The Kweim test is used in the differential diagnosis to exclude sarcoid.

25. **(D)** In the early stages of HIV infection, skin testing for tuberculin is intact; however, false-positive results occur because of infection by nontuberculous mycobacteria and false-negative results are common because of the immune disorder. Most patients with tuberculosis who are compliant can be treated on an outpatient basis.

26. **(B)** Bronchiectasis is caused by a congenital or acquired dilation of the segmental, subsegmental, or branches of the bronchi. Patients with B lymphocyte disorders are more likely to develop lower respiratory tract infection and bronchiectasis than those with impaired T-cell immunity. Treatment is aimed at obtaining maximal drainage. Resection may be indicated when the disease is localized and persistent symptoms and complications occur.

27. **(A)** Cystic fibrosis is an autosomal-recessive disorder of the exocrine glands and occurs in neonates who survive an episode of intestinal obstruction due to mucoviscidosis. Cystic fibrosis accounts for more than one-half of the cases of bronchiectasis seen today. Other causes include acute and chronic lung infections, humoral immunodeficiency, and localized bronchial obstruction (e.g., carcinoma). The basal segments of the lung, lingula, and right middle lobes are involved most frequently.

28. **(C)** Bronchogenic cysts are located in the mediastinum but are seen most frequently behind the carina. They have a thin wall, are lined by bronchial epithelium, and contain mucus. Bronchogenic cysts are usually asymptomatic, but symptoms may occur because of compression, with cough, wheezing, and possibly dysphagia. Bronchogenic cysts may become infected and rupture into surrounding organs. Cysts constitute 20% of mediastinal mass lesions. The most common mediastinal cyst is the pericardial cyst, which is found most often at the right costophrenic angle.

29. **(D)** Bronchopulmonary sequestration can be differentiated from a bronchogenic cyst in that it is composed of nonfunctioning lung tissue that is disconnected from the remaining lung; it has a separate blood supply. Glomus tumors

are rare tumors that arise in the middle ear or jugular bulb. Patients complain of tinnitus and hearing loss.

30. **(D)** There are three major openings of structures that penetrate the diaphragm at differing thoracic vertebra levels. The IVC enters at T8 (to the right of the midline), the esophagus at T10 (to the left of the midline), and the aorta at T12 in the midline.

31. **(A)** Funnel chest is the most important congenital chest wall deformity. It is usually present at birth, and there is marked asymmetry. The heart is displaced to the left. There is often a familial history, and associated congenital heart disease may frequently be encountered. Correction is recommended in asymptomatic patients with prominent deformity to avoid permanent cardiopulmonary changes. In flail chest, paradoxical respiration occurs as the chest wall deformity is sucked inward during inspiration. It occurs after extensive rib trauma where individual ribs are separated in two different sites.

32. **(A)** Any object that compromises the blood supply to the tracheal mucosa or cartilage can cause stenosis. When the mean intramural pressure exceeds 20–30 mmHg, damage may be anticipated. Riedel struma is a rare fibrosing thyroid condition, which must be differentiated from carcinoma and may cause severe tracheal stenosis. Achalasia is a neuromuscular defect at the lower end of the esophagus causing dysphagia, because of nonmechanical esophageal obstruction.

33. **(A)** On the left side, the pleural reflection deviates to the left anteriorly between the fourth and sixth costal cartilages to accommodate the cardiac notch. Although the right and left pleural reflections approach each other in the midline, there is no direct communication between the two sides.

34. **(D)** Frequently, a fracture cannot be seen on the chest x-ray; however, the patient should be treated for fracture, although none is seen on the x-ray. Pneumothorax may occur if more than one rib is involved, but a chest tube is indicated only if it is of substantial size or increasing in amount. Hemothorax usually occurs because of a tear in the intercostal or other intrathoracic vessels.

35. **(D)** A thoracoabdominal incision is still used occasionally where access to both the upper abdomen and posterior thoracic structures is required. The main reasons for less frequent use of this incision are poor healing of the divided costal margin, postoperative pain, and an increased risk of infection in both the thoracic and abdominal compartments.

36. **(B)** Sternal injuries usually involve the body or manubriosternal junction in a transverse direction and frequently cause displacement. Sternal injuries occur most commonly as a result of injury by steering wheel impact in car accidents. It is important to exclude cardiac and major vessel injury in such injuries.

37. **(B)** Most lesions of the trachea (except infiltrating adenoid cystic carcinoma) that cause tracheal stenosis should be resected when possible. In general, up to 50% of the trachea may be resected. Unequivocal postintubation stenosis is treated by surgical repair. Congenital tracheal stenosis should be treated by surgery if symptoms necessitate it.

38. **(B)** Patients with hyperparathyroidism develop demineralization, and 1.5% show osteitis fibrosa cystica. The presence of subperiosteal resorption of bone of the phalanges and lamina dura of the teeth are fairly diagnostic radiological findings of hyperparathyroidism. Chondromas account for 20% of benign tumors of the rib and occur at the costochondral junction. Osteochondromas arise from the cortex and usually occur in men. Eosinophilic granuloma results in a destructive lesion apparent on x-ray.

39. **(D)** Antibiotics and vigorous attempts to obtain bronchial drainage will treat the abscess adequately in the majority of cases. Lung abscesses commonly are associated with aspiration pneumonia, where the abscess is found posteriorly. In the presence of an unexplained lung abscess, bronchoscopy is essential to exclude a

foreign body or tumor that could cause bronchial obstruction.

40. **(B)** Branchial cleft cysts (Figure 9–4) arise from the second and third branchial clefts. Branchial cysts may become evident after an URTI and present as a mass anterior to the sternocleidomastoid muscle. Intraoperatively, they can be traced to pass between the internal and external carotid artery to the piriform sinus or tonsillar fossa.

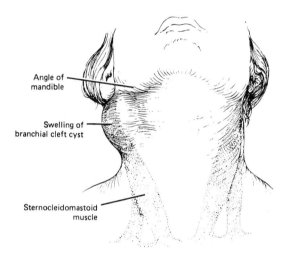

Figure 9–4. Branchial cyst. (Reproduced, with permission, from Lindner, HH: Clinical Anatomy, Appleton & Lange, 1989.)

41. **(C)** Cystic hygromas are relatively rare tumors. Most are encountered in the posterior triangle of the neck, but occasionally they are found in the mediastinum, axilla, or groin. They are often noted at birth and represent persistence of primary lymphatic buds. They extend into the surrounding tissues but are not associated with malignancy. Transillumination is a useful sign to diagnose this lesion.

42. **(D)** Females are affected by myasthenia gravis twice as commonly as males. It is an autoimmune disease that produces antibodies to acetylcholine receptors. The external ocular and other cranial muscles are often involved at an early stage. There is a deficiency in acetylcholine receptors, and thymectomy is often helpful.

43. **(D)** Squamous carcinoma of the lip comprises 15–20% of all malignant tumors of the oral cav-

ity. In approximately 30%, there is a clear association with heavy exposure to the sun. The incidence increases in those areas where there is a more southerly latitude, the air is dry, and the altitude is higher.

44. **(C)** If the lesion is treated early, patients will achieve a cure in most cases. The upper lip is involved in 10% of patients.

45. **(C)** Hyperkeratosis of the lip is a premalignant lesion and usually occurs in people exposed excessively to the sun. The mucosa undergoes metaplasia to keratosquamous epithelium. The lip becomes pale, thin, and fragile, with cracks and fissures, and is covered with a white base.

46. **(D)** Ameloblastoma is a benign tumor and usually occurs at the junction of the body and ramus of the mandible. Although it is a benign tumor, it recurs if inadequately excised. It is relatively radioresistant. Histologically, odontogenic epithelium is seen in connective tissue stroma with extensive areas of cystic degeneration.

47. **(E)** Papillary cystadenoma lymphomatosum is also called Warthin's tumor. It occurs mainly in men. The epithelial component is interspersed with lymphoid tissue that shows germinal centers. The most common tumor of the parotid gland is a pleomorphic adenoma, with papillary cystadenoma (although much less frequent) as the second most common tumor.

48. **(B)** The lingual nerve swings forward deep to the mylohyoid muscle and crosses twice over the submandibular (Wharton's) duct. The mandibular branch of the facial nerve (not listed in the answer choices) may accidentally be injured below the angle of the mandible (Figure 9–5). Injury to this branch causes serious facial deformity.

49. **(C)** Squamous cell carcinoma of the tongue frequently (40–60%) metastasizes to the lymph glands. Carcinoma of the tongue usually commences at the tip or side. The 5-year survival rate for carcinoma of the tongue is 40%, but it improves to 55% if lymph nodes are not involved.

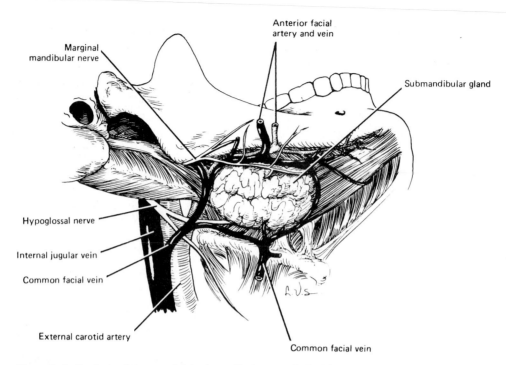

Marginal
mandibular nerve

Anterior facial
artery and vein

Submandibular gland

Hypoglossal nerve

Internal jugular vein

Common facial vein

External carotid artery

Common facial vein

Figure 9–5. Contents of the superficial submandibular area. An incision over the lower border of the mandible where it is crossed by the facial artery may sever the mandibular branch of the facial nerve and result in severe deformity. (Reproduced, with permission, from Lindner, HH: Clinical Anatomy, Appleton & Lange, 1989.)

50. (B) Carcinoma of the posterior third of the tongue is often detected late and carries a worse prognosis. Posterior-third tongue tumors are also called lymphoepitheliomas.

51. (A) Tumors of the hard palate usually arise from the minor salivary glands. Posterior-third tongue tumors are also called lymphoepitheliomas.

52. (A) Poorly differentiated squamous cell carcinoma of the floor of the mouth tends to be more invasive than better differentiated tumors. Poorer prognosis can be expected when invasion is larger than 9 mm, perineural invasion is noted, and lymph node metastasis is evident.

53. (C) Nasopharyngeal carcinoma is prevalent in China. It has been associated with high levels of Epstein–Barr virus titers. The most common sign is a neck mass, even when the primary lesion is microscopic. The first cranial nerve to be affected is the abducent (VI) and indicates cranial extension.

54. (D) Any object that compromises the blood supply to the tracheal mucosa or cartilage can cause stenosis. When the mean intramural pressure exceeds 20–30 mmHg over a prolonged period, damage occurs.

55. (A) Verrucous carcinoma is a low-grade malignancy and is seen more frequently in the southern part of the United States. It is found most commonly on the gingival–buccal junction in tobacco chewers. It is grayish white and exophytic. Radiation is associated with possible metastases. If not excised, the lesion tends to invade locally.

56. (D) Juvenile nasopharyngeal hemangiofibromas are rare nonmalignant tumors containing both fibrous and vascular tissue. They occur exclusively among boys.

57. (C) If the neck nodes are removed, some patients have surgically curable primary disease. In some series, as many as 20% remain free of disease for more than 5 years without any manifestation of a primary tumor. It is essential to search extensively for a primary source before labeling the lesion as a possible branchial cleft carcinoma, which is extremely rare.

58. **(D)** More than 80% of neck gland tumors arise from structures above the clavicle. The piriform fossa is lateral to the aryepiglottic folds and is a major site that a primary cancer may remain hidden from early detection. Twenty percent of neck gland tumors are primary and 80% represent metastatic disease.

59. **(D)** The response is transient, lasting only 2–3 months. The results of this type of therapy, combined with those of artery occlusion, radiotherapy, or other modes of chemotherapy, require further evaluation.

60. **(B)** The classic block dissection includes sternocleidomastoid muscle, the external and internal jugular veins, the spinal accessory nerve, the submandibular gland, and the lymphatic tissue of the lateral compartment of the neck. Procedures that preserve muscle, nerve, or vessels are called modified neck dissection.

61. **(B)** The chorda tympani (branch of the facial nerve) joins the lingual nerve in the infratemporal fossa to supply the anterior two-thirds of the tongue with taste fibers (cell stations in the geniculate ganglion of the facial nerve). It also contains the secretory parasympathetic fibers to the submandibular and sublingual glands.

62. **(D)** The thymus gland is removed in certain cases of myasthenia gravis. It is located in the anterior mediastinum and can be approached by a cervical or mediastinal approach. It arises from the third and fourth branchial arches. Pneumococcal infections are particularly likely to develop after splenectomy performed in children.

63. **(A)** The most common organisms isolated in acute pharyngitis are streptococci, virus, *Neisseria gonorrhoeae,* and mycoplasma.

64. **(C)** Odynophagia is a sensation of sharp retrosternal pain on swallowing. It is usually caused by severe erosive conditions such as *Candida,*

herpesvirus, and corrosive injury following caustic ingestion.

65. **(B)** The most common source of epistaxis is Kisselbach's vascular plexus on the anterior nasal septum. Predisposing factors include foreign bodies, forceful nose-blowing, nose-picking, rhinitis, and deviated septum.

66. **(D)** Carotid body tumor is the most common type of paraganglioma in the head and neck region, followed by the glomus jugular tumor. Carotid body tumor grows slowly, rarely metastasizes, and may secrete catecholamines. The tumor usually is supplied by the external carotid artery, and dissection to remove it off the carotid bifurcation may be difficult and cause bleeding. Malignancy occurs in 6% of patients.

67. **(A)** Otitis media is a bacterial infection of the mucosally lined middle ear contained in the temporal bone. Purulent material spreads to the mastoid air cells and apex of petrous bone if pneumatized. In children and adults the most common pathogens are *Streptococcus pneumoniae, Haemophilus influenzae,* and *S. pyogenes.*

68. **(E)** Bell's palsy (of the facial nerve) has been attributed to an inflammatory condition of the facial nerve at the site where it exits through the stylomastoid foramen. Its cause remains unclear, and recent studies indicate a possible association with reactivation of herpes simplex virus in some cases. Facial paresis usually comes on abruptly.

69. **(B)** Prospective nonrandomized evaluations of treatment duration of acute otitis media reveal no difference in outcome if given over 5-day, 7-day, or 10-day duration. However, 10-day treatment is indicated for children with history of acute otitis media within the preceding month.

70. **(A)** Neuroleptic anesthesia is the use of agents that suppress psychomotor activity. Droperidol produces marked sedation and tranquilization. The onset of action is 3–10 min after injection, but the full effect may not be noted until 30 min after injection. The sedative action lasts 2–4 hours. It potentiates the action of central nervous system

(CNS)-depressant drugs, can cause hypotension, and causes mild α-adrenergic blockade.

71. **(C)** The most common complication of thyroid and parathyroid surgery is iatrogenic injury to the recurrent laryngeal nerve, which can result in temporary (up to 7.1%) or permanent (up to 3.6%) paralysis of the vocal cord.

72. **(B)** Laryngomalacia is characterized by inspiratory stridor and is caused by redundant epiglottis and aryepiglottic folds in young children. The condition usually resolves without surgical intervention.

73. **(B)** Jet irrigation (e.g., *Water Pik*) should be avoided to remove cerumen impaction. Detergent ear drops (such as 3% hydrogen peroxide) may be used. Aqueous irrigation should be avoided if organic material is present, because further swelling will be induced.

74. **(A)** The presence of a nasogastric tube causes swelling and irritation of the nasal mucosa. This, in turn, may partly occlude drainage of the sinus into the meatus.

75. **(B)** Foreign bodies in the ear canal are more frequently encountered in children than adults. In general, foreign bodies in the ear are removed under microscopic control to avoid further injury.

76. **(D)** Rapid testing for streptococci with latex agglutination (LA) antigen test is much less sensitive than with solid-phase enzyme-linked immunoassay (ELISA).

77. **(B)** Pharyngeal (branchial arch) remnants account for many cysts or fistulas in the lateral neck. The associated tract can be found in various locations. Thyroglossal duct cysts associated with the decent of the thyroid gland are usually midline, extending as high as the base of tongue.

78. **(A)** Epistaxis in children and young adults usually arises from the anterior nasal septum (Kiesselbach's plexus). In elderly persons, however, spontaneous rupture of a sclerotic blood vessel in the posterior nasal septum is usually the cause of bleeding, especially in combination with hypertension.

79. **(A)** Tinnitus is the perception of abnormal noise in the ear or head. It is usually attributed to a sensory loss; pulsatile tinnitus occurs with conductive hearing loss and is due to carotid pulsation's becoming more apparent.

80. **(E)** Surgical drainage of otitis media (myringotomy) is performed in either chronic infections or severe infections. Complications of otitis media include mastoiditis and meningitis.

81. **(E)** These may be difficult to excise because of the focal nerve involvement by the hemangioma.

82. **(E)** Blowout fractures of the orbit exhibit all of the above-noted findings. Subcutaneous emphysema and periorbital ecchymosis are also frequently encountered. Treatment of most severe injuries is by surgical repair, often by a lower lid blepharoplasty incision.

83. **(C)** Unlike the other sinuses, the ethmoid sinus is well developed at birth. The maxillary and sphenoid sinuses continue to develop into puberty. Frontal sinusitis is usually not encountered prior to 6 years of age.

84. **(E)** Tympanostomy tube placement is performed through the external auditory canal with microscopic guidance. The tympanic membrane is directly visualized after clearing wax and debris from external auditory canal. Otorrhea is the most common sequela, requiring tube removal in 13.5% of long-term tubes and 0.9% of short-term tubes.

85. **(C)** The external laryngeal nerve supplies the cricothyroid muscle, which assists in tensing the cords.

86. **(A)** Scrofula is tuberculosis lymphadenitis. It may occur in immunocompromised hosts as well as in patients from underdeveloped countries. A chest x-ray must be obtained and a purified protein derivative (PPD) skin test must be

carried out. The response rate to antituberculous drugs is good, but excision of the residual lesion may be required.

87. **(D)** Mucor is an opportunistic mold that causes mucormycosis. At least 50% of reported cases are associated with uncontrolled diabetes, and many of the rest of the patients are immunosuppressed. It appears as black crusting in the nose and sinuses and spreads rapidly to involve the cerebrum. Biopsy reveals nonseptate hyphae, which confirms the diagnosis. Treatment is directed toward control for diabetic ketoacidosis and use of amphotericin B.

88. **(B)** Dermoid cysts arise along line of fusion of embryonic parts. In the floor of the mouth, the swelling forces the tongue upward. Alternatively, the swelling may occur below the mylohyoid muscle, where it gives the impression of a double chin. It is not a premalignant lesion. It has an epithelial lining and may contain secretions, sloughed-off cells, and hair.

89. **(D)** In Peutz–Jegher syndrome, pigmented melanin spots are found in the buccal and perineal region. The lesions are flat and greenish black in the buccal region and remain after puberty. Pigmentation is found inside the mouth, nostrils, palms, and feet. Usually at about 20–30 years of age, hamartomatous polyps are found in the small intestine, but other parts of the alimentary tract may also be involved. Adenocarcinoma develops in 23% of patients.

90. **(D)** Benign mixed tumor (pleomorphic adenoma) requires appropriate excision (superficial parotidectomy). If the tumor is shelled out, recurrence is likely. Approximately 80% of tumors of the salivary glands occur in the parotid gland.

91. **(B)** The trigeminal nerve exits from the foramen ovale to enter the infratemporal fossa. The motor mandibular division of cranial nerve V also exits through the same opening.

92. **(A)** If the thyroid gland is absent from the neck, it may be in the lingual position at the foramen cecum. Excision of this lesion from the tongue will require thyroid hormone replacement.

93. **(B)** Nasopharyngeal cancer is most closely associated with Epstein–Barr virus. This virus is also associated with infective mononucleosis and Burkitt's lymphoma.

94. **(E)** If the tumor should extend upward into the sphenoid bone, the cavernous sinus may be involved.

95. **(B)** The tip of the tongue drains into the submental lymph nodes, whereas, the side of the tongue drains into the submandibular lymph nodes.

96. **(G)** Dermoid cysts form along lines of fusion of embryological dermatomes of the skin. In the neck, they are commonly above the thyroid cartilage and may be classified as one of four varieties according to whether they are central in the midline or lateral and whether they are above or below the mylohyoid muscle.

97. **(G)** The thyroid develops from the foramen cecum in the tongue and descends to its definitive position in the neck. Failure of the tract to close may result in a thyroglossal duct cyst.

CHAPTER 10

Neurosurgery
Questions

Jose A. Torres-Gluck and Virany Huynh Hillard

DIRECTIONS (Questions 1 through 50): Each of the numbered items or incomplete statements in this section is followed by answers or by completions of the statement. Select the ONE lettered answer or completion that is BEST in each case.

1. A 43-year-old man experiences lower back pain after lifting a heavy object off the ground. The following morning, he notices that the pain has begun to radiate down the posterolateral aspect of the right leg and across the top of the foot to the big toe. The pain is severe, electric in quality, associated with paresthesia over the same distribution, and made worse by coughing. On examination, it is found that he has an area of diminished sensation to pinprick over the dorsum of the right foot and mild weakness in his right extensor hallucis longus muscle. The deep tendon reflexes are all intact. What is the most likely diagnosis?

    (A) lumbar spinal fracture with compression of the cauda equina
    (B) herniated lumbar disk on the right at the level of L4–L5
    (C) herniated lumbar disk on the left at the level of L4–L5
    (D) herniated lumbar disk on the right at the level of S1–S2
    (E) intermittent claudication

2. A 48-year-old woman has a lower back pain and hypoesthesia in the left S1 dermatomal distribution (left calf and lateral left foot). What is the most likely cause?

    (A) a lesion at the right L4–L5 interspace
    (B) pathology where the nerve exits the spinal canal immediately above the pedicle of S3 vertebra
    (C) a herniated nucleus pulposus
    (D) compression by the L5 lamina
    (E) a lesion outside the vertebral column

3. A 35-year-old secretary complains of severe pain in the neck that radiates down the right arm. The pain is electric in quality and affects specifically the radial aspect of the right forearm and the thumb. She also describes numbness and paresthesia over the same distribution. On physical examination, she is found to have an area of diminished sensation to pinprick over the right wrist and thumb. The right biceps tendon reflex is diminished, but there is no loss of muscle strength. She has right C5–C6 disk compression and radiculopathy affecting which of the following?

    (A) the right C4 root
    (B) the right C4 mixed spinal nerve
    (C) the right C4 anterior primary rami
    (D) the right C6 root
    (E) the right C6 spinal ganglion

Questions 4 and 5

A 47-year-old man presents to the emergency department after falling from his bicycle. He claims that his neck was suddenly and violently hyperflexed. Although he is currently complaining of neck pain, his chief complaint is weakness of the arms. On examination, he is found to have profound symmetric weakness of both hands and wrists. His biceps and triceps are moderately weak. The lower extremities are only minimally weak, and he is able to ambulate, albeit with some difficulty. His sensation to all modalities is within normal limits. Plain radiographs of his neck reveal no fracture or dislocation, but there is evidence of severe spondylosis with osteophytes narrowing the neural canal at C3–C4, C4–C5, and C5–C6.

4.   What is the most likely mechanism of injury?

   (A) brachial plexus injury
   (B) epidural hematoma
   (C) contusion of the spinal cord
   (D) external carotid artery occlusion
   (E) internal jugular vein occlusion

5.   What is this pattern of motor findings that results from this injury termed?

   (A) central cord syndrome
   (B) cervical radiculopathy
   (C) cauda equina syndrome
   (D) Lhermitte sign
   (E) Erb's palsy

Questions 6 and 7

A 57-year-old woman is referred to you for evaluation of difficulty with ambulation. Her chief complaint is weakness of her left leg that has been slowly progressive over the last 6 months. On neurologic examination, her mental status and cranial nerve findings are within normal limits. She has marked (grade 4–5) weakness of both her left leg and arm. On her left side, she has diminished sensation to light touch and vibration below the C5 dermatome. Sensation to pinprick and temperature are severely diminished on the right side below approximately the C8 dermatome. Her deep tendon reflexes and muscle tone are increased on the left.

6.   This pattern of neurologic deficits is which of the following?

   (A) spondylolisthesis
   (B) Brown–Sequard syndrome
   (C) central cord syndrome
   (D) Guillain–Barré syndrome
   (E) poliomyelitis

7.   This pattern of neurologic deficits is explained by injury to the spinal cord with damage to which of the following?

   (A) anterior horn cells
   (B) peripheral part
   (C) central canal
   (D) right half (right hemicord)
   (E) left half (left hemicord)

8.   A 73-year-old man presents for evaluation of weakness in his lower extremities and recurrent falls. On further questioning, the patient admits to having frequent spasms affecting both of his lower extremities. He also claims that his legs occasionally feel as if ants were crawling all over them. On neurological examination, he is found to have a slightly unstable gait and with minimal flexion of the knees. His strength is slightly but symmetrically diminished in both lower extremities and both triceps muscles. There is decreased sensation to vibration and light touch below approximately the level of the nipples bilaterally. In both lower extremities, muscle tone is markedly increased, and deep tendon reflexes are hyperactive. Babinski reflex is present bilaterally. What is the most likely diagnosis?

   (A) a thoracic spinal cord compression
   (B) a thoracic radiculopathy
   (C) a cervical myelopathy
   (D) cerebellar tumor
   (E) intracranial aneurysm

9.   An 87-year-old woman is referred to you for evaluation of lower back pain. It is exacerbated by walking or prolonged standing and occasionally made better by bending over. Physical examination reveals a thin elderly woman who

walks with a cane with her lower back moderately flexed. Motor power in her lower extremities is normal, but she has impaired sensation to light touch and vibration below the L4 dermatome bilaterally. Deep tendon reflexes are normal in her upper extremities but absent in both lower extremities. You refer her for magnetic resonance imaging (MRI) of the lumbosacral spine. What will be the most likely finding on this study?

(A) lumbar spinal stenosis

(B) a fracture of the odontoid process

(C) a herniated L3–L4 disk causing unilateral compression of the L4 root

(D) spinal cord compression at the level of L1 vertebra level

(E) spinal cord compression at the T1 vertebra level

10. A 33-year-old man is brought to the emergency department after being involved in a major motor vehicle accident. He is unable to move his legs and complains of severe pain in his mid- to lower back. On physical examination, he is found to have exquisite tenderness over some of the bony prominence of his lower back, but no gross physical deformity can be appreciated. On neurologic examination, flaccid paralysis of both lower extremities and complete anesthesia to all sensory modalities below approximately the L3 dermatome are noted. Catheterization of his bladder yields approximately 700 mL of urine. Plain radiographs of the spine reveal compression fracture in the body of L3 with greater than 50% of loss in its height. A computed tomography (CT) scan through this area reveals a burst fracture of the body of L3. There are large fragments of bone driven dorsally with an 80% canal compromise. What is the cause of weakness?

(A) compression of the conus medullaris

(B) compression of the spinal cord at the level of L3

(C) compression of the cauda equina

(D) rupture of the anterior spinal ligament

(E) associated epidural hemorrhage

Questions 11 and 12

A 17-year-old boy suffers a hyperextension injury of his neck when he jumps head-first into a shallow pool. He does not lose consciousness. He arrives at the emergency department holding his neck stiffly and complaining of severe neck pain. He says the pain is particularly severe whenever he tries to move his head. He says he has no neurologic symptoms such as weakness, numbness, or paresthesia. On physical examination, he is found to have no areas of ecchymosis or deformity on the cervical spine. He has exquisite pain on deep palpation of the bony prominence of the midcervical spine. There are no neurological signs. Routine plain radiographs (anteroposterior [AP], lateral, open-mouth view) of the cervical spine in the neutral position show no fracture or subluxation of the bony elements. There is, however, thickening of the pretracheal space ventral to the body of C6, suggesting soft-tissue swelling.

11. What would the next step in management involve?

(A) analgesics alone

(B) a hard cervical collar

(C) internal fixation of the cervical vertebra

(D) burr holes and traction

(E) plaster cast to face, neck, and thorax

12. What would be the most appropriate radiologic examination?

(A) plain lateral radiographs in flexion and extension to rule out occult ligamentous tear and instability of the cervical spine

(B) a CT scan of the cervical spine to rule out the possibility of a bony fracture not seen on plain radiographs

(C) lateral tomogram of the cervical spine to rule out the possibility of an occult fracture

(D) angiography

(E) ultrasound of the neck

Questions 13 and 14

A 63-year-old woman with a history of local inoperable breast cancer is referred to you for the evaluation of new-onset diplopia. Upon questioning, she admits that her diplopia occurs mostly when she attempts to look at objects in the distance and when she attempts to look toward the left side. In addition, she reports having severe headaches and an electric-type discomfort affecting her right deltoid region for approximately 3 weeks. On neurologic examination, she is found to have left abducens (sixth) nerve palsy; the rest of her cranial nerves are intact. She also has mild weakness of the right deltoid and a diminished biceps tendon jerk on the same side. Findings on an MRI of the brain with intravenous contrast are unremarkable.

13. In this patient, what would be the most likely site where metastasis occurs?

    (A) brain
    (B) orbital cavity
    (C) meninges
    (D) cerebellum
    (E) optic chiasm

14. What would the next step in management involve?

    (A) an MRI of the cervical spine to rule out metastatic deposits within the cervical roots
    (B) a CT scan of the brain with intravenous contrast
    (C) a lumbar puncture to measure opening pressure and obtain cerebrospinal fluid (CSF) for cytologic analysis
    (D) repeated breast biopsy
    (E) no further tests until further symptoms develop

15. A 57-year-old woman presents to the emergency department with new-onset seizures. She was witnessed by her husband to have a generalized seizure lasting approximately 1 minute. She has smoked 1 pack of cigarettes a day for over 40 years. In the past 3 months, she has lost 25 lbs in weight. On examination, she appears thin and nervous but findings on her neurologic examination are otherwise essentially within normal limits. Plain radiographs of the chest obtained in the emergency department show a 4-cm nodule in the upper lobe of her right lung. To exclude cerebral metastasis as a cause of her seizure, what should the next test requested be?

    (A) an electroencephalogram (EEG)
    (B) a CT scan of the brain with intravenous contrast
    (C) a spinal tap to measure opening pressure and obtain CSF for cytology
    (D) an MRI of the brain with intravenous contrast
    (E) Doppler ultrasound

Questions 16 and 17

A 58-year-old woman is admitted from the emergency department with a history of approximately 2 weeks of headache. She has a history of breast cancer. Her headache is severe, particularly in the mornings when she wakes up. It is accompanied by occasional vomiting. She says she experiences no focal weakness, numbness, or paresthesia. On physical examination, she is found to have a mild weakness of her left arm. An MRI of the brain with intravenous contrast reveals the presence of a neoplasm in the right motor cortex that is considered responsible for her weakness.

16. If the MRI shows multiple brain metastases, what should be the treatment required in addition to corticosteroids?

    (A) whole-brain radiotherapy
    (B) craniotomy to resect the lesion responsible for her left arm weakness
    (C) chemotherapy
    (D) placement of an Ommaya reservoir for use in treatment by intrathecal chemotherapy
    (E) no further treatment

17. If the MRI shows a single brain metastasis, what should be the next step in management?

    (A) whole-brain radiotherapy
    (B) craniotomy to resect the lesion responsible for her left arm weakness
    (C) chemotherapy
    (D) placement of an Ommaya reservoir for use in treatment by intrathecal chemotherapy
    (E) no further treatment

18. A 63-year-old woman presents with a several-week history of headaches and difficulties with speech. A sister who lives with her claims that her language "has recently not been making much sense" and that she is a bit confused. Her condition seems to be deteriorating. On neurologic examination, she has a moderately severe aphasia, with difficulty understanding language and following commands, and she makes frequent paraphasic errors when she speaks. There are no other motor or sensory deficits. An MRI with intravenous contrast reveals the presence of a ring-enhancing mass lesion within the substance of the left temporal lobe. The lesion is approximately 3 cm in greatest diameter, poorly demarcated from the surrounding brain, and surrounded by a moderate amount of cerebral edema. Findings on routine admission tests, including a chest x-ray and serum chemistry, are unremarkable. What is the most likely diagnosis?

(A) low-grade cerebral astrocytoma

(B) glioblastoma multiforme

(C) metastasis to the brain from an occult primary cancer

(D) meningioma

(E) glomus tumor

19. A 64-year-old man presents with headache and left-sided upper extremity weakness. The MRI findings suggest that this is a glioblastoma multiforme. This is because the tumor exhibits which of the following?

(A) It is regular in shape.

(B) It is well demarcated from surrounding brain tissue.

(C) It shows a ring pattern of enhancement with intravenous contrast and has a nonenhancing necrotic center.

(D) It shows an absence of surrounding white-matter edema.

(E) It arises from the carotid body.

20. A 63-year-old woman presents for workup to determine the reason for a gradual hearing loss over approximately 5 years and intermittent tinnitus over the last several months. Findings on physical and neurologic examination are entirely within normal limits, except for the presence of sensorineural hearing loss in the left ear.

She has no cranial nerve deficits. An MRI of the brain with gadolinium reveals the presence of an extra-axial tumor in the region of the left cerebella–pontine angle. What is the most likely diagnosis?

(A) epidermoid tumor (cholesteatoma)

(B) glioblastoma multiforme

(C) meningioma

(D) acoustic neuroma

(E) glomus tumor

Questions 21 and 22

A 4-year-old boy is brought to the emergency department with the complaint of approximately 2 weeks of headache and vomiting. He was seen in the emergency department 1 week earlier with the same complaints. At that time, his parents were told that the probable cause was a gastrointestinal virus, and the boy was sent home. His symptoms have not improved. On general examination, the child appears somewhat dehydrated and has a dry mouth and sunken eyes. His examination findings are also remarkable for the presence of bilateral papilledema and marked nystagmus. An MRI with intravenous contrast is obtained that reveals the presence of a 2-cm mass in the posterior fossa. The mass is entirely within the fourth ventricle and appears to be arising from the vermis of the cerebellum. It enhances uniformly with contrast. The lateral and third ventricles are moderately dilated with hydrocephalus.

21. What is the most likely diagnosis?

(A) acoustic neuroma

(B) craniopharyngioma

(C) medulloblastoma

(D) brain metastasis

(E) polycystic cerebellar astrocytoma

22. If at craniotomy the tumor found is not that listed in question 21 and the pathologist reports that it is a benign lesion, what is that lesion?

(A) ependymoma

(B) choroid plexus papilloma

(C) polycystic (cystic) cerebellar astrocytoma

(D) teratoma

(E) dermoid cyst

Questions 23 and 24

A 5-year-old girl undergoes debulking of a medullo-blastoma. She undergoes a repeat MRI of the brain with intravenous contrast, which shows a small amount of enhancement consistent with limited residual tumor. She is given a full course of radiotherapy to the posterior fossa and does very well for 6 weeks, until she experiences difficulty in walking. Physical examination at this time indicates moderate weakness of both lower extremities (particularly on the right side) but strength in her upper extremities and cranial nerves are normal. Her sensation to light touch and vibration are intact, but she has diminished sensation to pinprick throughout her left leg.

23. What should be the next step in management?

    (A) repeat the MRI of the brain to rule out an early recurrence

    (B) obtain a single-photon-emission CT (SPECT) scan of the brain to rule out the possibility of radiation-induced toxicity

    (C) begin treatment with chemotherapy for the residual tumor within the brain

    (D) obtain an MRI or myelogram of the entire spinal axis to rule out the possibility of "drop metastases" from the medullo-blastoma

    (E) obtain an ultrasound of the lumbar spine

24. What should treatment of this girl involve?

    (A) removal of recurrent medulloblastoma and neck dissection

    (B) ventriculoperitoneal shunt

    (C) repeat irradiation to the posterior cranial fossa

    (D) complete craniospinal irradiation with local boosts to the areas where tumor nodules are detected

    (E) cortisone alone

25. A 35-year-old man is brought to the hospital unconscious after being resuscitated in an ambulance from the site of a motor vehicle accident. No other history or information is available. On general inspection, he is found to have multiple bruises over his body and has a massively swollen left thigh. His vital signs are stable with a heart rate of 100 beats per minute (bpm) and a

blood pressure of 150/75 mmHg. He is obtunded and does not follow commands or open his eyes. He withdraws his left arm and leg from painful stimuli, but not his right. His left pupil is 3 mm in diameter, and it is sluggishly reactive to light, while his right is 5 mm in diameter and fixed. Corneal reflexes are present bilaterally. His pulse rate is 120 bpm and respiration rate is 40 breaths per minute. To avoid injury to his spinal cord by an unstable cervical spine, an order is issued to not perform testing of his doll's eye reflex. Intracranial hemorrhage causing increased intracranial pressure (ICP) is suspected, along with a right uncal herniation. What is the next step in management?

    (A) intubation of his airway for hyperventilation and administration of intravenous mannitol

    (B) immediate CT scanning of the brain to confirm the presence of the suspected intracranial hemorrhage

    (C) intubation of his airway for hyperventilation and intravenous administration of corticosteroids

    (D) immediately evacuation of the suspected intracranial hematoma

    (E) controlled hypoventilation

26. In the management of a 64-year-old woman struck by a car, mannitol is given to do which of the following?

    (A) increase CSF formation

    (B) increase the respiratory rate

    (C) increase the pulse rate

    (D) replace extensive fluid loss

    (E) lower raised ICP

27. A 17-year-old boy is brought to the emergency department after he was assaulted. Witnesses claim what he was hit on the head with a lead pipe, after which he was unconscious for several minutes. No seizure activity was witnessed. On arrival, he complains of a headache, particularly severe at the point where he was hit in the right frontoparietal region. On examination, he is found to have swelling and ecchymosis over this region. He is awake, alert, and fully oriented. A complete neurologic examination reveals no deficit. Plain radiographs of the skull show a lin-

ear, nondepressed skull fracture in the frontoparietal skull that crosses the groove of the medial meningeal artery. During the following hour, he becomes sleepier and begins to vomit. A repeat neurologic examination at that time reveals him to be lethargic but without weakness, numbness, paresthesia, or other focal deficit. What is the most likely cause of the neurologic deterioration?

(A) diffuse axonal injury

(B) Todd's phenomenon

(C) subdural hematoma

(D) epidural hematoma

(E) trigeminal ganglion hematoma

28. Following a sudden impact in an accident, the 34-year-old race car driver becomes unconscious and is admitted to the hospital. A CT scan is performed, and a right space-occupying lesion is noted (Figure 10–1). What is the most likely diagnosis?

(A) corpus callosum injury

(B) pituitary apoplexia

(C) acute subdural hematoma

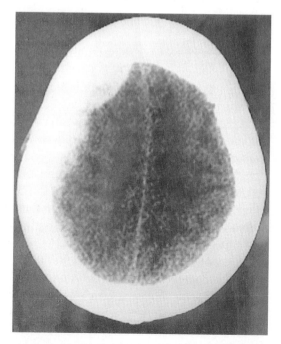

Figure 10–1. Horizontal computed tomography (CT) image through the head showing a high-density irregular layer covering the right hemispheres. (Reproduced, with permission, from Lindner, HH: Clinical Anatomy, Appleton & Lange, 1989.)

(D) acute epidural hematoma

(E) chronic subdural hematoma

29. A 44-year-old woman was brought to the emergency department after she was involved in a high-speed motor vehicle accident. She was extracted from the wreckage by paramedics. She was intubated at the site and rushed to the emergency department. On arrival, her blood pressure was 160/80 mmHg and heart rate was 100 bpm, and exam showed evidence of decerebrate rigidity. A CT scan of the head revealed small punctate hemorrhages in the corpus callosum and the midbrain tegmentum, but there was no mass effect on adjacent structures. The size of the ventricles was normal. This grave clinical presentation and these CT findings are most consistent with the diagnosis of which of the following?

(A) diffuse axonal injury (DAI)

(B) cerebral contusion

(C) cerebral concussion

(D) traumatic subarachnoid hemorrhage

(E) petrous temporal lobe fracture

30. A 43-year-old man presents to the emergency department after falling down a flight of stairs and landing on his head. He did not lose consciousness. He complains of severe headache, marked decreased acuity in hearing in the left ear, and a "runny nose" since the fall. On physical examination, he is found to have a left-sided Battle sign (an ecchymosis in the area of the left mastoid process) and hemotympanum. He has a constant dripping of a clear, watery fluid through his nose. Findings on his neurologic examination, other than the hearing loss, are completely normal. X-ray studies will reveal which of the following?

(A) a fracture of the cribriform plate with a CSF leak into the paranasal sinuses

(B) a skull-base fracture with a mucocele

(C) a temporal bone fracture with paradoxical rhinorrhea

(D) occipital bone fracture

(E) fracture of the maxillary antrum and greater wing of the sphenoid

31. A 52-year-old painter injured his lower back 3 weeks ago when he fell off his ladder. He presents for evaluation of abnormal findings on plain radiographs of his lumbar spine. His pain has subsided, and he is now asymptomatic. Physical examination reveals a dense tuft of hair in his lumbosacral region that has been present for as long as he can remember. There is no tenderness or palpable abnormality in his spine. Findings on his neurologic examination are unremarkable. The radiographs mentioned show absence of the spinous processes and laminae at the levels of L5 and S1, with their corresponding pedicle displaced and angled laterally. What is the diagnosis?

(A) an L5–S1 spondylolisthesis
(B) a burst fracture of L5 and S1
(C) spina bifida occulta
(D) spinal stenosis
(E) fracture of the vertebral bodies and nucleus pulposus

32. In the investigation of chronic back pain, a 72-year-old man is found on radiologic examination to have spondylolisthesis. The diagnosis is based upon disruption between two adjacent vertebra at which site?

(A) bodies and disks
(B) spinous process
(C) transverse process
(D) articular process
(E) pedicle

33. A baby is born with a 2.5- × 2.0-cm myelomeningocele in the mid- to lower lumbar region. Just hours after birth, he is rushed to the operating room (OR) for repair of this defect. Approximately 48 hours later, the baby is doing well, but it is noted that his head circumference has increased by 2 cm. On examination, the fontanelle is found to be slightly bulging and tense. On neurologic examination, the baby is awake but is found to have no spontaneous sensory or motor function below approximately the L3 dermatome. An ultrasound of the brain is obtained through the open fontanelle. This study shows an enlarged ventricular system, consistent with the presence of hydrocephalus.

What is the related abnormality responsible for the hydrocephalus?

(A) a fourth-ventricle ependymoma
(B) stenosis of the aqueduct of Sylvius
(C) amelia (failure of limbs to develop)
(D) Arnold–Chiari malformation
(E) nasopharyngeal hamartoma

34. A 4-month-old infant has undergone surgical treatment for meningomyeloencephalocele. A CT tomogram of head was made immediately after birth (see Figure 10–2). At birth, an operation was carried out in the posterior cranial fossa to partially replace brain cerebellar contents to an intracranial position. In investigations for progressive hydrocephalus, it is noted that there is herniation of the cerebellar tonsils through the foramen magnum, and a diagnosis of Arnold–Chiari syndrome is established. This syndrome may also include which of the following?

(A) fusion of the frontal lobes
(B) fusion of the temporal, parietal, and occipital lobes
(C) abnormal elongation of the medulla and lower cranial nerves
(D) partial or complete absence of the pituitary gland
(E) hypertrophy of cerebral lobes

35. During a regular visit to the pediatrician 1 week after birth, an infant's size and head circumference are recorded as being in the 75th percentile. Repeat measurement 1 month later still shows the size of the baby at the 75th percentile, but the baby's head circumference is now at the 95th percentile. The pediatrician notices that the baby's anterior fontanelle is tense and that the skull sutures are open. He obtains an MRI of the brain with intravenous contrast. This study shows the presence of greatly dilated lateral and third ventricles. The aqueduct of Sylvius cannot be easily visualized. The fourth ventricle is small. There are no lesions within the subarachnoid space or cerebral parenchyma. The appearance of the MRI is consistent with which of the following?

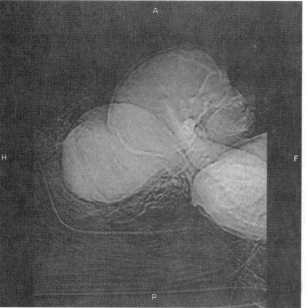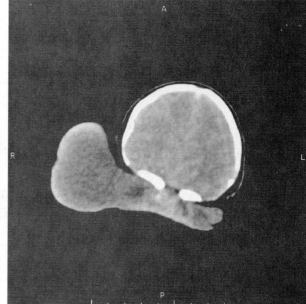

Figure 10–2. Tomogram from CT head taken 4 months previously (immediately after birth). Opening in the posterior cranial fossa showing brain and meninges protruding into sac (axial view).

(A) noncommunicating hydrocephalus

(B) communicating hydrocephalus

(C) normal-pressure hydrocephalus

(D) Arnold–Chiari malformation with herniation of the cerebellum into the foramen magnum

(E) anencephalus

36. A 64-year-old woman complains of severe headache and deterioration of mental status over the past several months. Her vision is normal. A CT scan reveals hydrocephalus, but the lumbar puncture pressure is unexpectedly low. What does she have?

(A) meningitis

(B) normal-pressure hydrocephalus

(C) sigmoid sinus thrombosis

(D) *Echinococcus*

(E) glioblastoma multiforme

37. A 23-year-old woman complains of progressive loss of vision. Investigations show normal findings on CT scan. A lumbar puncture shows elevation of pressure. What is the most likely diagnosis?

(A) pseudotumor cerebri

(B) corpus cavernous thrombosis

(C) cavernous sinus thrombosis

(D) retinoblastoma

(E) chordoma

38. During her eighth month of pregnancy, a 29-year-old woman is noted to have hydramnios. Further testing shows anencephalus. In this case hydramnios is caused by which of the following?

(A) impairment of the fetus's swallowing mechanism

(B) tumor of the fetus's brain

(C) a secretory peptide from the placenta

(D) excess antidiuretic hormone (ADH) from the fetus

(E) renal agenesis

39. A 28-year-old man presents with a history of chronic headache. The headache is intermittent, severe, poorly localized, and most often present when he arises in the morning. He suffered a severe blow to the head and sustained a skull fracture at the age of 15. Findings on his phys-

ical and neurologic examinations are within normal limits. An MRI of the brain with gadolinium reveals the presence of a large, nonenhancing extra-axial cyst in the region of the right temporal tip. This most likely represents which of the following?

(A) an arachnoid cyst

(B) a cystic astrocytoma

(C) Rathke's cleft cyst

(D) a Dandy–Walker cyst (failure of proper formation of the foramina of Lushka and Magendie)

(E) polycystic disease

40. A 15-year-old boy complains of right-sided weakness and gait impairment. A CT scan shows a large, nonenhancing cyst in the posterior cranial region, with an enhancing tumor nodule in the left cerebellum. What is the most likely diagnosis?

(A) an arachnoid cyst

(B) a cystic astrocytoma

(C) Rathke's cleft cyst

(D) glioblastoma multiforme

(E) a large sebaceous cyst

41. A 56-year-old woman presents with a history of several months of pain involving both hands. She describes the pain as electric and severe. It is localized to the palmar aspect of the first three digits of each hand and associated with numbness. The pain is particularly severe in the morning when she wakes up. She reports no weakness of the hands, but she says that sometimes objects fall off her hand because she cannot feel them. Physical examination reveals atrophy and weakness in the muscles of the thenar eminence bilaterally. She also has numbness in the distribution of the median nerve within the hands. You suspect carpal tunnel syndrome (CTS). Which is the best test to confirm this condition?

(A) an MRI of the hand to visualize an enlarged carpal ligament

(B) a nerve-conduction study to detect evidence of median nerve dysfunction in the hand

(C) an electromyogram (EMG) to quantify the degree of motor denervation in the muscles of the hand

(D) an x-ray of the hand

(E) none of the above

Questions 42–44

A 28-year-old police officer is brought to the emergency room by ambulance following a gunshot to the head. EMS reports that he was found unresponsive at the site of the shooting and was immersed in a pool of blood. There were no witnesses. On arrival to the emergency department, he is noted to have a bullet entry wound on the right frontal region without any exit wound. His blood pressure is 80/35, pulse rate 150/min, and on examination, he does not open his eyes or follow commands. He is unresponsive to deep painful stimuli such as testing by sternal rub. His pupils are dilated approximately 4 mm bilaterally, but sluggishly reactive. He is aggressively resuscitated with colloid and blood products. The blood pressure is now 140/75. There is improvement in his neurologic examination: 1 hour after admission, he withdraws his limbs from painful stimuli. A CT scan shows a small skull defect in the right frontal region, representing the bullet entry site. The bullet is lodged within the cerebral parenchyma, approximately 2 cm from the surface of the brain, and there is a trail of bone fragments along the bullet path. The bullet has not crossed the midline. There is a $2 \times 2 \times 2.5$-cm hematoma within the substance of the right frontal lobe with surrounding edema and subfalcian herniation.

42. Which item is *least* likely to be useful as a prognostic marker for subsequent recovery?

(A) neurologic examination upon presentation and early response

(B) the fact that the bullet did not cross the midline

(C) the presence of an intracerebral hematoma

(D) the presence of edema with sub-falcian herniation

(E) bullet crosses the midcoronal plane

43. What is the next step in management?

(A) administration of mannitol (1 g/kg) through a rapid IV infusion followed by the placement of an intracranial pressure monitor

(B) administration of mannitol (1 g/kg) through a rapid IV infusion followed by urgent craniotomy

(C) administration of mannitol (1 g/kg) through a rapid IV infusion followed by the placement of burr holes for emergent decompression of raised intracranial pressure

(D) no treatment should be administered, because the patient's prognosis is poor, and he is unlikely to survive

(E) anticoagulation

44. Intraoperative management of this patient should be avoidance of which of the following?

(A) placement of an intracranial pressure monitor

(B) performance of a wide craniotomy for evacuation of the intraparenchymal hematoma

(C) extensive debridement of all bullet and bone fragments

(D) reconstruction of the cranial defect caused by the bullet

(E) removal of necrotic brain material

Questions 45 and 46

A 54-year-old-man comes to the emergency department complaining of a severe headache for several hours. He describes the headache as the worst of his life. It started suddenly "like a firecracker had gone off" inside his head. He has had no loss of consciousness but has had several episodes of vomiting. General physical examination reveals a patient who is in severe distress due to the headache. His blood pressure is 180/70 mmHg, and his pulse racing at 120/min. He is afebrile. He has photophobia and gross neck rigidity. Neurologically, he is fully alert and oriented. He has a normal motor and sensory examination. His left pupil is 2 mm and briskly reactive to light; his right is 4.5 mm and fixed to both light and accommodation.

45. What is the most likely diagnosis?

(A) acute bacterial meningitis

(B) incipient uncal herniation due to an expanding lesion in the right temporal lobe

(C) acute subarachnoid hemorrhage from an anterior communicating artery aneurysm

(D) acute subarachnoid hemorrhage from a right posterior communicating aneurysm

(E) cavernous sinus thrombosis

46. What is the most appropriate test to establish the diagnosis?

(A) MRI of the brain with and without gadolinium

(B) CT scan of the brain without contrast

(C) a lumbar puncture

(D) an electroencephalogram

(E) optometry

47. Measures of unproved value in the management of this lesion include which of the following?

(A) control of blood pressure with analgesics and antihypertensive agents

(B) initiation of treatment with nimodipine for the prevention of cerebral vasospasm

(C) placement of a ventricular drain in an effort to remove the excess blood within the subarachnoid space

(D) performance of an urgent craniotomy to clip the aneurysm and, thus, exclude it from the cerebral circulation

(E) none of the above

48. A 43-year-old man is treated with pyridostigmine for facial, ocular, and pharyngeal weakness due to myasthenia gravis. Which statement is true of pyridostigmine?

(A) It is unrelated to neostigmine.

(B) It has far more side effects than neostigmine.

(C) Pyridostigmine and neostigmine reverse depolarizing neuromuscular blockade.

(D) It causes greater muscarinic effect than neostigmine.

(E) It is an anticholinesterase agent.

49. During anesthesia using a narcotic, thiopental, and N_2O, the respiratory response to a rising end-respiratory CO_2 tension is which of the following?

(A) depressed only by the narcotic

(B) depressed only by thiopental

(C) depressed progressively by the addition

of each agent

(D) depressed by the narcotic and thiopental, then elevated by N_2O

(E) Unchanged from control response

50. A plastic surgeon is performing a minor procedure on the face of an 18-year-old woman. She has a seizure that is attributed to the local anesthetic agent. Convulsion following an overdose of local anesthesia is best treated by which of the following?

(A) droperidol

(B) hydroxyzine (Vistaril)

(C) diazepam (Valium)

(D) fentanyl

(E) ketamine

Answers and Explanations

1. **(B)** The patient has a right-sided L5 radiculopathy, most likely resulting from a disk herniation at the right L4–L5 interspace. The key to this diagnosis is in understanding the dermatomal anatomy of the lower extremity. The L5 dermatomal distribution involves the lateral calf and the dorsomedial aspect of the foot. The dermatome also typically includes the big toe.

2. **(C)** Thoracic, lumbar, and sacral nerves exit off the spinal canal immediately below the pedicle of the corresponding numbered vertebra. The left S1 root, for example, passes immediately dorsal to the L5–S1 disk, where it can be susceptible to compression by a herniated nucleus pulposus. The root then swings laterally to exit immediately caudal to the left L5 pedicle. For a correlation between level of disk herniation and the root affected, see the table below.

Level of herniation	Root affected
L1–L2	L2
L2–L3	L3
L3–L4	L4
L4–L5	L5
L5–S1	S1

3. **(D)** This patient has radiculopathy of her right C6 root. To make this diagnosis, it is essential to understand the dermatomal anatomy of the upper extremity. The C6 dermatome includes the radial aspect of the distal forearm and hand. The C4 dermatomes include the deltoid region. The biceps tendon jerk is mediated by the C5 and C6 roots.

4. **(C)** The mechanism of injury was a contusion to the cervical spinal cord. This probably occurred when the violent hyperflexion of the neck caused the cervical cord to bump against the osteophytic ridges of the spine. The typical clinical picture of a spinal cord contusion is a central cord syndrome.

5. **(A)** The central spinal cord syndrome describes the following pattern of weakness: (a) weakness in upper extremity > weakness in lower extremity; (b) weakness in distal muscles > weakness in proximal muscles and limb girdle. This results from the distribution of motor fibers within the corticospinal tracts of the cervical cord. Fibers supplying the upper extremity and more proximal muscles are more centrally located and, thus, more susceptible to dysfunction from a central injury. Within the spinal cord, sensory fibers are more peripherally located and, thus, less frequently affected. Sensory deficits, when present, are often variable and inconsistent. A Lhermitte sign or syndrome also results from stenosis of the cervical canal, causing compression of the spinal cord. The patient develops severe numbness and paresthesia of the upper extremities as the result of sustained hyperextension of the neck.

6. **(B)** Brown–Sequard syndrome (Figure 10–3) describes: (a) weakness of muscle *ipsilaterally* below the spinal cord lesion, (b) impaired sensation to light touch and vibration *ipsilaterally* below the spinal cord lesion; and (c) impaired sensation to pain and temperature *contralaterally* below the spinal cord lesion.

7. **(E)** The motor deficit is on the left ipsilateral side. Brown–Sequard syndrome is caused by unilateral injury or dysfunction following hemisections of the spinal cord. In the human nervous system, motor and sensory functions

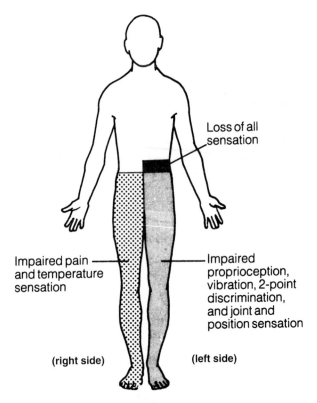

Figure 10–3. Brown–Sequard syndrome. The lesion depicted here is at a lower spinal cord level than that described in the text. (Reproduced, with permission, from Lindner, HH: Clinical Anatomy, Appleton & Lange, 1989.)

Loss of all sensation

Impaired pain and temperature sensation

Impaired proprioception, vibration, 2-point discrimination, and joint and position sensation

(right side)   (left side)

on one side of the body are under the direct control of the opposite side of the brain. All major motor and sensory tracts decussate. The decussation of the various tracts occurs at different levels of the neuraxis.

8. **(C)** On subsequent MRI of the cervicothoracic spine, this patient is found to have severe spondylosis at multiple levels of the spine. There is spinal cord compression by a large osteophyte at the level of C6–C7. The patient has all the signs and symptoms of cervical spinal cord dysfunction. The weakness affecting the triceps muscles in addition to the lower extremities indicates that the lesion is above the level of the thoracic cord. Absence of similar symptoms on the face as well as the absence of cranial nerve abnormalities indicate that the lesion is not intracranial. The diffuseness of the symptoms as well as the fact that they are associated with increased reflexes and tone indicate that the problem lies within the CNS (upper motor neuron) rather than the peripheral nervous system (lower motor neuron).

9. **(A)** The clinical presentation indicates a lower motor neuron lesion. The clinical diagnosis is neurologic claudication secondary to lumbar spinal stenosis, which is commonly seen in elderly persons in whom (as a consequence of wear and tear over the years) bony structures of the lumbar spine hypertrophy and develop osteophytes. These bony changes, in turn, lead to stenosis of the spinal canal and intervertebral foramina. Thus, the result is compression and dysfunction of multiple lumbosacral nerve roots bilaterally. Bending over opens the lumbar canal and relieves the stenosis.

10. **(C)** This patient has suffered a traumatic fracture of L3 in which bony fragments were displaced dorsally to compress the cauda equina at that level. It is important to remember that the spinal cord does not extend along the entire length of the spine. The conus medullaris, the most caudal tip of the spinal cord, ends in 98% of people at or above L2 vertebrae. Thus, it is highly unlikely for an L3 fracture to cause compression of the spinal cord or conus medullaris.

11. **(B)** The most appropriate step is to place him in a hard cervical collar to protect his neck and obtain plain lateral radiographs in flexion and extension. In this boy, the continuous neck pain and the prevertebral swelling on the plain radiographs are strongly suggestive of an injury to the ligamentous structures of the cervical spine. A severe ligamentous tear can lead to instability of the spine from excessive movement between adjacent vertebrae. Ligamentous injury must be ruled out by obtaining lateral radiographs in flexion and extension to demonstrate any excessive movement between adjacent vertebrae. This excessive movement, if missed, can result in compression of the cervical spinal cord and a serious neurologic deficit. These studies require supervision by appropriate specialist consultants.

12. **(A)** A CT scan of the cervical spine is more sensitive for fractures of the spine than are plain radiographs. Because CT images are in the axial plane, only one vertebral body can be seen at a time. This makes CT scanning entirely inadequate to rule out all but large subluxation resulting from the most major ligamen-

tous disruptions. Sagittal MRI of the cervical spine in this case may show swelling or hematoma within the soft tissues of the spine. MRI, however, is poor in demonstrating bony anatomy and detail. Furthermore, without flexion and extension of the neck, an MRI of the cervical spine is no better in showing bony instability than plain radiographs in the neutral position.

13. **(C)** Meningeal carcinomatosis results when malignant cells gain access to the CSF and are able to disseminate within it. Cells most commonly adhere to and affect the neural structures traversing the CSF, such as cranial nerves and peripheral nerve roots. Cells cause dysfunction at multiple sites of the CNS. This patient has a left abducens nerve palsy and a right C5 radiculopathy, making the diagnosis of meningeal carcinomatosis highly likely.

14. **(C)** In the presence of meningeal carcinomatosis (also called carcinomatous meningitis), the lumbar puncture CSF examination may reveal elevated protein and positive cytology. The sensitivity of MRI to detect small tumor deposits within the intracranial compartment is much greater than that of a CT scan. Thus, a CT scan is unlikely to be helpful in this clinical scenario.

15. **(D)** An adult with new onset seizures is considered to have a brain tumor until proved otherwise. The best test available to detect metastatic deposits in the brain is the MRI with intravenous contrast. MRI is exquisitely sensitive in diagnosing brain metastases, sometimes detecting them by the brain edema they induce even when the lesion itself is too small to be seen. The EEG may likely show the presence of seizure activity and even localize it to a particular region of the brain; it will not, however, answer the question of what pathologic process is responsible. Also, in this case, because a mass lesion is expected, performing a spinal tap is relatively contraindicated for the fear of inducing uncal herniation in a patient who may have increased intracranial pressure (ICP).

16. **(A)** The optimal management of any intracranial neoplasm includes use of corticosteroids. These significantly diminish the amount of tumor-induced brain edema and are remarkably effective in ameliorating symptoms caused by CNS neoplasms. The current recommendation for the treatment of multiple brain metastases is treatment with a full course of fractionated radiation to the whole brain. This is geared to treat all visible lesions within the parenchyma as well as those that may still be too small to be detected. Intrathecal chemotherapy is effective in treating meningeal carcinomatosis, where the primary site of involvement is the meninges and the surface of the brain. The two available agents for this modality of treatment have very poor penetration into deeper regions of the brain when administered intrathecally.

17. **(B)** Surgical resection is recommended only for cases involving a single brain metastasis that is surgically accessible in patients with a reasonable life expectancy. It is also relatively indicated in patients with multiple brain lesions in whom one particular lesion is imminently life-threatening. Intravenous chemotherapy has, unfortunately, yielded poor results in the treatment of brain metastases. This is particularly so in this patient, because her tumors are already likely to be resistant to the chemotherapeutic agents with which she has already been treated.

18. **(B)** Glioblastoma multiforme is a highly malignant neoplasm, arising from glial cells or their precursors within the CNS. It is the most common of all primary malignancies of the CNS and its peak incidence is within the fifth to seventh decade of life. A low-grade astrocytoma is a tumor derived from glial cells of astrocytes. Figure 10–4 shows a large cystic giant astrocytoma on T2 weighted MRI where fluid is shown as a white area with midline shift (not glioblastoma multiforme presented in this question).

19. **(C)** Glioblastoma multiforme grows rapidly, and the tumor often contains a necrotic core that occurs as its growth surpasses its blood supply. Additional features on MRI include irregular shape, poor demarcation from surrounding brain tissue, and the presence of variable amount of surrounding white-matter edema.

20. **(D)** This cerebella–pontine angle tumor is most likely an acoustic neuroma. This is the most commonly encountered neoplasm in this region. It

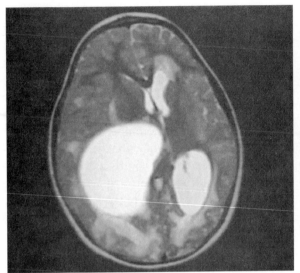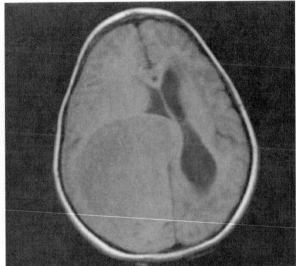

Figure 10–4. Large cystic giant astrocytoma on T2 weighted MRI where fluid is shown as a white area. Midline shift.

arises from the Schwann cells that form the myelin sheath of the vestibular division of the eighth cranial nerve (hence a more accurate name is vestibular schwannoma). This tumor typically arises within the internal acoustic canal and growths in the direction of least resistance: through the meatus into the cerebella–pontine angle cistern.

21. **(C)** An astute neurologist once said that in neurologic diagnosis, as in real estate, location is everything. He alluded to the fact that in the diagnosis of neurologic ailments, one can often generate lists of possible diagnoses based solely on the location of the lesion in question. With unusual exceptions, each location within the CNS is likely to be associated with a certain type of neoplasm. The medulloblastoma (also called a primitive neuroectodermal tumor or PNET) is a highly aggressive and rapidly growing tumor that most often arises within the cerebellar vermis. It usually grows locally as a roughly spherical mass to bulge into and obliterate the adjacent fourth ventricle. Ependymoma or choroid plexus papilloma should also be considered in the differential diagnosis.

22. **(B)** Choroid plexus papillomas are benign tumors of the CNS that arise from the cells that

form the choroid plexus. These tumors can be found wherever choroid plexus is present, including the lateral and fourth ventricles. They cause symptoms of increased ICP, most commonly by causing massive degrees of hydrocephalus. This can be from two mechanisms: obstruction of normal CSF pathways or production by the tumor of excessive volumes of CSF. (Remember that CSF is produced mainly by the choroid plexus.) Ependymomas are also highly malignant tumors usually found in the fourth ventricle of children. Its precursor cell is the ependymal cell that lines the ventricular system. As medulloblastomas, these tumors are highly aggressive and fast growing. Contrary to the former, however, ependymomas tend to arise from the floor of the fourth ventricle (the dorsal surface of the brain stem).

23. **(D)** Obtain an MRI or myelogram of the entire spinal axis to rule out the possibility of "drop metastases" from the medulloblastoma. The constellation of emerging new symptoms points toward spinal cord dysfunction; the most likely cause is the presence of drop metastases from the medulloblastoma. Primary CNS neoplasms rarely metastasize outside of their site of origin. Exceptions to this statement include both medulloblastoma and ependymoma. These tumors

shed viable cells into the CSF, where they are transferred to such distant areas as the intracranial or, more commonly, the spinal subarachnoid space. There they can lodge and replicate to form tumor nodules that can compress adjacent neural structures. The test of choice for diagnosing the presence of these drop metastases is a MRI of the spine with intravenous contrast or a myelogram.

24. **(D)** Treatment of drop metastases consists primarily of complete craniospinal irradiation with local boosts to the areas where tumor nodules are detected. Chemotherapy, particularly a combination of procarbazine, (lomustine), CCNU, and vincristine (PCV), is usually given to treat disease that is locally recurrent after maximal irradiation. Radiation-induced toxicity or radionecrosis is highly unlikely to be the cause of these newly developed symptoms. The first reason for this is that the child's new symptoms and findings appear to be exclusively spinal in origin. Second, radiation-induced necrosis, a feared complication of CNS irradiation, is never observed in such a short interval after completing treatment.

25. **(A)** Intubation will accomplish two purposes. First, it will protect the airway and prevent the possibility of aspiration. Second, it will allow controlled hyperventilation (P_{CO_2} of 25–30 mmHg), which causes cerebral vasoconstriction, which, in turn, transiently lowers ICP and reduces intracranial intravascular blood volume. Mannitol will reduce intracerebral pressure and volume. The role of corticosteroids in the management of cerebral trauma is controversial at best. Their advocates propose that corticosteroids work by reducing the amount of traumatically induced brain edema. Even these investigators concur that their effect is not immediate and that they take at least 4–6 hours to work. The subdural space is between the inner layer of dura and the arachnoid.

26. **(E)** Mannitol is a complex sugar that remains in the intravascular space because of its high molecular weight. When it is given in large doses (1–2 g/kg of body weight), water is extracted from the cerebral interstitium by its osmotic effect, causing reduction in total brain volume. Both these measures are temporizing steps to allow enough time for definitive diagnosis and treatment to take place. The effect of hyperventilation on ICP rapidly wears off after a few hours. Over time, mannitol will diffuse into the cerebral interstitium, losing its effectiveness and even exacerbating cerebral edema. A note of caution, however: mannitol is an osmotic diuretic and as such must be given with extreme caution in the setting of hypotension due to excessive blood loss.

27. **(D)** This is the classic presentation of an acute epidural hematoma: transient traumatic loss of consciousness, followed by a lucid interval and then by neurologic deterioration. Epidural hematomas are frequently associated with linear skull fractures, which cause injury to the middle meningeal artery located immediately deep to the overlying fracture. They are more common in younger individuals, because in younger people, the dura mater is less firmly adherent to the inner table of the skull. Todd's phenomenon is a transient focal weakness or paralysis that results after a seizure. The particular pattern of weakness is often a clue to the site of the seizure focus within the brain.

28. **(C)** Acute subdural hematomas occur most commonly when violent accelerations or deceleration injuries of the head cause tearing of the bridging veins within the subdural potential space. They generally imply a much more severe injury to the brain itself than in the case of their epidural counterpart. For this reason, they are associated with cerebral contusions in over 30% of cases.

29. **(A)** This entity is caused by sharp accelerations or decelerations of the head and its contents as seen in high-speed motor vehicle accidents. During impact, shock waves are generated that are able to travel through the semisolid substance of the brain. These shock waves penetrate and cause shear and stretch injury to multiple deep axonal tracts. DAI represents a severe diffuse injury to the entire brain. For this reason, victims present with marked neurological dysfunction. CT scan typically shows no evidence

or reason to suspect increased ICP; it merely shows punctate hemorrhages in many of the tracts that are affected.

30. **(C)** The presence of a Battle sign and hemotympanum is highly suggestive of the possibility of a left temporal bone fracture. When this occurs, it is common for the dura mater at this site to be torn. This leads to leakage of CSF into the mastoid air cells and middle ear. CSF is subsequently able to reach the nasopharynx via the eustachian tube, a phenomenon called paradoxical rhinorrhea, which is a serious but usually self-limiting condition. Most cases of traumatic CSF leaks heal spontaneously within approximately 1 week. Patients require close in-hospital observation, however, because bacterial meningitis readily occurs in the presence of CSF leakage to the outside.

31. **(C)** Spina bifida occulta does not cause symptoms and is frequently found incidentally in the workup of other conditions. The presence of a tuft of hair and the radiographic abnormalities described above are consistent with the diagnosis of spina bifida occulta. This is a congenital abnormality that results from abnormalities in the development of mesodermal elements (sclerotome) that form the dorsal elements of the lumbosacral spine. A burst fracture of the spine is found after acute excessive axial loading of the spine. The features of such a fracture are reduced height of the affected vertebral body and displacement of bony fragments centrifugally in the axial plane (hence the term *burst*).

32. **(D)** Spondylolisthesis occurs when there is disruption, most often by a fracture, of the pars intra-articularis of the L5 vertebra. The pars is the bony element that is found between the ascending facets of L5 (that articulate with the L4 vertebra) and the descending facets of L5 (that articulate with S1). The functional result of this disruption is that the descending facets are "floating" and not able to function in stabilizing the L5–S1 joint. If this becomes progressive, then anterior subluxation of the L5 vertebral body with respect to that of S1 occurs.

33. **(D)** There is a high degree of correlation in the occurrence of defects in neural tube closure and

Arnold–Chiari malformations, and all babies born with one should be examined for the other. Development of communicating hydrocephalus is a feature of a type-2 Arnold–Chiari abnormality. Stenosis of the aqueduct of Sylvius and the presence of an ependymoma in the fourth ventricles are other reasons for the development of hydrocephalus in children. There is, however, no incidental correlation between these and defects of neural tube closure.

34. **(C)** Abnormal elongation of the medulla and lower cranial nerves may be evident in Arnold–Chiari syndrome. Additional features include fusion of the corpora quadrigemina, leading to a "beaked" tectum; partial or complete absence of the corpus callosum; and microgyria. The corpora quadragemina are relay stations for hearing (inferior corpora quadragemina) and the light reflex (superior copora quadragemina), and they form the posterior surface of the midbrain.

35. **(A)** Noncommunicating hydrocephalus is defined as hydrocephalus caused by obstruction of CSF flow by and obstruction within the ventricular system. In this case, the ventricular system is dilated upstream from the obstruction caused by stenosis of the aqueduct of Sylvius and collapsed distally. Communicating hydrocephalus occurs when the obstruction to CSF flow occurs within the subarachnoid space or at the level of its resorption into the bloodstream by the arachnoid granulations. In this case, all ventricles are dilated proportionately.

36. **(B)** Normal-pressure hydrocephalus is a condition seen in the elderly in which there is symmetrical enlargement the entire ventricular system. When patients with this condition are studied by lumbar puncture, it is found that despite ventriculomegaly, the ICP is abnormally low. This syndrome presents with a characteristic triad of symptoms: dementia, ataxia, and urinary incontinence.

37. **(A)** Pseudotumor cerebri is a condition that most commonly occurs in young adults, particularly in females. In this condition, ICP as measured by a lumbar puncture is elevated, while

the size of the cerebral ventricles on imaging studies is small or normal. It is a generally progressive condition that causes headache and damage to the optic nerve, sometimes leading to loss of peripheral vision and blindness.

38. **(A)** This abnormality is relatively common and occurs in 1 of 1,000 pregnancies. It occurs four times more commonly in whites than blacks and four times more commonly in female fetuses than in male fetuses. The abnormality can be identified on an x-ray, because the vault of the skull is absent. Anencephalus is caused by failure of the cephalic part of the neural tube to close off.

39. **(A)** This cystic structure is an arachnoid cyst. These are CSF-filled cysts that occur when leaves of arachnoidal tissue fuse, trapping CSF within them. These cysts slowly grow over time, sometimes attaining very large size. They cause symptoms by virtue of their large size, as they are able to compress adjacent structures. Patients with these cysts most commonly present with a history of chronic headache. Neurologic symptoms or deficits are unusual. Patients with arachnoid cysts frequently give a history of severe blows to the head and skull fractures, perhaps implying head trauma as a causative agent. The most common locations of arachnoid cysts are the middle cranial fossa, the cerebella–pontine angle, and the suprasellar area. Dandy–Walker cysts are the result of an intrauterine developmental abnormality in which there is failure of proper formation of the foramina of Lushka and Magendie. As a consequence, the main egress of CSF out of the ventricular system is obstructed, leading to hydrocephalus and a massively enlarged, cystlike fourth ventricle.

40. **(B)** Cystic astrocytomas are neoplasms of the CNS. They usually consist of a large, non-enhancing cyst on the wall of which is an enhancing tumor nodule. They are most commonly found within the substance of the cerebellar hemispheres of children and young adults. A Rathke's cleft cyst is a remnant of the embryologic Rathke pouch. These are found within the sella turcica.

41. **(B)** CTS is a condition in which the median nerve is compressed at the level of the wrist by a thickened carpal flexor retinaculum. This leads to numbness and painful paresthesia along the median nerve distribution within the hand. It also causes weakness and atrophy of the thenar muscles within the hand innervated by the superficial recurrent branch of the median nerve. Once there is clinical suspicion, the best diagnostic test to confirm the presence of CTS is a nerve-conduction study. This study often shows a block or delay in conduction of the median nerve at the level of the carpal tunnel. Conduction within all branches of the ulnar nerve should be normal. This test is often also useful in distinguishing between CTS and the possibility of a C6 radiculopathy.

42. **(A)** The best prognostic indicator of survival and outcome in patients with missile wounds to the brain is the mental status and level of responsiveness after proper resuscitation. His initial poor neurologic grade can be attributed to cerebral injury itself or to cerebral hypoperfusion in a patient with clear hemodynamic shock. Initial presentation is, thus, of little value in judging the prognosis for these types of injuries. Other prognostic factors that have been identified as important in predicting the outcome of gunshot wounds to the head include:

a) path of the bullet. A missile that crosses the midline or the midcoronal plane is associated with a much worse outcome than one that stays unilaterally.
b) the presence of an intracranial hematoma of greater than $2 \times 2 \times 2$ cm > is ironically a positive prognosticator, because it represents a mass lesion that can be causing intracranial hypertension and can be more readily evacuated via a craniotomy.

43. **(B)** A markedly diminished level of consciousness coupled by a CT scan that shows a hematoma, edema and subfalcian herniation indicate that the patient is suffering from intracranial hypertension. Hyperventilation and mannitol are quick and effective ways to reduce intracranial pressure temporarily. However, these measures are only temporary, and the patient needs urgent decompression by craniotomy. Placement of burr holes in the emergency room is of

no value in the management of these injuries. Placement of an ICP monitor may be helpful for the postoperative period, but is likely to be of limited help without prior craniotomy.

44. **(C)** The ideal intraoperative management of this patient would begin by performance of a wide craniotomy through which the intracerebral hematoma can be evacuated. Necrotic brain tissue if left alone is likely to worsen the occurrence of cerebral edema postoperatively, and for that reason, every measure should be taken to debride it as thoroughly as possible. Easily accessible bone and bullet fragments can also be removed. Bone and bullet fragments that are deeply located and difficult to locate should be left intact. Persistence in their removal often leads to a greater risk of brain injury by intraoperative manipulation and dissection. If problems with raised intracranial pressure are expected, placement of a suitable ICP monitoring device is highly recommended as part of the surgical procedure.

45. **(D)** This is the classic history for acute subarachnoid hemorrhage: the acute onset of a massive headache. The acuity should suggest nothing other than a vascular phenomenon. Furthermore, the presence of a right occulomotor nerve palsy strongly suggests bleeding from an aneurysm of the right posterior communicating artery. Anatomically, most posterior communicating aneurysms point their domes laterally and inferiorly, in the direction toward the occulomotor nerve. In general, when the dome of the aneurysm ruptures, the jet of blood injures the adjacent nerve. In this situation, the lesion results in complete occulomotor nerve palsy with a fixed dilated pupil. It is a neurosurgic dogma that complete occulomotor palsy should be regarded as a ruptured posterior communicating artery aneurysm until proved otherwise. Acute bacterial meningitis also presents with headache and meningism. The onset of the symptoms is, however, much more gradual, and high fever is usually present.

46. **(B)** The best test in the diagnosis of an acute subarachnoid hemorrhage is a nonenhanced CT of the brain. In this study, subarachnoid blood can easily be seen as a hyperdense substance filling the otherwise hypodense cisterns of the subarachnoid space. Its sensitivity is greater 95%, but sensitivity falls to 50% by 1 week after the hemorrhage. Lumbar puncture can also be used to diagnose subarachnoid hemorrhage, but it is an invasive procedure that should be reserved for cases in which the suspicion of such hemorrhage remains following a negative CT scan. MRI (with or without gadolinium), despite its exquisite sensitivity for the diagnosis of intracerebral lesions, is notoriously poor in its ability to detect acute blood within the subarachnoid space. EEG is of no value for the diagnosis of an acute subarachnoid hemorrhage.

47. **(C)** Soon after the blood fills the subarachnoid cisterns it clots. Thus, it is not amenable for treatment that requires its removal by a small catheter. Furthermore, aggressive ventricular drainage can suddenly lower ICP. Lower ICP in the face of an unchanged pressure within the aneurysm lumen can predispose to rebleeding. This argument also applies to aggressive CSF drainage from a spinal tap. Further steps geared toward reducing the chance or recurrent aneurysmal bleeding include lowering arterial blood pressure to normal levels in an effort to reduce the pressure within the the aneurismal lumen. The aneurysm must be urgently obliterated by either clipping via craniotomy or embolization. In the patient presented here with a broad-necked aneurysm, the former is preferred. The cerebroselective calcium-channel blocker nimodipine is well accepted for its role in counteracting the ischemic effects of cerebral vasospasm, a common delayed sequelae of aneurysmal subarachnoid hemorrhage.

48. **(E)** Neostigmine and pyridostigmine are both anticholinesterase agents and can be used in the reversal of nondepolarizing muscle relaxants.

Pyridostigmine causes less muscarinic effect than does neostigmine. The effect of pyridostigmine is more prolonged and produces fewer secretions and less severe bradycardia.

49. **(C)** Both narcotics and thiopental depress respiration, and the addition of N_2O further augments this depressant action. Thus, the response to hypercapnea is diminished.

50. **(C)** Diazepam is a benzodiazepine derivative that seems to have a calming effect on part of the limbic system, the thalamus, and hypothalamus. It should be injected slowly (< 1 mg/min) into a larger vein to avoid phlebitis and local irritation.

CHAPTER 11

Surgical Endocrinology, Skin, and Wound Healing
Questions

C. Gene Cayten, Haroon Durrani, and Simon Wapnick

DIRECTIONS (Questions 1 through 59): Each of the numbered items or incomplete statements in this section is followed by answers or by completions of the statement. Select the ONE lettered answer or completion that is BEST in each case.

1. A 64-year-old woman develops prominent features of the fingers, mouth, and nose. She has diabetes and hypertension. A computed tomography (CT) scan shows that she has a pituitary tumor. What test would indicate the exact cause of her disease?

    (A) prolactin level assessment
    (B) cerebral angiography
    (C) pituitary growth hormone assay
    (D) lumbar puncture
    (E) x-ray of the hands and face

2. A 53-year-old woman with visual symptoms is shown on magnetic resonance imaging (MRI) to have a pituitary lesion that is approximately 3 cm in height and is eroding the sella turcica. A full endocrinologic evaluation has shown the tumor is not hormonally active. What will ophthalmic examination reveal?

    (A) pronounced difficulty with upward gaze
    (B) homonymous hemianopsia
    (C) unilateral isolated blindness
    (D) bitemporal hemianopsia
    (E) miosis

3. A 58-year-old homeless man is admitted to the neurologic institute for evaluation of severe headaches. He is not coherent and cannot give a clear history. An x-ray of his skull demonstrates marked erosion of the sphenoid bone extending to the sphenoid sinus, and a CT scan demonstrates upward extension of the tumor. In evaluation, which function of the endocrine system will be found to have remained within the normal range?

    (A) oxytocin
    (B) parathormone
    (C) cortisone
    (D) thyroid-stimulating hormone (TSH) or thyrotropin
    (E) luteinizing hormone (LH)

4. After removal of both adrenal glands for adrenal hyperplasia in 1966, a 48-year-old banker was placed on steroids. After surgery, she developed marked pigmentation of the skin. What procedure most likely would have avoided these changes?

    (A) removal of thyroid-stimulating hormone-releasing factor (TSHRF), which arises from the hypothalamus
    (B) transection of the pituitary stalk
    (C) administration of an increased dose of hydrocortisone
    (D) administration of aspirin
    (E) trans-sphenoidal ablation of the pituitary

Questions 5 through 7

A 36-year-old woman presents with a several-month history of headache. The headache is sometimes severe but improves with analgesics. Further questioning also reveals a 3-month history of galactorrhea. Findings on physical and neurologic examinations are completely normal. An MRI of the brain with contrast reveals a small microadenoma within the sella turcica. Blood tests indicate a markedly elevated prolactin level.

5. What is the next step in management of this lesion?

   (A) immediate surgery to decompress the pituitary gland and rule out the possibility of malignancy
   (B) administration of bromocriptine and re-evaluation in 3 months
   (C) limited-field radiation to the pituitary gland
   (D) administration of thyroxin and cortisone
   (E) none of the above

6. What statement is true of hyperprolactinemia?

   (A) It is caused by dopamine agonists (Bromocriptin).
   (B) It is increased in pregnancy.
   (C) It increases ovulation.
   (D) It increases FSH release.
   (E) It occurs with level severance of hypothalamic hypophyseal tract.

7. Which statement is true of prolactin?

   (A) It is secreted by the hypothalamus.
   (B) It is stimulated by dopamine.
   (C) It is inhibited by thyrotropin-releasing hormone.
   (D) It inhibits secretion of electrolytes from breast tissue.
   (E) It is influenced by substances passing in the hypothalamic hypophyseal portal system.

Questions 8 through 11

A 47-year-old male physician had noted weight gain of 25 lbs, which was mainly in the face, shoulders, and trunk. His extremities had become thin. He complained of weakness. On examination, his blood pressure was 190/100. He had a moon face appearance and showed purple striae in the lower abdomen. His fasting blood sugar was elevated. Cushing's syndrome was diagnosed.

8. Cushing's disease is characterized by which of the following?

   (A) pituitary tumor
   (B) adrenal adenoma
   (C) adrenal carcinoma
   (D) ectopic adrenal tumor
   (E) administration of steroids

9. Adrenal cortex hormone release causes which of the following?

   (A) decreased cardiac output
   (B) hypokalaemia
   (C) hypoglycemia
   (D) protein anabolism
   (E) increase lipogenesis

10. Because of severe medical problems, surgery is contraindicated. What would further treatment be?

   (A) ketoconazole
   (B) bromocriptine
   (C) α blockers
   (D) cholecalciferol

11. His serum cortisol level is elevated but is suppressed following the administration of dexamethasone 10 mg orally. What is the most likely diagnosis?

   (A) Addison's syndrome
   (B) adrenal carcinoma
   (C) Cushing's disease
   (D) acromegaly
   (E) pineal gland tumor

Questions 12 and 13

A 48-year-old woman with known hypopituitarism lapses into a coma.

12. The cause of the coma may be aggravated by which of the following?

    (A) increased sensitivity to cortisone
    (B) increased sensitivity to insulin
    (C) paracetamol
    (D) hyperthyroidism
    (E) dermoid cyst of the ovary.

13. What is the initial step in management?

    (A) resuscitation with hypertonic saline solution
    (B) fluid and saline replacement
    (C) administration of a large dose of insulin
    (D) plasmapheresis
    (E) administration of thyroxin

14. A 24-year-old man has severe polyuria and polydipsia. His blood and urinary sugar levels are normal. He is diagnosed as having diabetes insipidus. What is true of diabetes insipidus?

    (A) It is a common entity.
    (B) It is characterized by urine with a specific gravity of 1.010.
    (C) It may occur after skull fracture.
    (D) It is characterized by urine containing an excess of solutes.
    (E) It usually shows hypercalcemia.

15. A 48-year-old woman with a known pituitary macroadenoma (greater than 1 cm) presents with a sudden onset of severe headache and diplopia. On examination, she is found to be lethargic but arousable to voice. She follows commands and has no focal motor deficits. Cranial nerve examination reveals bilateral oculomotor (third) nerve palsies. An emergency CT scan of the brain reveals that the size of the pituitary lesion is enlarged (when compared to her last imaging study), and there is evidence of acute bleeding within the tumor. What is the most likely diagnosis?

    (A) hemorrhage from an intracranial aneurysm
    (B) pituitary apoplexy
    (C) hemorrhage from an arteriovenous malformation (AVM)
    (D) Sheehan's pituitary necrosis

16. A 63-year-old woman has been bleeding from an internal carotid artery aneurysm into the cavernous sinus. In the cavernous sinus, which is the most likely nerve to be affected and show a neurologic lesion?

    (A) oculomotor (third) nerve
    (B) trochlear (fourth) nerve
    (C) aducens (sixth) nerve
    (D) ophthalmic nerve (the first division of the trigeminal nerve)
    (E) the maxillary nerve (the second division of the trigeminal nerve)

Questions 17 and 18

A 48-year-old heavy cigarette smoker is diagnosed as having inoperable oat-cell carcinoma of the lung with extension through the suprapleural membrane into the neck. His serum sodium level is markedly reduced to 104 mEq/L, and his urinary osmolarity is elevated. There is a gradual decrease in consciousness.

17. What is the diagnosis?

    (A) hypercalcemia
    (B) hyperosmolar syndrome
    (C) syndrome of inappropriate secretion of antidiuretic hormone (SIADH)
    (D) diabetes mellitus
    (E) carcinoid syndrome

18. What would be the most appropriate treatment?

    (A) intravenous administration of saline
    (B) administration of doxycycline and fluid restriction
    (C) renal dialysis
    (D) peritoneal dialysis
    (E) administration of lactose

19. A 40-year-old man is admitted with a thyroid swelling that has been increasing in size over the past 6 months. He has a lymph node removed from the right side of his neck that reveals adenocarcinoma with psammoma bodies. What is the primary lesion?

    (A) papillary carcinoma of the thyroid
    (B) follicular carcinoma of the thyroid
    (C) medullary carcinoma
    (D) anaplastic carcinoma
    (E) carcinosarcoma

20. After undergoing surgery for follicular thyroid carcinoma, a 48-year-old man asked what his expected prognosis is. What is the 10-year survival rate for papillary and follicular carcinoma of the thyroid?

    (A) <20%
    (B) 25%–30%
    (C) 40%–50%
    (D) 70%–80%
    (E) Over 95%

21. A 10-year-old boy is noted to have coarse facial features, small stature, and dry skin. He is mentally retarded. What are investigations likely to reveal?

    (A) pituitary dwarfism
    (B) microcephaly and micrognathia
    (C) prematurity
    (D) cretinism
    (E) diabetes mellitus

22. A 25-year-old woman complains of intermittent vague right upper quadrant (RUQ) pain. She has been on oral contraceptive tablets for 6 years. A CT scan of her abdomen shows multiple low-density solid masses occupying the entire right lobe of the liver as well as most of the left lobe. What is the best treatment for this patient?

    (A) hepatic embolization
    (B) discontinuation of oral contraceptives and a repeat of the CT scan of the abdomen in 3–6 months
    (C) CT-guided percutaneous needle biopsy of several liver masses

    (D) laparoscopic biopsy of the liver masses and cholecystectomy

23. A 52-year-old man is reported to have a hepatic adenoma. He most likely has which of the following?

    (A) associated neurofibromatosis
    (B) received methotestosterone
    (C) Cushing's syndrome
    (D) hepatic encephalopathy
    (E) pancreatitis

24. Which is true of islet-cell tumors of the pancreas producing insulinoma?

    (A) They arise from α cells.
    (B) They usually appear in elderly persons.
    (C) They are characterized by the inability to sweat.
    (D) They can cause coma and convulsions.
    (E) They result in dislike of food.

25. What is true of the cells in the islet responsible for insulin release?

    (A) They are α cells.
    (B) They are composed 40% of the islet cells.
    (C) They are found mainly in the periphery of the islets.
    (D) They stimulate polypeptide secretion.
    (E) They stimulate protein syntheses and inhibit glycogenolysis.

26. A 22-year-old female is noted on CT scan to have a hamartoma of the hypothalamus. What is true in a hypothalamic lesion?

    (A) Serum prolactin levels will increase.
    (B) Amenorrhea will improve.
    (C) Serum prolactin levels will decrease.
    (D) Serum TSH levels will increase.

27. A 33-year-old man undergoes an uneventful trans-sphenoidal resection of a 2.5-cm non-secreting pituitary adenoma. Postoperatively, he is kept in an intensive care unit (ICU) for careful monitoring of his urine output. By the second postoperative day, he is no longer receiving intravenous fluid or pain medication and is on a liberal diet. During his third post-

operative day, however, his urine output sharply rises to over 250 mL/h. His urine is highly dilute with a specific gravity (SG) of 1,000. Routine laboratory tests show a serum sodium of 153 g% and an osmolarity of 303 g%. What is the most likely cause for his diuresis?

(A) nephrogenic diabetes insipidus
(B) diabetic ketoacidosis
(C) SIADH
(D) diabetes insipidus
(E) acute tubular necrosis (ATN)

28. A 50-year-old female is admitted to hospital for muscle weakness. Her serum calcium is elevated to 13 mg. What is found in evaluating the possible cause?

(A) Primary hyperparathyroidism is secondary to hypocalcemia.
(B) Secondary hyperparathyroidism is often due to renal disease.
(C) Secondary hypoparathyroidism has a low serum calcium and low PTH.
(D) Secondary hypararathyroidism shows autonomous parathyroid hyperfunction.
(E) Primary hyerparathyroidism is characterized by stimulation of osteoblastic activity and inhibiting osteoclastic activity.

29. On further examination, a breast lump is found. What does hypercalcemia of malignancy show?

(A) osteoblastic activity on history
(B) elevated cAMP in urine
(C) elevated PTH
(D) elevated PTH related peptide

Questions 30 through 32

A 56-year-old male watchmaker is admitted to hospital with features of acute appendicitis. A small McBurney incision is made, and a 1-cm swelling at the distal end of the appendix is identified. Appendectomy is performed, and histologic examination reveals a carcinoid tumor. No other lesions are identified on exploration through the incision.

30. What is true of appendiceal carcinoid?

(A) It is the most common type of intestinal carcinoid tumor.

(B) It is associated with high levels of 5 hydroxy-indolacetic acid 5 HIAA levels in urine.
(C) It is regarded as a benign adenoma.
(D) It is frequently associated with the carcinoid syndrome.
(E) Early metastases to liver occurs in most cases.

31. What is true of the carcinoid syndrome?

(A) It may occur with a small tumor located to the ileum.
(B) It occurs only if extensive hepatic metastasis are present.
(C) It effectively responds to chemotherapeutic agents.
(D) It may respond to selective agents that inhibit synthesis of metabolic products.
(E) It presents with left-sided heart lesions.

32. In the absence of hepatic metastasis, the onset of carcinoid syndrome should indicate investigation of the primary site to be located where?

(A) islet cells of the pancreas
(B) ventral hypothalamus
(C) median eminence of the diencephalons
(D) tracheal bifurcation
(E) obex of the fourth ventricle

Questions 33 through 38

A 38-year-old healthy male athlete undergoes repair of an epigastric hernia under local anesthesia. The defect in the linea alba is closed with nonabsorbable sutures and the skin by subcuticular sutures. The patient is discharged 4 hours after surgery.

33. The inflammatory response of wound healing is characterized by which of the following?

(A) fibroplasia
(B) endothelial cell proliferation
(C) wound contraction by myofibroblasts
(D) capillary vessels that are more permeable to plasma proteins
(E) acellular collagen

34. The initial inflammatory phase is characterized by which of the following?

    (A) neutrophils essential for this phase to occur
    (B) initial changes will occur following discharge from hospital (12–16 hours after creation of the wound)
    (C) will proceed normally if monocytes are absent
    (D) is highlighted by initial vasoconstriction immediately following incision in the skin

35. The vascular response immediately following injury within 10–15 minutes is characterized by which by the following?

    (A) catecholamine-induced vasoconstriction
    (B) vagal release of acetylcholine
    (C) serotonin
    (D) kallikrein
    (E) inhibition of coagulation cascade.

36. During the inflammatory response, clot formation occurs. What is true in this process?

    (A) platelets are excluded, because they cannot penetrate capillaries.
    (B) The clot inhibits angiogenesis.
    (C) Thrombin stimulates monocytes and platelets.
    (D) Thrombin inhibits endothelial cell formation and platelets.
    (E) Thrombin inhibits release of monocytes and fibroblasts.

37. The proliferative (second) phase of wound healing is characterized by which of the following?

    (A) entry of monocytes
    (B) absence of basal epithelial cell proliferation
    (C) fibroblastic proliferation, release of collagen, and formation of the interstitial matrix
    (D) disappearance of fibroblasts from the scar
    (E) remodeling of skin layers

38. Phase of maturation (third phase of wound healing) is characterized by which of the following?

    (A) keloid formation
    (B) proliferation of monocytes

    (C) proliferation of macrophages
    (D) remodeling of tissue
    (E) epithelialization

39. A 30-year-old female with exompholos and hyperthyroidism underwent subtotal thyroidectomy 6 months previously. After surgery, she developed hoarseness, which on indirect laryngoscopy, was shown to be attributable to left recurrent laryngeal nerve injury. She was advised to undergo Teflon injection into the affected vocal cord. What will be the result of Teflon injection?

    (A) It will cause the vocal cord to abduct further.
    (B) It will result in chronic granulomatous reaction.
    (C) It will result in wound contraction.
    (D) It will inhibits macrophages.
    (E) It will increase leukocytosis.

Questions 40 and 41

An 8-year-old schoolgirl fell on her left elbow and sustained a partial-thickness abrasion on her left elbow.

40. What is true of epithelialization?

    (A) It only occurs in burns.
    (B) It will occur if all layers of epidermis are removed.
    (C) It is inhibited near wound edge.
    (D) It will be complete within 48 hours.
    (E) It occurs form hair follicles in deeper dermal layer.

41. Which is true of regenerated epithelium?

    (A) It contains more basal cells than normal epidermis.
    (B) It is characterised by rete pegs and projections to underlying dermis.
    (C) It is thicker at the wound edge than in the center.
    (D) Keratinization does not subsequently form.

42. What is true of collagen formation?

    (A) It commences 7 days after injury.

(B) It constitutes 5% of body proteins and 10% of protein in scar tissue.

(C) It shows increased rate of synthesis for up to 8 weeks after injury.

(D) It is stimulated by glucocorticoids.

(E) It shows an increase in type III collagen.

Questions 43 and 44

A 43-year-old window cleaner fell off a scaffold. He sustained an open wound on the right leg. Debridement was carried out in the emergency department, and the edges of the wound were left open. The wound measures 4 × 6 cm.

43. What is true of wound contraction?

(A) It occurs within 12 hours of injury.

(B) It is more prominent over the tibia than gluteal region.

(C) It is accelerated if wound excised 3 days after injury.

(D) It accounts for excessive fibrous tissue formation and fixation of tissue around a joint.

(E) It is experimentally less affected by excision of tissue from center of wound rather than at the periphery.

44. Which factor is least likely to inhibit wound contraction?

(A) radiation

(B) cytolytic drug

(C) transformation growth factor β

(D) full-thickness skin graft

(E) external splints

45. A 43-year-old male undergoes a total proctocolectomy for ulcerative colitis. The terminal ileum is brought out on the anterior abdominal wall as an end (Brooks) ileostomy. What is necessary to obtain optimal healing?

(A) The ileostomy should be circular rather than square.

(B) The seromuscular layer is sutured to the epithelium of the skin to avoid inflammatory changes.

(C) The ileostomy must be constructed to avoid fixing the mesentery.

(D) The mesentery of the ileal loop should be widely cut to increase its mobility.

Questions 46 and 47

A 64-year-old male is to undergo an elective laparotomy procedure. The proposed wound is considered as "clean–contaminated."

46. This term implies an infection rate of which of the following?

(A) 1%

(B) 2%

(C) 9%

(D) 15%

(E) 30%

47. The wound characteristic indicates which of the following?

(A) entry of intestinal or urinary tract without significant spillage

(B) gross spillage from intestinal tract

(C) no entry of intestinal tract

(D) entry into infected tissue

(E) drainage of an abscess

Questions 48 and 49

A 56-year-old male is burned while sleeping in his home. His right upper and lower extremity and the anterior aspect of the upper chest have extensive second-degree burns.

48. A second-degree burn is characterized by which of the following?

(A) coagulative necrosis extending to subcutaneous fat

(B) pearly white appearance

(C) anaesthetic

(D) erythema and bullae formation

(E) requires immediate skin grafting

49. The extent of the burn is calculated to represent what percentage of body surface area?

    (A) 10%
    (B) 20%
    (C) 30%
    (D) 40%
    (E) 50%

50. Following initial resuscitation, based upon the Parkland formula, the patient was resuscitated with Ringer's lactate solution at 800 mL/h. Further assessment after 6 hours reveals oliguria. What should the next step in management be?

    (A) continue with increased amount of lactated Ringer's solution
    (B) plasma
    (C) diuretics to improve urine flow
    (D) colloid solution

51. After a period of resuscitation, management of this patient should include which of the following?

    (A) tangential excision of all eschar until bleeding encountered
    (B) split-thickness graft if wound grows β-hemolytic streptococci
    (C) use of cadaver allograft when required
    (D) avoid use of porcine xenograft
    (E) chest x-ray useful for diagnosis of inhalation injury

52. List the layers of skin from most superficial to the deepest layer adjacent to the dermis: (a) basal layer; (b) granular layer; (c) prickle layer; and (d) stratum corneum.

    (A) a b c d
    (B) d b a c
    (C) d c b a
    (D) c a b d
    (E) c a d b

53. A 12-year-old boy has multiple skin lesions that are diagnosed as Von Recklinghausen's syndrome (NF 1). What is true of this condition?

    (A) It does not show other malignant lesions.
    (B) It is autosomal recessive.

(C) It is associated with optic nerve gliomas.
(D) It is characterized by A–V malformation.
(E) It is associated with dermoid.

54. A 29-year-old female swimmer develops a pigmented lesion on the right thigh. With reference to a pigmented lesion, there is an increased risk of developing melanoma if it is identified with which of the following?

    (A) Hutchinson's freckle (lentigo maligna)
    (B) freckle involving basal layer of skin
    (C) congenital nevocellular nevi
    (D) hemangioma
    (E) tophi

55. A 67-year-old business executive and tennis player has a basal cell carcinoma removed from the right cheek. What is true of basal cell carcinoma?

    (A) It may show a flat ulcer.
    (B) It may metastasise to lymph nodes.
    (C) It may metastasize to remote skin areas.
    (D) It is found exclusively in the head and neck.
    (E) It is best treated by topical 5-fluoruracil (5-FU).

56. A 38-year-old female undergoes removal of a 2 × 1-cm skin lesion shown to be a melanoma. It is reported as Clark Level 1, which implies what?

    (A) It is superficial to the basement membrane.
    (B) It is 1 mm in thickness.
    (C) It has nodal involvement.
    (D) It involves the papillary layer.
    (E) It involves the reticular dermis.

57. A 49-year-old male postman had undergone several operations to excise recurrent infections in both axillary lesions and perianal region. The lesions are hydradenitis supperativa. Which is true of these?

    (A) They arise from stratum corneum of skin.
    (B) They are noninflammatory conditions.
    (C) They always require surgical intervention.
    (D) They frequently involve the scalp.
    (E) They are usually caused by staphylococci and streptococci.

58. In preparation for an operation, the skin of the right groin is cleaned with an antiseptic solution that effectively does which of the following?

    (A) destroys aerobic organisms

    (B) destroys anaerobic organisms

    (C) destroys both anaerobic and aerobic organisms

    (D) destroys or prevents growth of pathogenic organisms

    (E) destroys pathogenic organisms on instruments

59. Following excision of a lipoma, a 38-year-old female with HIV develops methicillin-resistant *S. aureus* (MRSA) wound infection. What is true of MRSA?

    (A) It has become infrequent in clean operations.

    (B) It is a nosocomial infection.

    (C) It is resistant to methicillin.

    (D) It is more virulent the methicillin-sensitive *S. aureus.*

    (E) It is characterized by inability to produce coagulates.

DIRECTIONS (Questions 60 through 65): The matching questions in this section consist of a list of lettered options followed by numbered items. For each numbered item, select the appropriate lettered option(s). Each lettered option may be selected once, more than once, or not at all. EACH ITEM WILL STATE THE NUMBER OF OPTIONS TO SELECT. CHOOSE EXACTLY THIS NUMBER.

Questions 60 through 62

    (A) ganglion

    (B) dermoid

    (C) epidermal inclusion cyst

    (D) keratosis

    (E) trichilemmal cyst

    (F) neurofibroma

    (G) harmartoma

    (H) pilonidal cyst

60. Congenital skin lesion is which of the above? SELECT THREE.

61. What is the most common cystic lesion of the skin? SELECT ONLY ONE.

62. A 43-year-old male developed partial weakness of the right lower extremity with sensory loss mainly of the opposite lower extremity. He underwent a thoracotomy to remove a left-sided posterior mediastinal mass that partly involved the adjacent intervertebral foramen and spinal cord. What was the diagnosis? SELECT TWO.

Questions 63 through 65

    (A) Type I collagen

    (B) Type II collagen

    (C) Type III collagen

    (D) Type IV collagen

    (E) Type V collagen

63. What is noted in nearly all tissue and constitutes more than 80% of collagen found in skin? SELECT ONLY ONE.

64. What is increased in early phase of wound healing? SELECT ONLY ONE.

65. What is prominent in cartilage? SELECT ONLY ONE.

Answers and Explanations

1. **(C)** Acromegaly occurs in older patients, whereas gigantism is seen in younger individuals in whom bone growth occurs before epiphyseal closure. Acromegaly is due to a pituitary basophil tumor.

2. **(D)** Compression of the optic chiasm classically leads to diminished vision in both temporal hemifields (bitemporal hemianopsia). Because the lens of the eye inverts the image projected on the retina, temporal vision is subserved by the medial half of this structure and nasal vision by the lateral half. All fibers from the retina are somatotopically distributed in such a way that nasal fibers are medially located. Nasal retinal fibers from each retina, carrying visual information about both temporal hemifields, cross to the contralateral optic tract and occipital lobe via the optic chiasm. Compression of this latter structure causes dysfunction of decussating fibers, leading to the characteristic picture of bitemporal hemianopsia. Disruption of visual fibers after the decussation has occurred (i.e., in the optic tracts or occipital lobes) leads to homonymous visual field deficit.

3. **(B)** The secretion of parathormone from the parathyroid glands is released by a fall in serum calcium and is not directly under pituitary control. The anterior pituitary releases ACTH, TSH, gonadotropins, LH, FSH, growth hormone, lactogenic hormone (prolactin), and MSH. The posterior lobe and hypothalamus release the peptides ADH and vasopressin.

4. **(E)** MSH is thought to be responsible for hyperpigmentation of the skin after adrenalectomy. In Cushing's syndrome, the correct treatment is pituitary ablation by a surgical approach, unless the primary pathology is due to an adenoma or carcinoma of the adrenal gland, which requires adrenal gland resection. MSH is released at the same time as ACTH. After bilateral adrenalectomy, the inhibitory effect of cortisol is removed, and MSH and ACTH are secreted in excess.

5. **(B)** This patient has features consistent with an increased prolactin level associated with local pressure on dural structures caused by the presence of a tumor. Her symptoms are neither life-threatening nor irreversible, and this type of pituitary tumor is rarely malignant. Surgical intervention can be considered at a later date if her symptoms progress despite the bromocriptine. Bromocriptine is a dopamine agonist which secondarily diminishes production and release of prolactin. Prolactinomas are similarly affected by circulating levels of dopamine. In the majority of prolactinomas, not only does bromocriptine suppress prolactin synthesis, but it also causes the tumor to shrink dramatically in size.

6. **(E)** This is the explanation given following trauma. Removal of the inhibitory action of dopa leads to galactorrhea. Prolactin causes synthesis of lactose, casein, and lipids in the breast.

7. **(E)** The hypothalamus releases dopamine prolactin inhibiting factor (PIF) that inhibits prolactin from the lactotrophs of the anterior pituitary gland. Dopamine formed in the median eminence of the hypothalamus is released into the hypophyseal portal system to reach the anterior pituitary. Prolactin inhibits Gn RH (and, therefore, FSH) secretion. This results in failure of ovulation.

8. **(A)** The term Cushing's disease refers to the presence of an anterior pituitary gland tumor that releases ACTH. The term syndrome refers to the endogenous release of cortisol. Patients with an adrenal gland tumor or carcinoma will have low levels of ACTH due to the inhibitory effect of excess cortisol release.

9. **(B)** In patients with adrenal cortical adenoma and carcinoma there is also release of aldosterone, which lowers serum K^+ due to secretion by the principal cells of the kidney. Aldosterone also causes increased Na^+ reabsorption with increased extracellular fluid blood volume, and cardiac output. Cortisol increases muscle wasting due to a protein catabolic effect and decreases lipogenesis. There is gluconeogenesis.

10. **(A)** The first step in adrenocortical synthesis is catalyzed by cholesterol desmolase enzyme. Ketoconazole inhibits this enzyme. Ketoconazole thus inhibits the conversion of cholesterol to pregnenolone.

11. **(C)** This entity is caused by overproduction of ACTH by a pituitary adenoma. In Cushing's disease, ACTH production by the pituitary tumor is uncontrolled and unrelated to serum cortisol levels. In the majority of such adenomas, however, ACTH production can be suppressed by administration of a larger dose of dexamethasone. It is by this mechanism that the serum cortisol is diminished in the patient described after administration of this drug. In Cushing's syndrome, due to an adrenal tumor, cortisol is independent of circulating cortisol. In these cases, production is unhindered even by the administration of the lower dose of dexamethasone. Addison's disease is due to underproduction of cortisol, as steroid synthesis and release by the adrenal gland is inadequate. Acromegaly results from overproduction of growth hormone by the pituitary gland.

12. **(B)** Patients with hypopituitarism are sensitive to insulin. Coma is treated similarly to Addison's crisis. These patients have a deficiency of cortisol and require supplementation of this hormone, as well as of thyroid hormone. Women may require estrogen and men androgen at a later stage.

13. **(B)** Thyroid hormone should be given cautiously in small amounts and only after cortisol has been replaced. Spontaneous hypoglycemia, water intoxication, hypothyroidism, and ventilatory failure must be avoided or corrected, because these factors promote shock and coma associated with hypopituitarism.

14. **(C)** Diabetes insipidus is a relatively rare disease. The changes are brought about by the removal or marked reduction in secretion of ADH by the posterior pituitary. The condition is characterized by excessive thirst and polyuria of 5–20 L/d. The specific gravity of urine is low (1.002–1.003). Sugar, blood, and protein are absent from the urine. Diabetes insipidus occurs after operations in the skull region (such as those for craniopharyngioma), encephalitis, meningitis, syphilis, and base-of-skull fractures. If fluids are withheld or hypertonic saline is administered, plasma osmolarity increases without a fall in urine flow. The abnormality can be corrected by injecting vasopressin.

15. **(B)** In this entity, sudden severe bleeding occurs within a pituitary adenoma. The tumor–hematoma complex expands along the path of least resistance, which is laterally toward the cavernous sinuses. It causes compression and injury to the neural structures within this sinus. Sheehan's pituitary necrosis is avascular necrosis of the pituitary gland itself. It is unrelated to the presence of an adenoma. The most common scenario in which Sheehan's occurs is in the context of hypotension due to excessive blood loss during delivery. Bleeding from an intracranial aneurysm or AVM is likely to cause a subarachnoid, intracerebral, or intraventricular hemorrhage. These are unlikely to bleed into the contents of the sella turcica.

16. **(C)** The abducens is the closest structure immediately lateral to the internal carotid artery in its course through the cavernous sinus. Lateral rectus palsy takes place with inability to abduct the eye on the affected side.

17. **(C)** The carcinoma, usually like the case described here (oat cell), secretes ADH inappropriately. The characteristic features should be sought in a patient showing unexplained

changes in mental status with marked hypo-natremia despite the fact that serum osmolarity is not reduced.

18. **(B)** Fluids and saline must be restricted until the serum sodium level is increased, because attempts to replace hyponatremia aggravate the condition. Doxycycline frequently offers the beneficial effect of correcting hyponatremia.

19. **(A)** Psammoma bodies are shown as tiny cal-cified lesions on x-ray. Papillary carcinomas account for 50% of thyroid malignancies. Car-cinosarcoma is seen in the stomach but not in the thyroid.

20. **(D)** Follicular carcinoma accounts for 20% of malignant lesions in the thyroid. If the tumor has not spread beyond the capsule, 10-year sur-vival exceeds 85%. Papillary carcinoma tends to spread via the lymphatics.

21. **(D)** In cretinism, there is usually a genetic de-fect (Mendelian recessive) causing a deficiency in one of the enzymes responsible for thyroid hormone release. There is an associated goiter, and TSH levels will be increased. It is imperative to diagnose early to avoid mental retardation.

22. **(B)** The CT scan findings for this patient plus the history of prolonged use of oral contracep-tives are characteristic of hepatocellular ade-noma. Because the tumor extensively involves both the right and left lobes of the liver, oral contraceptive use must be discontinued, and the patient must be observed for 3–6 months. Significant reduction in size of the adenoma has been noted in many cases after cessation of oral contraceptive use. If there is no regression of lesions, then liver transplantation should be recommended.

23. **(B)** Hepatic adenoma occurs mainly in female patients taking oral contraceptive drugs. It may develop in male patients receiving methotestos-terone and occurs in about 60% of individuals with type 1 or 3 glycogen storage disease.

24. **(D)** The Whipple triad includes: (a) symptoms of hypoglycemia evoked by fasting; (b) blood sugar lower than 50 mg during an attack; and (c) favorable response to intravenous glucose. This condition may cause sweating, anxiety, and a sensation of hunger. It is confirmed by finding elevated insulin levels during an attack. The pathology may be caused by hyperplasia (nes-bestioma in children), adenoma, or carcinoma.

25. **(E)** The β cells are the most numerous cells in the islet, are located mainly in the center of the islet and cause release of insulin. The α cells release glucagons, and the β cells (also called PP cells) release insulin. PP inhibits exocrine secretion from the pancreas and is under vagal control

26. **(C)** Serum prolactin levels will decrease. Within the pituitary gland, synthesis and production of prolactin is regulated by hypothalamic produc-tion of dopamine. When secretion of this endo-genous catecholamine by the hypothalamus is increased, the anterior pituitary is stimulated to increase its production of prolactin.

27. **(D)** This entity is characterized by the produc-tion of a large volume of dilute urine despite concomitant dehydration. In this patient, the low urinary specific gravity attests to the low solute content of this body fluid. The occurrence of high serum sodium and osmolarity indicate that the patient has become hemoconcentrated as the result of dehydration.

28. **(B)** Secondary hyperparathyroidism is often due to renal disease. Although PTH is ele-vated, serum Ca is frequently normal or low. It is considered a compensatory response to the hyperphosphatemia with reduction in vi-tamin D_3 (1,25-dehydroxy), in renal disease or malabsorption in intestinal disease. Tertiary hyperparathyroidism refers to secondary hyper-parathyroidism in which parathyroid hyper-secretion of PTH has become autonomous. PTH is characterized by stimulation of osteoblastic activity and inhibition of osteoclastic activity.

29. **(D)** The cAMP in urine is elevated in primary hyperathyroidism. Histology shows osteoclustic activity. Hypercalcemia in malignancy occurs most commonly in carcinoma of the breast, lung, kidney, neuroendocrine tumors, multiple myeloma, leukemia and lymphoma.

30. **(A)** The appendix is the most frequent, and the ileum the second most common site affected by carcinoid tumor. The tumor arises from the Kulschitsky cells (Argentaffin) cells located at the base of the intestinal mucosa. Appendiceal carcinoids are much less likely to metastasise to the liver. In ileal carcinoids, diameter 1–2 cm have nodal metastasise in >80% of cases as compared to a similar size lesion in the appendix where <40% have nodal metastases. Less than 10% of patients with intestinal carcinoid tumors present with the carcinoid syndrome. The carcinoid syndrome arising from an intestinal primary tumor only occurs in the presence of hepatic metastases.

31. **(D)** The liver inactivates secretion of the metabolic active agents. The carcinoid syndrome arising from an intestinal primary tumor only occurs following extensive hepatic metastasis. The syndrome is characterized by diarrhea, intermittent flushing of the skin, and right- (not left-) sided cardiac lesions. Favorable response has been seen with the antiserotonergic drug methysergide, for flushing, α adrenergic drugs for diarrhea, and palliation with streptozoticin and 5FU.

32. **(D)** The cells that undergo neoplastic transformation in the bronchial mucosa release the active metabolic substances into the pulmonary veins; therefore, right-sided cardiac lesions do not occur, as they do in those patients with hepatic metastasis. Furthermore, these lesions may produce the syndrome at a much earlier stage, because the metabolic pathway is not inactivated by early passage through the liver. The obex is the inferior apex of the fourth ventricle. Carcinoid syndrome is not a feature of islet cell tumor of the pancreas and is not associated with Zollinger–Ellison syndrome or plurigladular syndrome.

33. **(D)** The initial response to wound healing is characterized by the inflammatory response. The inflammatory response is followed by the proliferative and then the phase of maturation.

34. **(D)** This short (10-minute) period of vasoconstriction is followed by vasodilation and increased vascular permeability. Vasoactive substances [histamine, kinins (bradykinin and kallidin)], platelet-derived growth factor (PDGF), and C_5 compliment are chemotactic and attract neutrophils into the wound. However, wound healing proceeds normally in noninfected wounds even though leukocytes are absent. Monocytes are essential for both phagocytes and initiating the second (fibroblastic) phase of wound healing.

35. **(A)** The immediate response to injury is characterized by sympathetic, norepinephrine circulating catecholamine (epinephrine) and such other substances as prostaglandins released from injured tissue.

36. **(C)** Prothrombin is converted to thrombin, which activates fibrinogen to fibrin. The clot acts as a scaffold to allow entry of fibroblasts. Platelets release numerous factors, such as transforming growth factor beta (TGF-β), platelet-derived growth factor (PDGF) fibronectin, von Willebrand factor, and serotonin. The clot stimulates angiogenesis. Thrombin stimulates: (a) endothelial cells; (b) fibroblasts; (c) monocytes; and (d) platelets.

37. **(C)** The fibroblastic response follows the initial inflammatory response. On the third day after creation of the wound, fibroblasts proliferate to form collagen. During this phase, endothelial cells proliferate to form new vessels. Wound contraction is taking place.

38. **(D)** The phase of maturation follows the proliferative (fibroplasia) phase. Approximately 3 weeks after the incision is made, fibroblasts and macrophages are removed, and a relatively acellular collagen is found.

39. **(B)** Teflon is an inert material used frequently in surgical procedures. Following wound healing, a fibrous capsule is formed that surrounds the Teflon injected in to the vocal cord. The Teflon induces a chronic granulomatous reaction, which, in turn, stimulates fibrous tissue formation. These changes result in close apposition of the vocal cords and, hence, improved phonation. Wound contraction refers to constant changes in early wound healing that reduce the diameter of the inflicted wound.

40. (E) In addition to growth from hair follicles, epithelialization occurs from sweat glands and sebaceous glands located in the dermis. In a finely coapted wound, epithelialization is complete within 48 hours of injury.

41. (C) Basal cells migrate along collagen fibers as a monolayer (contact guidance) until they reach other epithelial cells. Migration is halted at this point of contact (contact inhibition). Now epithelial proliferation occurs, and different layers form. Regenerated epithelial tissue lacks rete pegs and underlying projections into the dermis.

42. (E) Collagen synthesis is increased for 2–4 weeks after injury and then shows a decrease rate of formation. Glucocorticoids inhibits and TGF β facilitates collagen formation. Collagen constitutes 25% of body protein and 50% of scar tissue protein.

43. (E) Wound contraction refers to the decrease in diameter of an open wound. It commences on about the 4th day after injury and continues at a relatively rapid rate (½ to 1 mm/d). It is maximal in areas where tissue laxity exists. Wound contraction should not be confused with wound contracture where scar formation over a joint interferes with mobility. Experimentally, it less affected by excision of tissue from the center of the wound, rather than at the periphery.

44. (D) Following the application of a full-thickness graft, contraction at the site of the recipient site is maximally inhibited by a full-thickness and to a lesser extent by the partial-thickness graft.

45. (A) The ileostomy should be circular rather than square to avoid excessive stenosis of the stoma. Wound healing by a square incision results in a greater degree of stenosis than by an equivalent circular stoma. Failure to close the gap between the ileal loop on the abdominal wall may lead to subsequent internal herniation. It is critical to ensure that the ileal stump is not devascularized.

46. (C) In a clean wound, the anticipated infection rate should be 1.5–5%, in a "contaminated" wound, 15%, and a "dirty wound," 30–40%.

47. (A) If spillage is substantial or infected tissue has entered, the wound is classified as "contaminated." "Dirty" wounds are used for drainage of an abscess or debridement of infected tissue.

48. (D) In a second-degree burn, the skin appendages in the dermis are minimally destroyed (superficial partial thickness) or more extensively destroyed (deep partial thickness). In a third-degree (full-thickness) burn, all of the dermis (with skin appendages) are destroyed, and the lesion extends to the subcutaneous fat layer.

49. (D) In calculating burn surface area, the rule of "9" assigns 9% to each upper extremity, 18% to each lower extremity, and 9% to the head and neck. The trunk and abdomen (36%) is divided into four equal parts (9% each). Thus, upper trunk anteriorly would be 9%.

50. (A) Continue with increased amount of lactated Ringer's solution. Urine flow should be 0.5–1.0 mL/kg/h. Patients exposed to inhalation on burns, and those admitted following alcoholic intoxication require additional fluids. In general, for second and third-degree burns, the Parkland formula is used to administer 4 mL/kg weight of patient × percentage of area of burn. Half of the calculated amount is given within 8 hours and the remainder during the subsequent 16 hours.

51. (C) Use cadaver allograft when required. Tangential excision of the skin (to secure a bleeding surface) is done with a guarded dermatome. However, because of possible extensive blood loss, it should be limited to an area less than 20% of the total body surface area. The presence of bacteria growth more than 10^5 organisms/cm^2 or growth of β hemolytic streptococci should contraindicate split-skin-thickness grafting.

52. (C) The stratum corneum consists mainly of dead cells and keratin.

53. (C) It is inherited as a autosomal dominant disorder and noted in nearly 1/5,000 births. The NF-1 gene encodes a protein neurofibromin that plays a role in neuroectodermal differentiation and cardiac development.

54. **(C)** Most melanoma arise from nondysplastic nevi. Congenital nevocellular nevi found in about 1/100 births have a 3–5% lifetime risk of undergoing malignant change. Dysplastic (a typical) nevi may be familial and predisposed to malignancy. Hutchinson freckle occurs mainly in older patients.

55. **(A)** The surface of a basal cell carcinoma has a shiny appearance with telangiectasia. Ulcer formation may occur; hence, the name *rodent ulcer*. Although treatments with 5 FU, cryosurgery, or electrodessication are effective in treatment, surgical excision offers the best results and ensures an accurate diagnosis.

56. **(A)** Level II involves papillary layer III between papillar and reticular layer, IV the reticular layer, and V the subcutaneous fat. The Breslow classification utilizes differences in the thickness of the tumor.

57. **(E)** Usually caused by staphylococci and streptococci. Hydradenitis supperativa is an infection of the apocrine glands and surrounding subcutaneous tissue and fascia, which most commonly involves the axilla, groin, perineum, and perianal region. The periumbilical and areola region may be involved. In milder cases, local hygienic measures and tetracycline may be adequate; in more severe cases, wide excision is indicated.

58. **(D)** To destroy all organisms (including spores) sterilization by dry heat, radiation, chemicals, or pressurized steam is required. Antiseptic solutions are used to clean the skin where it destroys or reduces growth of organisms (but not spores).

59. **(B)** It is a nosocomial infection *S. aerus* but not *S. epidermidis* produces coagulage. Methicillin-resistant *S. aurens* responds to vancomysin and (if appropriately treated) is not considered a more virulent strain than methicillin-sensitive *S. aureus*.

60. **(B, G, H)** Dermoid cysts occur along lines of embryological tissue fusion, such as the midline of the abdomen, nose, chin, sacral region, and occipital region. Hamartoma is attributable to misfiring of tissue arrangement of tissue. Pilonidal cyst is caused by to the persistence of a congenital coccygeal sinus and characterized by the ingrowth of hair.

61. **(C)** Epidermal inclusion cyst is the most common cyst encountered in skin. It contains creamy material and is differentiated from a sebaceous cyst, which has a punctum and a trichilemmal cyst (usually on the scalp) that does not have a granular layer.

62. **(F, G)** Neurofibromata are hamartomas and form part of von Recklinghausen syndrome. The thoracotomy referred to an operation to remove a dumbbell enlarged neurofibroma that involved an intercostals nerve in the posterior mediastinum and the intervertebral foramen. The lesion could involve the spinal cord. Neurofibroma are associated with café-au-lait spots, plexiform neurofibroma, elephantiasis of a limb, and, in some cases, malignant transformation. Benign neurofibroma are hamartomas and not neoplastic.

63. **(A)** Collagen types are differentiated by differences in their polypeptide chains. Type I collagen comprises 90% of normal skin protein.

64. **(C)** Type III collagen is noted to be increased in the early phase of wound healing. Type III collagen is also prominent in embryonic collagen. Incision of embryonic tissue results in less scar tissue with a finer scar than in adult tissue. Type IV collagen is found in basement membrane.

65. **(B)** Both types II and XI are prominent in cartilage. Type V is prominent in smooth muscle.

CHAPTER 12

Practice Test
Questions

Jaroslaw Bilaniuk, C. Gene Cayten, and Simon Wapnick

DIRECTIONS (Questions 1 through 80): Each of the numbered items or incomplete statements in this section is followed by answers or by completions of the statement. Select the ONE lettered answer or completion that is BEST in each case.

1. As part of a hepatic resection, the right phrenic nerve is cut as it passes through which of the following?

   (A) caval opening
   (B) aortic opening
   (C) esophageal opening
   (D) right crus of the diaphragm
   (E) left crus of the diaphragm

Questions 2 and 3

An 18-year-old woman has a known history of polycystic kidney disease of 3 years' duration. A computed tomography (CT) scan of the abdomen shows multiple multiloculated cystic lesions involving most of the parenchyma of the left lobe of the liver (Figure 12–1). The spleen is also slightly enlarged.

2. The patient is most likely to manifest which of the following?

   (A) multiple lipoma
   (B) hemiplegia
   (C) teratoma
   (D) pancreatic pseudocyst
   (E) syndactyly

3. What is the most appropriate definitive treatment or advice for the management of this patient?

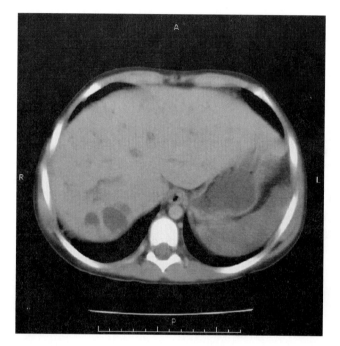

Figure 12–1. CT scan of abdomen. Patient with polycystic kidneys had previously undergone nephrectomy. Note multiple cystic lesions in liver.

   (A) administration of diuretics and repeated paracentesis
   (B) percutaneous chemical sclerosis of the liver cysts
   (C) resection of the large dominant cyst and fenestration of the smaller multiloculated cysts
   (D) exchange transfusion

4. A 25-year-old woman complains of intermittent vague right upper quadrant (RUQ) pain. She has been on oral contraceptive tablets for 6 years. A CT scan of her abdomen shows multiple low-density solid masses occupying the entire right lobe of her liver as well as most of the left lobe. What is the best treatment for this patient?

(A) hepatic embolization
(B) discontinuation of oral contraceptives and a repeated CT scan of her abdomen in 3–6 months
(C) CT-guided percutaneous needle biopsy of several liver masses
(D) laparoscopic biopsy of the liver masses and cholecystectomy
(E) gold therapy parenterally

5. After using contraceptives for 12 years, a 36-year-old woman is noted on clinical examination to have an enlarged mass in her liver. Hepatic adenoma is considered in the differential diagnosis. Which test would be most useful to confirm this diagnosis?

(A) Hepatic angiography
(B) Technetium scan
(C) Percutaneous needle biopsy of the liver mass
(D) Laparoscopic biopsy
(E) CT scan of the abdomen

Questions 6 and 7

A 76-year-old woman undergoes successful endoscopic stenting of the common bile duct (CBD) for obstructive jaundice secondary to an inoperable cholangiocarcinoma. Two weeks later, she consults her physician because of a fever of 102°F, general malaise, nausea, and RUQ discomfort. On physical examination, icteric sclera and RUQ tenderness are noted. Laboratory test results show leukocytosis, anemia, and an elevated serum bilirubin level. Chest x-ray shows no acute infiltrate, but the right diaphragm is elevated.

6. What is the most likely diagnosis?

(A) cholangitis
(B) liver abscess
(C) acute calculous cholecystitis

(D) liver metastasis
(E) pneumonia

7. What is the best ancillary procedure to diagnose the condition discussed?

(A) a liver scan
(B) ultrasound
(C) CT
(D) magnetic resonance imaging (MRI)
(E) endoscopic cholangiography

8. A 78-year-old woman develops a liver abscess following stent drainage of jaundice. What is the preferred therapy?

(A) oral administration of antibiotics
(B) aspiration of abscess
(C) CT-guided percutaneous drainage alone
(D) administration of antibiotics and CT-guided percutaneous drainage
(E) surgical drainage

9. A 64-year-old diabetic man undergoes stent insertion for inoperable biliary obstruction due to cancer. Three months after the procedure, he complains of pruritus, icterus, and intermittent fever. What is the most likely diagnosis?

(A) polycystic disease of the liver
(B) ascending cholangitis
(C) hemolytic anemia
(D) cholecystitis
(E) pyelonephritis

10. A 42-year-old man with abdominal pain is evaluated to exclude the presence of gallbladder disease. In addition to a HIDA scan and ultrasound of the gallbladder, an oral cholecystogram is ordered. What is this likely to visualize?

(A) fine details of the intrahepatic ducts
(B) biliary tree in obstructive jaundice (bilirubin > 4 mg/dL)
(C) gallbladder in obstructive jaundice (bilirubin > 4 mg/dL)
(D) gallbladder in renal disease
(E) gallbladder in cholecystitis

11. A 35-year-old man presents with a bleeding duodenal ulcer documented by endoscopy. The patient is somewhat unstable, and bleeding does not stop despite transfusing 8 units of blood. What is the most appropriate surgical therapy?

   (A) further blood transfusion alone
   (B) oversewing the ulcer alone
   (C) oversewing the ulcer and performing a gastrojejunostomy
   (D) oversewing the ulcer and performing a vagotomy and pyloroplasty
   (E) oversewing the ulcer and performing a proximal gastrectomy

12. After suffering a complication from colon surgery, a 64-year-old man learns that the organisms found in the wound are due to colonization. What does colonization after antibiotic therapy imply?

   (A) Fungi are present in the colon.
   (B) Small-bowel contents are evident in the colon.
   (C) The colon mucosa undergoes small-bowel villi proliferation.
   (D) There is an alteration in flora, with overgrowth of virulent organisms.
   (E) Bacteroides outnumber *Escherichia coli.*

13. A 48-year-old man presents with an intraabdominal abscess consequent to leakage from a bowel anastomosis. Where and why does mortality due to postoperative sepsis with intra-abdominal abscess increase?

   (A) in younger patients
   (B) when a single organ is involved
   (C) by percutaneous drainage
   (D) if multiple abscesses occur
   (E) all of the above

14. After undergoing a gynecologic operation, a 36-year-old patient developed β-streptococcal septicemia. Which is true of β-Streptococcal infection?

   (A) It does not spread rapidly along lymphatic channels.
   (B) It is mainly resistant to penicillin?

   (C) It may spread rapidly through tissue planes.
   (D) It is unlikely to cause overwhelming infection from an intravenous site.
   (E) It commonly causes urinary tract infection (UTI).

15. A 44-year-old man develops intra-abdominal sepsis after undergoing difficult bowel resection and anastomosis. He is initially given ceftizoxime sodium (Cefizox), which is ineffective because of overgrowth of which of the following?

   (A) *Pseudomonas*
   (B) *Staphylococcus aureus*
   (C) *Neisseria gonorrhoeae*
   (D) *Bacteroides fragilis*
   (E) *Haemophilus influenzae*

16. A 64-year-old man is noted on CT scan to have a liver abscess. He is diagnosed as more likely to have a pyogenic than amebic liver abscess. Why?

   (A) He emigrated from Mexico.
   (B) Jaundice is absent.
   (C) He has associated diarrhea.
   (D) He has a history of biliary tract disease.
   (E) There is a rapid response to metronidazole.

17. What is true of *Candida* sepsis?

   (A) It carries a relatively low mortality risk.
   (B) It is treated with actinomycin.
   (C) It can be partly prevented by ketoconazole.
   (D) It is caused by spore-forming organisms.
   (E) It is seen usually in conditions not requiring antibiotics.

18. A 43-year-old man had a previous injury to his wrist. The ulnar nerve was severed, as indicated by which of the following?

   (A) claw hand involving the ring and little fingers
   (B) claw hand involving the index and middle fingers
   (C) atrophy of the thenar muscles
   (D) absent sensation in the index finger
   (E) inability to flex the distal phalanx of the index finger

19. After falling on the pavement, a 72-year-old woman is found to have a fracture of the radius and ulna (Colles' fracture). What is true of this fracture?

    (A) The fall occurs on the dorsum of the wrist.
    (B) Open reduction is most commonly indicated.
    (C) Younger men are generally affected.
    (D) The distal radial metaphysis is displaced dorsally.
    (E) The ulnar shaft is fractured proximally.

20. An 83-year-old retired navy general is scheduled to undergo aortoiliac bypass surgery for intermittent claudication. The factor(s) that would most likely cause concern because of the potential for development of cardiac complications is (are):

    (A) signs of left ventricular failure
    (B) the patient's advanced age (>80 years) and jugular venous distention
    (C) history of angina and myocardial infarction (MI) 6 months previously
    (D) left ejection fraction of over 50%
    (E) aortic stenosis

Questions 21 and 22

A 24-year-old bank clerk is admitted to the hospital with left-sided blindness. She had emigrated from Africa and had been treated for sickle-cell disease. Examination reveals bleeding into the posterior (vitreous) chamber of the eye. Funduscopy cannot be done because of the presence of blood inside the eye.

21. What should be the next step in management?

    (A) needle aspiration of the anterior chamber of the eye
    (B) exploration of the posterior chamber
    (C) administration of cortisone
    (D) administration of steroids
    (E) observation

22. The patient should be advised that repeated crisis may occur with which of the following?

    (A) alkalosis
    (B) moderate warmth
    (C) pregnancy

    (D) anemia
    (E) oxygen administration

23. Autotransfusion of blood by use of the Cell Saver in an emergency situation may be preferable to use of banked blood autotransfusion. Why?

    (A) It increases potassium levels.
    (B) It is always available.
    (C) It reduces the risk of bacterial infections.
    (D) It reduces changes in coagulation parameters.
    (E) It can be encouraged in the face of bowel laceration.

24. A 62-year-old woman underwent a modified mastectomy operation 5 years ago. One month before hospital admission, she undergoes repeated paracentesis of her left pleural cavity for a malignant effusion. The effusion recurred, as seen on x-ray, and she complains of dyspnea. What would appropriate therapy include?

    (A) diuretic therapy
    (B) a salt-free diet
    (C) a low-albumin diet
    (D) thoracoscopy, removal of fluid, and injection of talc into the left pleural cavity
    (E) thoracotomy and pneumonectomy

25. A 43-year-old man sustains a fracture of the tibia. There are no neurologic or muscular lesions noted on careful examination. An above-knee cast is applied. After 6 weeks, the plaster is removed. It is noted that he has a foot drop and is unable to extend his ankle because of pressure injury to which of the following?

    (A) posterior tibial nerve
    (B) saphenous nerve
    (C) femoral nerve
    (D) deep fibula (peroneal) nerve
    (E) nerve to the soleus muscle

26. A 62-year-old woman with multiple myeloma is given pamidronate calcium biphosphonate. This treatment has been shown to do what?

    (A) increase survival
    (B) improve quality of life and protect against skeletal fractures

(C) stimulate osteoclast

(D) increase hypercalcemia

(E) replace chemotherapy

27. A 34-year-old man is admitted to the hospital with a diagnosis of appendicitis. On examination, he is found to have mild tenderness in the right iliac fossa, and a mass is palpated in this region. The white blood cell (WBC) count was 12,000, his pulse rate is 82 beats per minute, and his temperature is 100°F. A CT scan of the abdomen confirms the presence of a fecolith (Figure 12–2A), and an MRI shows fluid accumulation in a distended appendix (Figure 12–2B). What is the next step in management?

(A) administration of laxatives to treat constipation

(B) intravenous administration of fluids and antibiotics—nothing by mouth

(C) intravenous administration of fluids and antibiotics—nothing by mouth, and elective appendectomy

(D) emergency right hemicolectomy

(E) ileotransverse colostomy

28. In treating the complications of vomiting caused by chemotherapy given to a 48-year-old man with cancer of the stomach, the physician chooses a dopamine-inhibitor drug. A CT scan of the lung reveals metastatic disease and a CT scan of the abdomen shows extensive splenic metastasis (Figures 12–3A and 12-3B). What drug is selected?

(A) antihistaminic

(B) a benzodiazepine

(C) a phenothiazine

(D) a cannabinoid

(E) a corticosteroid

29. A newborn is found to have a meningocele. What is true in this neural tube defect?

(A) Neural arches are fused.

(B) Maternal α-fetoprotein levels are low.

(C) Amniotic α-fetoprotein levels are low.

(D) Intake of valproic acid during pregnancy may be a causative factor.

(E) Folic acid causes defects.

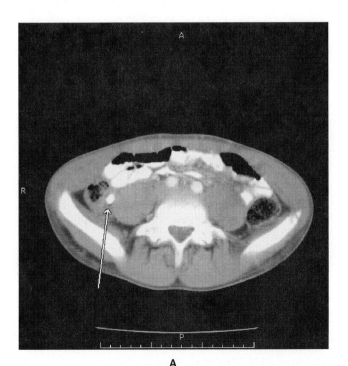

A

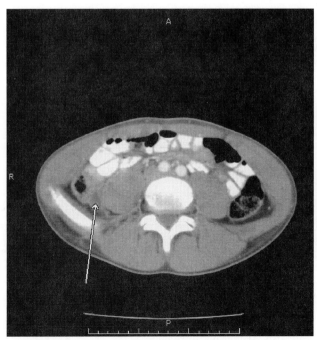

B

Figure 12–2. CT scan of the abdomen confirms the presence of a fecolith (Figure 12–2A), and a CT shows fluid accumulation in a distended appendix (Figure 12–2B).

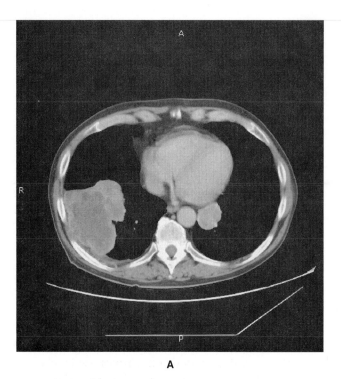

A

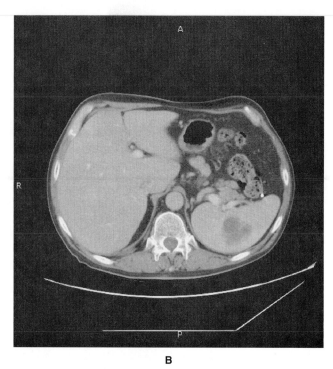

B

Figure 12–3. CT scan of the lung **(A)** reveals metastasis and CT scan of the abdomen shows splenic involvement **(B)**.

30. A recently arrived 62-year-old emigrant from Greece complains of upper abdominal pain and fever. Ultrasound reveals a large liver cyst that, on serological testing, is shown to be hydatid disease. What should he undergo?

   (A) cortisone therapy
   (B) percutaneous drainage
   (C) laparotomy and open drainage
   (D) laparotomy and needle aspiration
   (E) laparotomy and excision of cyst and perioperative albedazole.

31. A 34-year-old woman with Crohn's disease has undergone her fifth operation with small-bowel resection. She has hemoglobin of 7 g%. An upper GI series shows an apple-core lesion due to adenocarcinoma of the small bowel (Figure 12–4). What is the most likely cause of her anemia?

   (A) erythropoietin deficiency
   (B) thyroid overactivity
   (C) megaloblastic anemia
   (D) aplastic anemia
   (E) inability to absorb fat-soluble vitamins

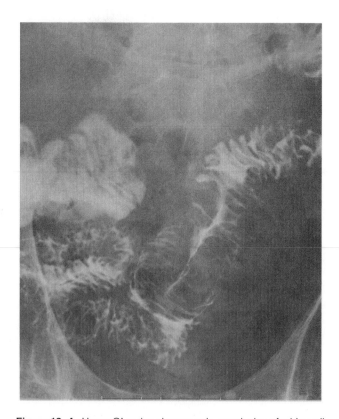

Figure 12–4. Upper GI series shows apple-core lesion of mid small bowel.

32. The risk of developing deep vein thrombosis (DVT) after surgery is not altered if the patient has which of the following?

    (A) a history of DVT
    (B) varicose veins
    (C) had a cancer operation
    (D) used oral contraceptives
    (E) ulcerative colitis

33. Unexplained thrombosis is likely to occur with increased frequency in which of the following?

    (A) paroxysmal nocturnal hemoglobinuria
    (B) neurofibromatosis
    (C) fibrinogen deficiency
    (D) condom use
    (E) excess antithrombin III levels

34. A 42-year-old man who has consumed several bottles of whiskey weekly for the past 20 years presents with hematemesis due to gastric varices. After appropriate resuscitation surgery is undertaken, what should he undergo?

    (A) total gastrectomy
    (B) splenectomy
    (C) portal vein ligation
    (D) hepatic vein ligation
    (E) placement of an emergency portacaval shunt

35. A 12-year-old boy is admitted to the hospital with severe abdominal pain. He is noted to have slight jaundice. His hematocrit is 30, and reticulocytes are evident in a peripheral smear. His father underwent a splenectomy at age 25. Which test would clarify the cause of anemia?

    (A) barium enema
    (B) hemoglobin electrophoresis
    (C) serum iron
    (D) Coombs' test
    (E) red blood cell (RBC) osmotic fragility test

36. A 58-year-old woman has a gastric ulcer, achlorhydria, and vibration sense loss in the lower extremities. She has a megaloblastic anemia. What test would help support a diagnosis of pernicious anemia?

    (A) response to injection of radioactive B_{12}
    (B) endoscopic retrograde cholangiopancreatography (ERCP)
    (C) prothrombin time (PT)
    (D) radiolabeled B_{12} given orally
    (E) response to trial of folic acid

37. A 34-year-old occupational therapist with a 12-year history of Crohn's disease is admitted for excision of a right cecal mass. She underwent a major resection of more than 1.5 m of terminal ileum 5 years previously. Her hematocrit is 22, and a peripheral blood smear shows macro-ovalocytes and hypersegmented neutrophils. Before surgery, what is the most likely cause of her anemia?

    (A) low serum B_{12} and RBC folate level
    (B) positive Coombs's test results
    (C) elevated lactate dehydrogenase levels (LDH) and positive findings on Ham (acidified serum) test
    (D) elevated gastrin levels and loss of vibration sense
    (E) her body's response to intravenous iron

38. A black ambulance driver presents with upper extremity pain, abdominal pain, jaundice, and splenomegaly. He appears cyanotic and gives a history of chronic obstructive pulmonary disease (COPD). X-rays show osteomyelitis, which, on needle aspiration, grows *Salmonella*. He has mild jaundice and a nonhealing ulcer on the left leg. His mother had anemia and died after suffering a stroke. His hematocrit is 28, and his blood shows sickle cells. What should treatment do and not do?

    (A) not include antibiotic treatment of osteomyelitis
    (B) always include blood transfusion when his hematocrit is less than 30
    (C) include administration of folic acid
    (D) avoid the use of nasal oxygen
    (E) include intravenous iron

39. A 62-year-old woman with metastatic cancer has mild chronic renal disease. Renal excretion of antineoplastic drugs is least likely to be affected by which of the following?

    (A) nonsteroidal anti-inflammatory drugs (NSAIDs)
    (B) probenecid
    (C) aspirin
    (D) alkalinizing urine
    (E) vitamin C

40. A 62-year-old farmer receives chemotherapy for cancer of the head and neck. He develops classic multidrug resistance (MDR) to which of the following?

    (A) alkylating agents
    (B) antimetabolites
    (C) bleomycin
    (D) vinca alkaloid
    (E) cyclosporine

41. A black physiotherapist who emigrated from Nigeria is placed on nitrofurantoin and sulfonamides before a urologic operation. Examination reveals jaundice. His hemoglobin is 9.5 mg with reticulocytosis. Male members of his family had glucose-6-phosphate dehydrogenase (G6PD)-deficiency anemia. What is true in this condition?

    (A) B_{12} and folate must be avoided.
    (B) Nitrofurantoin and sulfonamides must be avoided.
    (C) Thyroid medication is indicated.
    (D) Gastrin levels are low.

42. Laparoscopy in abdominal trauma may be indicated in which of the following?

    (A) to exclude diaphragmatic injury
    (B) in patients with multiple previous abdominal operations
    (C) if there is limited cardiovascular reserve
    (D) if severe diffuse peritonitis exists
    (E) in hemodynamically unstable patients

43. The most common cause of diaphragmatic injury is which of the following?

    (A) iatrogenic injury
    (B) a subphrenic inflammatory process
    (C) dehiscence of a surgical operation
    (D) blunt trauma
    (E) penetrating trauma

Questions 44 and 45

A 42-year-old woman presents with a 3-cm breast mass of 3 months' duration. Mammography shows microcalcification and features suggestive of malignancy.

44. The diagnosis is confirmed by which of the following?

    (A) needle biopsy
    (B) open biopsy from the edge
    (C) mammography
    (D) lymph node biopsy
    (E) thermography

45. If cancer is present, the patient will allow the surgeon to perform only a segmental resection without axillary node resection. Her risk of developing subsequent disease in the breast after lumpectomy alone is which of the following?

    (A) 5%
    (B) 15%
    (C) 30%
    (D) 50%
    (E) 75%

46. Nitrous oxide is most commonly used as an anesthetic agent in which procedures?

    (A) for minor surgical procedures
    (B) for office procedures
    (C) for induction
    (D) as an analgesic in conjunction with an inhalation anesthetic agent
    (E) for oral surgery

47. In the anesthetic programs for general surgery operations, intravenous anesthetics are frequently used. What is the major disadvantage of intravenous anesthetic agents?

(A) their extremely low lipid solubility

(B) the difficulty in maintaining a predictable level of anesthesia

(C) that they cannot provide the depth of anesthesia available with inhalation agents

(D) that they cost more than inhalation agents

(E) that their duration of action is very short

48. In determining the safety of a local anesthetic agent for use by a patient undergoing removal of a sebaceous cyst, the surgeon inquired concerning the metabolism of procaine, which is initially detoxified by which of the following?

(A) pseudocholinesterase hydrolysis

(B) conjugation with glucuronic acid in the liver

(C) oxidation

(D) excretion through the liver

(E) reduction in the liver

49. A 45-year-old male is admitted to the emergency department subsequent to a high-speed motor vehicle accident. He was reportedly driving while intoxicated with alcohol and hit the embankment of an overpass. Examination reveals an unconscious male with a swollen neck and inspiratory stridor. Oxygen saturation is rapidly decreasing. What is the first concern?

(A) Immobilize the neck to avoid further neurologic injury.

(B) Obtain a whole body CT scan to assess full extent of injury.

(C) Call an otolaryngologist to evaluate the airway further.

(D) Perform a cricothyrotomy.

(E) Locate family members to obtain consent for any possible surgical intervention.

50. A 28-year-old woman has new-onset hypertension and a bruit on abdominal examination. An arteriogram shows fibromuscular dysplasia (FMD) of the right renal artery. What is the best treatment option?

(A) aortorenal saphenous vein bypass

(B) patch angioplasty of the renal artery

(C) percutaneous transluminal angioplasty

(D) transaortic renal endarterectomy

(E) hepatorenal bypass

Questions 51 and 52

A 42-year-old woman undergoes hysterectomy under spinal anesthesia. She develops severe respiratory distress after completion of the procedure.

51. What is the most common cause of respiratory arrest during administration of spinal anesthesia?

(A) paralysis of the intercostal muscle

(B) paralysis of the diaphragm (phrenic nerves)

(C) centrally induced mechanism secondary to decreased cardiac output

(D) diffusion of anesthetic to the level of the pons

(E) diffusion of anesthetic to the level of the medulla

52. What is the most important factor in the development of spinal headaches after spinal anesthesia?

(A) the level of the anesthesia

(B) the gauge of the needle used

(C) the closing pressure after injection of tetracaine

(D) advanced age—it occurs most often in the elderly

(E) patient's sex—it occurs most often in males

Questions 53 through 55

A 35-year-old man is brought to the emergency department after having been assaulted. A witness claims that he was hit on the head with a baseball bat and that after the blow he was unconscious for approximately 10 minutes. The patient has a large bruise behind the left ear (Battle sign)—the site of impact being just a few centimeters above that. He is a little somnolesent but responds to questions and follows commands appropriately and accurately. He has no neurologic deficit other than mild weakness throughout the entire left half of the face. Inspection reveals dripping of a blood-tinged fluid coming from the patient's nose, which occurs particularly after attempts to rise from the recumbent position. A CT scan of the brain with bone windows shows no injury to the brain itself. There is a linear, nondepressed fracture transversely on the left petrous bone. There is opacification of the ipsilateral mastoid air cells, and there is a small amount of air intracranially at the tip of the left temporal fossa. The diagnosis of a traumatic CSF leak is obvious.

53. The most likely site of injury leading to cerebro-spinal fluid rhinorrhea is an occult fracture in the frontal basal skull of which of the following?

    (A) semicircular canal
    (B) cavernous sinus
    (C) eustachian auditory tube
    (D) odontoid process
    (E) superior orbital fissure

54. Weakness of the left side of the face is due to an injury of the left facial nerve as it courses through the petrous temporal bone. The patient will manifest which of the following?

    (A) absent gag reflex
    (B) dilated pupil (mydriasis)
    (C) a bad taste sensation over the posterior third of the tongue
    (D) deafness
    (E) dryness of the cornea

55. Which of following treatments should be recommended?

    (A) Trendelenberg position (lowering the head of the bed)

    (B) urgent craniotomy to repair leakage of the CSF
    (C) lumbar spinal drainage if the leakage persists
    (D) encourage mobilization
    (E) insertion of a nasopharyngeal ribbon.

56. A young couple has been unsuccessful in conceiving a child over a 4-month period. The 28-year-old wife had been extensively investi-gated by a female reproductive specialist, and no abnormalities were detected. The husband, who initially refused to undergo semen analy-sis now agreed to this investigation, which re-vealed a low volume and azotemia. FSH level is normal. What is the most likely diagnosis?

    (A) bilateral testicular atrophy
    (B) congenital absence of the vas deferens
    (C) hydrocele
    (D) varicocele
    (E) emotional disturbance

57. In evaluating a breast lesion in a female athlete, the surgeon notes that the tumor is in the ante-rior axillary line. To which site does the lateral edge of normal breast tissue extend?

    (A) the lateral edge of the pectoralis major muscle
    (B) the medial edge of the pectoralis minor muscle
    (C) cover the medial third of the serratus anterior muscle
    (D) the semispinalis capitis
    (E) the posterior axillary fold

58. During a modified radical mastectomy opera-tion, the axilla is exposed. The first structure (i.e., inferior in the axilla) that is likely to be injured is which of the following?

    (A) accessory nerve
    (B) phrenic nerve
    (C) axillary vein
    (D) axillary artery
    (E) suprascapular vessels

59. Injury to the long thoracic nerve (C5–C7) to the serratus anterior muscle during breast surgery is likely to cause which of the following?

    (A) increase in muscle size
    (B) winging of the scapula
    (C) inability to abduct the shoulder
    (D) paralysis of underlying intercostal muscles
    (E) sensory loss in the axilla

60. In evaluating a bloody discharge from the nipple, what will be found?

    (A) Secretions drain from the nipple by multiple openings.
    (B) The most common cause of bloody nipple discharge is intraductal papilloma.
    (C) Milky or clear discharge may be due to a pituitary tumor.
    (D) Bloody nipple discharge may be associated with cancer.
    (E) All of the above will be found.

61. A 64-year-old man is shot through the vertebral column at the C6 level. The left half of his spinal cord is severed. What will examination reveal?

    (A) decreased knee jerk on the left
    (B) decreased ankle jerk on the right
    (C) loss of sensation over the radial aspect of the left upper extremity and decreased biceps reflex (C6)
    (D) impaired sensation to vibration of the right arm
    (E) impaired sensation to pain and temperature in the left leg

62. A 74-year-old man presents with severe constant pain in the lower extremities associated with numbness and paresthesia of the plantar and lateral aspect of both feet. It is aggravated by walking or prolonged standing and occasionally made better by lying down. A magnetic resonance image (MRI) shows lumbar stenosis. He will have which of the following?

    (A) spasticity
    (B) hyperreflexia
    (C) vertebral artery occlusion
    (D) multiple roots involved bilaterally
    (E) cancer is inevitably found

63. A 9-year-old boy has a 70% body surface area (BSA) burn that requires daily debridement in the Hubbard tank. To ease the pain of this debridement, what is the best selection?

    (A) diazepam (Valium) and morphine
    (B) innovar
    (C) thiopental (Pentothal)
    (D) nitrous oxide
    (E) ketamine (Ketalar)

64. A 12-year-old boy has anemia. He was previously diagnosed as having sickle-cell disease. Diagnostic features on x-ray include which of the following?

    (A) "bossing" of the frontal and parietal lobes
    (B) stricture of the esophagus
    (C) hair "on end"
    (D) loss of midmetacarpal constriction
    (E) osteosclerotic lesion of the pelvis

65. An 83-year-old retired scientist has inoperable prostatic cancer. His prostate-specific antigen (PSA) levels begin to increase, and x-rays of his pelvis reveal metastatic bone disease. What is the characteristic feature of prostatic metastasis?

    (A) "bossing" of the frontal and parietal lobes
    (B) osteoblastic lesions
    (B) osteopetrosis and vascular necrosis of the head of the femur
    (D) fracture
    (E) onion peel lesion

66. A 62-year-old man develops abdominal pain after eating. An arteriogram reveals absence of blood flow in the celiac artery. Collateral branches supply the stomach through which of the following?

    (A) intercostal arteries
    (B) right renal artery
    (C) superior mesenteric artery
    (D) inferior epigastric artery
    (E) left colic artery

67. A 33-year-old man is involved in a motor vehicle accident. At operation, hepatic laceration and severe bleeding are noted. Which of the following would be relatively well tolerated by the patient?

    (A) persistent hepatic bleeding
    (B) portacaval shunt
    (C) portal vein ligation
    (D) hepatic arterial ligation
    (E) esophageal variceal bleeding

68. In evaluation of a patient who had previous surgery, acid secretion studies are performed. In the normal individual, what does gastrin do?

    (A) It decreases basal (baseline) acid.
    (B) It causes basal acid to remain constant.
    (C) It causes basal acid to rise substantially within 1 hour.
    (D) It causes a rise in basal acid after a latent period of 6 hours.
    (E) It causes a fall and then a rise in basal acid.

69. In fluid replacement following a 20% BSA burn, the fluid requirement for the initial 24 hour period is dependent on which of the following?

    (A) patient's weight
    (B) serum Na
    (C) CO level
    (D) acid base status
    (E) lactate level

70. A 20-year-old man with a duodenal ulcer complains of pain when eating food as well as during the early hours of the morning. During the cephalic phase of digestion, the stomach is stimulated by which of the following?

    (A) olfactory nerve
    (B) right glossopharyngeal nerve
    (C) sympathetic chain
    (D) left splanchnic nerve
    (E) vagus nerve

71. A 43-year-old woman has had multiple operations related to complications from sigmoid diverticulitis. She is placed on hyperalimentation. She is given albumin intravenously, because her serum albumin is 2 g%. The introduction of albumin would do what?

    (A) increase osmosis
    (B) increase the freezing point of the fluid
    (C) decrease the boiling point of water
    (D) make cells swell
    (E) none of the above

72. In assessing oxygen diffusion across the alveolus, the net rate of diffusion (J), expressed in moles or grams per unit of time, is figured as follows:

$$J = (D)(A)(C)/B$$

where A is the area of the membrane, B is the thickness of the membrane, C is the concentration difference across the membrane, and D is the diffusing coefficient of the diffusing solute in the membrane. A 43-year-old man who has smoked over two packs of cigarettes per day since age 11 undergoes a total left pneumonectomy. The net rate of diffusion is reduced because of a decrease in which of the following?

    (A) concentration thickness across the membrane
    (B) increase in diffusing coefficient of the diffusing solute in the membrane
    (C) area increase is alveolar
    (D) increased pulmonary flow
    (E) all of the above

73. A 42-year-old construction worker noted a swelling in the right submandibuler region. Biopsy reveals malignancy, and surgical excision is advised. The patient is informed that one of the risks of this operation is which of the following?

    (A) Horner's syndrome
    (B) excessive sweating in the temporal region
    (C) deformity of the angle of the mouth
    (D) submandibular duct calculus
    (E) trismus

74. A 33-year-old man treated for lymphoma has increased levels of uric acid. In this situation there is which of the following?

    (A) increased secretion of uric acid by the kidneys

(B) increased production of uric acid in the body

(C) hypercalcemia

(D) severe disease in the proximal inter-phalangeal (PIP) joints

(E) all of the above

75. In osteoarthritis, there is which of the following?

(A) degeneration of cartilage

(B) slipped epiphysis

(C) symmetrical polyarthritis and marked inflammatory synovitis

(D) always a history of trauma

(E) usually a prescription for colchicine

76. A 12-year-old boy is admitted to the hospital with a tentative diagnosis of osteomyelitis of the distal radius. What is found in this condition?

(A) Tenderness is characteristically minimal.

(B) There is an abscess in the soft tissue over the radius.

(C) Hematogenous penicillin-resistant *S. aureus* infection is likely to be present.

(D) Fracture of the bone is always present.

(E) There is tenosynovitis of the flexor tendons.

77. After sustaining an injury to the thigh, a 23-year-old woman develops severe pain due to sympathetic overactivity (causalgia). After the sympathetic nerve to the lower extremity is cut (to relieve pain), the leg will show which of the following?

(A) increased sweating

(B) decreased sweating

(C) bowleg

(D) brittle nails and damage to the skin (trophic changes)

(E) myasthenia gravis

78. A student develops Bell's palsy of the facial nerve. During examination, she may also be found to have which of the following?

(A) loss of sensation in the skin over the cheek

(B) loss of sensation in the skin over the upper lip

(C) loss of cornea sensation

(D) dryness and damage to the cornea

(E) absent pupil reflex

79. A fracture of the femur occurs through the diaphysis of the femur. This injury involves which of the following?

(A) head of the femur

(B) acetabulum

(C) midshaft

(D) medial condyle

(E) anterior cruciate ligament

80. A 14-year-old boy is seen by his physician because of pain in the right hip. He is noted to have a limp on walking. His symptoms gradually developed over the past 3 months. The most likely cause of his symptoms is which of the following?

(A) Volkmann's ischemia

(B) congenital dislocation of the hip

(C) slipped capital femoral epiphysis

(D) fracture of the proximal end of the fibula

(D) referred from a prostate lesion

DIRECTIONS (Questions 81 through 98): Each set of matching questions in this section consists of a list of lettered options followed by several numbered items. For each numbered item, select the appropriate lettered option(s). Each lettered option may be selected once, more than once, or not at all. EACH ITEM WILL STATE THE NUMBER OF OPTIONS TO SELECT. CHOOSE EXACTLY THIS NUMBER.

Question 81

(A) spina bifida occulta

(B) a patch of hair

(C) disk lesion overlying L4–L5

(D) spondylolisthesis

(E) mainly thoracic region symptoms

(F) mental retardation in most cases

(G) meningocele

(H) meningomyelocele

81. A baby, born with a neural tube defect, with spina bifida cystica has what? SELECT TWO.

Question 82

(A) blood group AB

(B) Lewis antigen

(C) excess of pepsinogen

(D) excess gastrin

(E) excess of gastric volume

(F) Rh incompatibility

(G) blood group A

(H) blood group antigen in tissue fluids

(I) blood group O

82. Secretor status implies what? SELECT ONLY ONE.

Question 83

(A) pituitary ablation by surgery

(B) pituitary suppression with luteinizing hormone (LH) agonists

(C) prostatectomy

(D) cyclophosphamide (Endoxana)

(E) methotrexate

(F) thyroidectomy

(G) toxoids

(H) aromatase inhibitors (Anastrazol)

(I) parathyroidectomy

83. A 45-year-old man with abdominal pain, kidney stones, and peptic ulcer disease may very likely require which? SELECT ONLY ONE.

Question 84

(A) mucinous cystadenocarcinoma

(B) serous cystadenocarcinoma

(C) corpus luteum cyst

(D) dermoid cyst

(E) benign serous cyst

(F) pseudocyst

(G) endometriosis cyst

(H) hydatid cyst

84. The most common cyst in the ovary in a premenopausal patient is which? SELECT ONLY ONE.

Question 85

(A) Is a condition in which it is safe to leave microscopic disease at the cut edges.

(B) Shows favorable response to radiotherapy.

(C) Has a 5-year survival rate of about 12%.

(D) Rates are increased in patients with duodenal ulcer.

(E) Rates are increased in patients with gastric ulcer.

(F) Is a condition in which extensive removal of drainage lymph nodes should not be done.

(G) Is associated with hyperchlorhydria.

(H) Is associated with diverticulitis.

85. Gastric cancer is or behaves in which way? SELECT TWO.

Question 86

(A) Decreases basal (baseline) acid.

(B) Causes amylase elevation.

(C) Causes basal acid to rise substantially within 1 hour.

(D) Causes a rise in basal acid after a latent period of 6 hours.

(E) Causes lipase release.

(F) Passes into the portal system to the stomach and intestinal mucosa.

(G) Is proteolytic.

(H) Is a potent enzyme.

86. What is true of pepsinogen? SELECT TWO.

Questions 87 through 91

(A) double aortic arch

(B) tetralogy of Fallot

(C) ductus arteriosus

(D) coarctation of the aorta

(E) tricuspid atresia

(F) umbilical caput medusae

(G) neurofibromatosis (von Recklinghausen's disease)

(H) noncyanotic atrial septal defect (ASD)

(I) spider nevi

(J) femoral arteriovenous (AV) fistula

(K) AV fistula of the vertebral system

(L) "beading" (notching of ribs)

87. Cerebrovascular accidents result from which? SELECT TWO.

88. Tracheal compression and right recurrent laryngeal nerve originating in the superior mediastinum are features of which? SELECT ONLY ONE.

89. Differential pressure in the right arm and right leg is caused by which? SELECT ONLY ONE.

90. A child was born with congenital heart disease. The mother had rubella during pregnancy. The child has what? SELECT ONLY ONE.

91. Hypoplasia of the right ventricle occurs in which? SELECT ONLY ONE.

Questions 92 and 93

   (A) thoracic duct
   (B) thoracic vertebra level T8
   (C) thoracic vertebra level T12
   (D) thoracic vertebra level L2
   (E) right phrenic nerve
   (F) inferior vena cava (IVC)
   (G) esophagus
   (H) vagus nerves
   (I) azygos vein

92. The membranous portion of the diaphragm involves which? SELECT THREE.

93. Which pass through the diaphragm at the T10 level? SELECT TWO.

Question 94

   (A) antrum
   (B) gallbladder contraction
   (C) increased metabolic rate
   (D) bicarbonate secretion
   (E) intrinsic factor release
   (F) pancreas
   (G) jejunum
   (H) ileum
   (I) liver
   (J) stomach

94. Removal of which feature or organ is incompatible with survival unless transplantation is performed? SELECT ONLY ONE.

Questions 95 through 97

   (A) It would be stimulated by hot food placed at the tip of the tongue.
   (B) It controls static balance.
   (C) It responds to changes in oxygen in the blood.
   (D) It passes inferior to the frontal lobe.
   (E) It controls pupil constriction.
   (F) It controls afferent impulse of the light reflex.
   (G) It controls afferent impulse of the pupillary reflex.
   (H) It controls vision at the side of the eye.
   (I) It provides parasympathetic control in the region of the appendix.
   (J) It turns the neck to the opposite side.
   (K) It causes hyperacuism.
   (L) It causes tears to emerge from the eyes when trying to answer a difficult question.
   (M) It produces toothache in the region of lower incisors.
   (N) It produces bradycardia.
   (O) It controls taste in the posterior third of the tongue.
   (P) If damaged, it causes perceptive hearing loss.

95. What is true of cranial nerve II? SELECT THREE.

96. What is true of cranial nerve VIII? SELECT TWO.

97. What is true of cranial nerve IX? SELECT TWO.

Question 98

   (A) skin on the anterior aspect of the thigh
   (B) ankle jerk
   (C) knee jerk
   (D) eversion (peroneus) of the ankle
   (E) skin on the posterior aspect of the thigh
   (F) cremaster reflex
   (G) abduction of the thigh
   (H) bulbocavernosus

98. Tumor with spinal segment S1 involvement causes loss of which? SELECT TWO.

Answers and Explanations

1. **(A)** The phrenic nerve passes through the inferior caval opening to supply the diaphragm from its inferior aspect. There are three major large openings in the diaphragm: the IVC at T8 (with the right phrenic nerve), esophagus at T10 (with vagi nerves), and the aorta at T12 (the thoracic duct and azygos vein usually pass through the aortic opening).

2. **(B)** Cerebral aneurysm occurs in about 10% of patients with polycystic liver disease. In infancy, polycystic liver disease is commonly associated with congenital hepatic fibrosis inherited as an autosomal-recessive disorder. In adults, polycystic kidney disease is commonly associated with polycystic liver disease as an autosomal-dominant trait.

3. **(C)** Resection of the large dominant cyst and fenestration of the smaller multiloculated cysts is the most appropriate definitive treatment recommended for extensive polycystic disease. This procedure can be carried out only if at least two functional anatomic hepatic segments can be maintained.

4. **(B)** The CT scan findings of this patient plus the history of prolonged use of oral contraceptives are characteristic in hepatocellular adenoma. Because the tumor extensively involves both the right and left lobes of the liver, oral contraceptive use must be discontinued, and the patient must be observed for 3–6 months. Significant reduction in size of the adenoma has been noted in many cases after cessation of oral contraceptive use. If there is no regression of lesions, then liver transplantation should be recommended.

5. **(E)** The CT scan findings in a patient who has taken oral contraceptives for a long period of time are fairly typical of a hepatocellular adenoma. The CT scan reveals low-density solid mass(es). Biopsies done percutaneously or laparoscopically present a real risk of bleeding. Hepatic angiography may strengthen the diagnosis by showing areas of hypovascularity secondary to necrosis or hemorrhage surrounded by tortuous or encased vessel. It is an invasive ancillary test with known complications and will not give the patient added benefits in terms of therapeutic options at this time. The incidence of hepatic adenoma is directly proportional to both the duration of usage and the dosage of oral contraceptive.

6. **(B)** Fever, jaundice, RUQ pain with tenderness, and leukocytosis are symptoms common to both cholangitis and liver abscess. Elevation of the right diaphragm on chest x-ray favors a diagnosis of a liver abscess. Because of the popularity of treating patients with cholangiocarcinoma with long-term indwelling stents, the incidence of complications due to pyogenic abscess has also increased.

7. **(C)** Although liver scan and ultrasound are about 85% accurate in detecting liver abscess(es), they have been largely replaced by CT scan, which can detect lesions less than 1 cm in diameter and can accurately define underlying biliary pathology. ERCP is an invasive procedure with known complications. Furthermore, if the CBD is completely obstructed, lesions above the obstruction will not be detected.

8. **(D)** Administration of antibiotics and CT-guided percutaneous drainage of a liver abscess (consequent to biliary stenting) can be achieved with lower morbidity and mortality. Most pyogenic liver abscesses harbor multiple organisms (*E. coli*, *Klebsiella*, *Proteus*, *Streptococcus*, and anaerobes). Broad-spectrum antibiotics should be empirically started before the specific organism has been identified and before sensitivities are known. Closed aspiration of a liver abscess without drainage is inadequate in providing a more rapid resolution of the condition.

9. **(B)** Ascending cholangitis is a common complication for patients undergoing stent drainage of the obstructed biliary tree. Such patients may develop complete occlusion of the CBD stent with bacterial biofilm leading to cholangitis with subsequent liver abscess. Acute cholecystitis will manifest as jaundice if a stone is dislodged into the CBD.

10. **(D)** Renal disease should not influence visualization of the gallbladder. The oral cholecystogram depends on the administration of Telepaque tablets, which are then concentrated by the gallbladder if the mucosa is healthy. In cholecystitis, the gallbladder cannot concentrate the dye. This test has been replaced by ultrasound and HIDA scanning.

11. **(D)** For the patient who is unstable and has a pyloric or duodenal ulcer, oversewing the ulcer and closing the pyloric incision as a pyloroplasty and performing a vagotomy is the procedure of choice because of its low operative mortality. However, this procedure carries a higher recurrence rate. Major resections, such as antrectomy and subtotal gastrectomy are contraindicated in the unstable patient. At endoscopy biopsies for *H. pylori* should be taken and, if positive, treatment designed to eradicate *H. pylori* should be started. Eradication of *H. pylori* reduces the recurrence rate of bleeding.

12. **(D)** There is an alteration in flora, with overgrowth of virulent organisms. The inappropriate administration of antibiotics leads to this complication. Colonization implies that virulent organisms (originally present in small amounts) now proliferate rapidly because of removal of other bacteria.

13. **(D)** CT scan predicts abscess in 80% of cases, and ultrasound predicts abscess in 70% of cases. Mortality in patients over 60 years of age is 86%, as compared to 20% in younger patients. Multiple abscesses carry a mortality of 50%, as compared to 15% for a single abscess. The presence of multiorgan failure (MOF) has a much higher mortality (50% vs. 6%).

14. **(C)** It is unclear why patients develop overwhelming infection at certain times. A surgical wound must be examined if a high fever occurs.

15. **(A)** Ceftizoxime (Cefizox) is not effective against many strains of *Pseudomonas*. If the drug is used, a higher dosage may be indicated, and the antibiotic should be changed if a quick response does not occur. Complications may occur in patients who are allergic to penicillin.

16. **(D)** He has a history of biliary tract disease. Pyogenic abscess occurs after abdominal sepsis, biliary tract surgery, and septicemia. Amebic liver abscess is not commonly encountered in the United States. Amebic liver abscess should be considered, however, if the patient has recently visited a tropical country or if abdominal pain and diarrhea are present. Metronidazole (Flagyl) is most effective in treating amebic abscess, and laparotomy should be avoided when possible unless complications specifically indicating intervention are present.

17. **(C)** *Candida* sepsis is an important clinical problem in burn units and intensive care units (ICUs) and in patients with immunosuppression. *Candida albicans* is dimorphic, and both yeast and mycelial forms are seen in infected tissues. Ketoconazole is given by mouth; it cannot be given in liver disease or in a nonacid environment. The main treatment of *Candida* sepsis is administration of amphotericin B. Actinomycin is an antibiotic that has antineoplastic action.

18. **(A)** The lumbrical muscles arise from the flexor digitorum profundus tendons at a level distal

to the small bones in the hand. The hypothenar muscles are on the ulnar side, and the thenar muscles are on the thumb side of the hand. The medial two lumbrical muscles are paralyzed, and this leads to the typical deformity.

19. **(D)** The distal radial metaphysis is displaced dorsally. This fracture was described by Colles over 150 years ago. The impact is caused by a fall on the flexor surface of the wrist. The distal segment is displaced dorsally. The reverse injury, involving a fall on the extensor surface of the wrist and flexor deformity, is a Smith fracture. Colles's fracture occurs more commonly in older women. The styloid of the ulna—not the shaft of this bone—is fractured.

20. **(A)** The single most serious prognostic sign for adverse changes after vascular surgery is the presence of congestive cardiac failure. Every effort must be made to correct pulmonary congestion and improve left ventricular function before undertaking elective procedures. Myocardial infarction (MI) occurring within 3 weeks before operation carries a high mortality rate.

21. **(E)** Sickle-cell disease typically affects small arterioles and causes acute and chronic clinical manifestations. After an interval of a few days, an ophthalmologist should re-examine the patient to determine the next step in treatment.

22. **(A)** Treatment of sickle-cell disease is aimed at minimizing the precipitating factors, such as hypoxemia and alkalosis. Analgesics are required to treat the acute attack.

23. **(D)** Autotransfusion cannot be used when the blood is collected from an open field that is contaminated by infection or intestinal perforation.

24. **(D)** If this method is unsuccessful, then fluid drained into the peritoneal cavity by a shunt could be considered.

25. **(D)** The common fibula (peroneal) nerve divides into the superficial fibula (peroneal) nerve, which supplies the fibula (peroneal) compartment, and the deep fibula (peroneal) nerve, which supplies the extensor compartment of the leg. This injury may occur because of a fracture of the proximal fibula or because of compression of the nerve by a tightly applied plaster cast in this region.

26. **(B)** In multiple myeloma, pamidronate calcium biphosphonate has been found to be useful as an adjunctive treatment, reducing the incidence of skeletal fractures.

27. **(C)** In the presence of a well-localized mass, it is safer to introduce conservative treatment and carefully examine the patient to ensure that the mass is resolving on a daily basis. Elective appendectomy after 6 weeks is recommended to avoid recurrence.

28. **(C)** Phenothiazine derivatives act by reducing synaptic transmission of dopamine on the chemotherapeutic trigger zone (CTZ).

29. **(D)** Intake of valproic acid during pregnancy may be a causative factor. Neural tube defects may be detected *in utero* by ultrasound or by amniotic fluid and maternal serum elevation of α-fetoprotein. Folic acid may reduce the incidence; whereas, valproic acid, hypervitamin A, and hyperthermia are etiologic factors linked to neural tube defect.

30. **(E)** During the operative procedure, care must be taken to avoid spilling fluid from the cyst, which contains daughter scoleces. Perioperative treatment with albendazole should be started to help protect against any operative spillage of cyst contents. Recommended course is albendazole (10 mg/kg) for 1 week. If spillage occurs, treatment should continue for 1 month postoperatively.

31. **(C)** The distal ileum is the site of absorption of vitamin B12 following release of intrinsic factor from the gastric mucosa.

32. **(B)** Uncomplicated varicose veins do not increase the rate of postoperative complications.

33. **(A)** Other conditions or medications that may predispose patients to increased risk of thrombosis include antithrombin deficiency, lupus anticoagulant, dysfibrinogenemia, and oral contraceptives.

34. **(B)** The most common causes of gastric varices in patients with splenic vein thrombosis occur following pancreatitis and malignancy.

35. **(E)** The clinical finding of a positive family history suggests autosomal-dominant hereditary spherocytosis. The diagnosis is confirmed by the presence of spherocytes in the peripheral blood and the abnormal osmotic fragility of their RBCs in dilute saline. In childhood, pigmented biliary tract stones and hemolytic anemia may be present.

36. **(D)** The Schilling test is performed by giving radiolabeled B_{12} orally (after saturating the B_{12} stores by intramuscular B_{12}). In pernicious anemia, less than 3% of the label is found in the 24-hour urine collection ($N > 7\%$). Hemoglobin electrophoresis will detect defects in α- or β-globin chain synthesis, as seen in thalassemia (Mediterranean anemia).

37. **(A)** In patients with Crohn's disease and in those who have undergone distal (ileal) small-bowel resection, both folic acid and vitamin B_{12} levels are reduced and cause a macrocytic anemia: mean corpuscular volume (MCV) of over 110 fL, abnormal smear (macro-ovalocytes, anisocytosis, and poikilocytosis).

38. **(C)** Eight percent of American blacks have the HbS gene and 1 in 400 have the disease. Symptoms may appear in the first year of life if associated infection or hypersensitive drugs are administered.

39. **(A)** NSAIDs may decrease renal blood flow. Probenecid and aspirin inhibit excretion of methotrexate and increase the alkalinization effect that methotrexate has on excretion.

40. **(D)** The hallmark of classical MDR is the development of cross-resistance to several drugs after exposure to a single drug, such as dactinomycin, anthracycline, vinca alkaloid, and doxorubicin. The mechanism is a glycoprotein transmitter (Pgp) that occurs as a result of the MDR1 gene. Cyclosporine and verapamil block the effect of Pgp.

41. **(B)** Nitrofurantoin and sulfonamides must be avoided. In this condition, G6PD deficiency occurs. There is a failure to form glutathione, which detoxifies H_2O_2 and prevents hemoglobin from becoming oxidized to form denatured hemoglobin.

42. **(A)** Laparoscopy in abdominal trauma is indicated in the management of select patients with intra-abdominal injuries. It may minimize intra-operative intervention in select patients with penetrating wounds to the abdomen.

43. **(E)** Penetrating injuries are the most common cause of diaphragmatic injuries and twice more common than those resulting from blunt trauma. Both types of diaphragmatic injuries require surgical repair. An x-ray may reveal the stomach or viscera above the diaphragm. Diaphragmatic injuries occur in 3% of all abdominal injuries.

44. **(A)** In general, a needle biopsy or needle-aspiration cytology is performed as an outpatient procedure. Establishment of the diagnosis before hospital admission enables the surgeon to discuss surgical options before anesthesia is given. Excision biopsy is performed if the biopsy fails to confirm the diagnosis of a suspicious lesion.

45. **(D)** The biology of individual malignant tumors varies among different people. The size of the lesion, presence of nodal or metastatic disease, and presence of estrogen-negative status adversely affect prognosis. Fifteen percent of patients will survive 5 years even with no further treatment of the breast cancer.

46. **(D)** Nitrous oxide is a relatively satisfactory analgesic agent. The advantage of nitrous oxide over other analgesic agents is the relative absence of respiratory and circulatory depression. Nitrous oxide will allow reduction of the amount of other combined anesthetic agents required. Nitrous oxide cannot be used alone to obtain complete anesthesia without inducing hypoxia. Local anesthesia is used more frequently as an office procedure and for minor hospital procedures than is nitrous oxide.

47. **(B)** Intravenous agents are used mainly for induction of anesthesia. Thiobarbiturate is used commonly as a single agent, but combined analgesic, hypnotic, sedative, and amnesia-type agents also are frequently used. Induction is rapid. The main limitation of intravenous anesthesia is that respiratory depression may occur before adequate anesthesia. This situation may be particularly complicated if an endotracheal tube cannot be introduced successfully.

48. **(A)** Procaine (Novocain) is a benzoic acid ethyl ester. Ester-type local anesthetic agents are hydrolyzed initially by pseudocholinesterase in the plasma and the liver. This differs from the amide group of anesthetics, which are metabolized in the liver before renal excretion.

49. **(D)** Blunt trauma to the neck is the most frequent cause of injury to the larynx. Rapid accumulation of blood, usually in supraglottic portions, can produce rapid laryngeal obstruction. A tear in the mucosal lining of the larynx and pharynx causes subcutaneous emphysema. The initial treatment is establishment of an adequate airway. Physicians should familiarize themselves with this technique. All clinics and doctors' offices should have the essential equipment required to perform this procedure should such an emergency arise.

50. **(C)** Among all causes of renovascular hypertension, FMD responds best to angioplasty. Results of PTA for FMD are similar to those of bypass. PTA has lower morbidity, causes less discomfort, and is less expensive. Recurrence can be treated by repeated PTA.

51. **(C)** Spinal anesthesia induces venous vasodilation because of sympathetic blockade. Venous pooling can seriously impair venous return. It is the sympathetic blockade and not somatic nerve blockade that is responsible for the vasomotor and respiratory changes. It is important to ensure that volume depletion is corrected before induction of spinal anesthesia, because venous return and, hence, cardiac output are diminished. These changes are aggravated by keeping the head raised.

52. **(B)** Spinal headaches are reported more commonly by women and younger obstetric patients. These headaches are often relieved by intravenous fluid and mild analgesics. The use of a 25-gauge needle decreases this complication to as low as 2%, as compared to 20% if a wider-gauge needle is used.

53. **(C)** This is paradoxical rhinorrhea. CSF leaks through a fracture in the temporal bone (with a local dural laceration) into the mastoid air cells and middle ear. Because of the communication of the middle ear with the nasopharynx through the Eustachian tube, CSF enters the nasopharynx and may exit through the nose In the case of a small leak, there may be no more than the complaint of a postnasal drip or an unusual salty taste in the back of the mouth. In more severe cases, one can experience a frank constant drip of CSF through the nose. In this case, the evidence for the site of the leak being the temporal fracture is compelling: the presence of a petrous fracture, the opacification of the normally aereated mastoid air cells, and the presence of air in the middle fossa.

54. **(E)** After the facial nerve leaves the brainstem, it exits the skull through the internal acoustic meatus. Subsequently, it has a long and tortuous intraosseous pathway through the petrous bone that makes it particularly vulnerable to injury when the petrous bone itself had undergone a fracture. Nondisplaced fractures can result in a contusion of the nerve; whereas, displaced fractures can result in a complete transection of the nerve before it exits the skull through the stylomastoid foramen. Hyperacustism occurs if the facial nerve lesion is proximal to innervation of the stapes muscle. Severance of the accompanying chorda tympany nerve will result in loss of taste sensation in the anterior two-thirds of the tongue.

55. **(C)** Upward of 95% of CSF leaks that are caused by nonpenetrating trauma will heal without the need for surgery. Optimal conservative management in these cases consists of head elevation geared toward reducing the pressure of CSF and, thus, its tendency to leak out of the head. In the case of more persistent leaks, serial spinal

taps or a lumbar drain can be employed. A lumbar drain places a small silicone tube into the lumbar subarachnoid space through a spinal needle. CSF can be drained through it in a controlled fashion. Only a minority of patients with nonpenetrating CSF leaks will develop meningitis or eventually need surgery to repair the leak.

56. **(B)** In congenital absence of the vas deferens, mutation of the cystic fibrosis transmembrane receptor gene (CFTg) occurs. The epididymis vas deferens, seminal vesicle, membranous urethra, part of the trigone of the bladder, and ureter arise from the mesonephric duct. In the presence of a normal FSH level, testicular biopsy would most likely confirm normal sperm formation. In the presence of a Sertoli cell tumor, spermatozoa are unlikely to form, and the FSH level is elevated.

57. **(C)** The breast tissue extends over the medial margin of the serratus anterior muscle. The nerve to the serratus anterior lies on the lateral aspect of this muscle and may be accidentally injured during breast surgery.

58. **(C)** Injury to the axillary vein may contribute to complications of swelling and edema of the extremity in the subsequent follow-up period.

59. **(B)** The serratus anterior is the main muscle used for protraction of the scapula (as in punching). It also assists the trapezius in rotation of the scapula upward.

60. **(E)** Secretions drain from the nipple by multiple openings. Blood drainage from the nipple is usually caused by a benign papilloma, but malignancy must be excluded. The most common cause of a bloody nipple discharge is intraductal papilloma (approx. 45%). In about 10% of cases, an underlying carcinoma is detected. Prolactinoma of the pituitary gland may be responsible for clear or milky discharge (frequently bilateral). This may be diagnosed by an elevated prolactin level.

61. **(C)** In the spinal segments of the same site of injury, there is a lower motor neuron deficit due to injury to the spinal roots. Ascending sensory fibers in the dorsal columns, controlling the sensation of light touch and vibration, decussate in the medial lemniscus within the substance of the lower medulla.

62. **(D)** Symptoms, although not always perfectly symmetric, are almost invariably bilateral. Symptoms are usually accompanied by diminished tone and reflexes and the absence of upper motor neuron features of spasticity, hyper-reflexia, and upgoing toes.

63. **(E)** Ketamine is a neuroleptic agent (it suppresses psychomotor activity). It often provides adequate analgesia without respiratory or cardiorespiratory depression. It may increase laryngospasm and raise intracranial pressure (ICP). In adults, its main disadvantage is that it may induce hallucinations (emergence reactions), which occur in 12% of patients, manifesting as dreamlike states, confusion, excitement, and possible irrational behavior.

64. **(A)** "Bossing" of the frontal and parietal lobes is a characteristic feature in sickle-cell disease. The skull bones show increased changes around the coronal and sagittal suture.

65. **(B)** Patients with metastatic bone disease from prostatic cancer may survive for several years after diagnosis is established.

66. **(C)** The superior mesenteric artery will supply the inferior pancreaticoduodenal branch, which will form collateral branches with the superior pancreaticoduodenal branch from the celiac axis branch (gastroduodenal).

67. **(D)** Hepatic arterial ligation is often well tolerated. It reduces hepatic blood flow and, thus, decreases portal pressure. As in many other sites, the effect of proximal ligation is less drastic than that of distal ligation, because collaterals beyond the obstruction supply the definitive organ. Hepatic ligation should be avoided in the presence of obstructive jaundice or portal vein obstruction.

68. **(C)** After gastrin or histamine administration, there is an increase in acid secretion to between 20 and 60 mEq/h, with a mean value in this group significantly higher than in normal

individuals or gastric ulcer patients. The rise in acid secretion after injection of gastrin is known as the augmented value. Basal acid output is usually 0.5–15 mEq/h.

69. **(A)** In burns, the Parkland formula is used to calculate initial fluid management. Fluid requirement = 4 × weight (kg) × % 2nd and 3rd degree BSA. Half this volume is given over the first 8 hours from time of the burn and the other half over the next 16 hours. After the initial 24-h period, clinical parameters are used to guide fluid management.

70. **(E)** Both the right and left vagi contribute to the cephalic, gastric, and intestinal phase of acid secretion. The left vagus contributes predominantly to the anterior and the right to the posterior vagus nerve as they enter the abdominal cavity.

71. **(A)** Albumin increases osmotic pressure and, therefore, selectively facilitates the transportation of fluid to the intravascular compartment and decreases the intracellular fluid. The osmotic pressure of fluid may be measured by the decrease in freezing point and/or the increase of the fluid containing this substance.

72. **(A)** One of the critical factors in determining the extent of pneumonectomy would depend on judgment to provide adequate available residual diffusion membrane surface for gaseous exchange.

73. **(C)** The mandibular branch of the facial nerve may pass below the margin of the mandible (15% of cases). Injury to the nerve will result in considerable deformity of the lower facial muscles including paralysis of those acting on the angle of the mouth and lower lip.

74. **(B)** The numerous causes of gout can conveniently be divided into overproduction of uric acid and undersecretion of uric acid by the kidneys. Hyperuricemia results from increased cellular turnover in patients with lymphoma.

75. **(A)** Osteoarthritis is characteristically a non-inflammatory condition with normal WBC count in joint fluid; rheumatoid arthritis causes a symmetrical polyarthritis and marked inflammatory synovitis with an increase in the fluid WBC count.

76. **(C)** Hematogenous penicillin-resistant *S. aureus* infection is likely to be present. Osteomyelitis may also be caused by compound fractures and infection of the soft tissues surrounding the periosteum.

77. **(B)** If causalgia does not respond to medical therapy, pain may be relieved by sympathectomy. Sympathectomy was once recommended to treat the trophic skin changes in peripheral vascular disease but is rarely indicated for this situation.

78. **(D)** The palpebral portion of the orbicularis oculi muscle closes the eye. Damage to the facial nerve causes inability to close the eye, and serious dryness of the conjunctiva may cause blindness.

79. **(C)** The physis is the growing cartilaginous portion of the bone. The diaphysis is toward the center and the epiphysis toward the ends of the bone.

80. **(C)** It is important to recognize this entity on x-ray. Treatment must be carried out to avoid further slipping of the joint epiphysis, because arthritis may result in neglected cases. Unlike fractures of the head of the femur occurring in older persons, the condition is unlikely to lead to necrosis of the femoral head.

81. **(G, H)** Meningomyelocele implies that nerve tissue is present together with overlying meninges (usually in the lower region). Spina bifida cystica indicates the presence of meninges alone (meningocele) or in combination with spinal cord tissue (meningomyelocele).

82. **(H)** Secretors have an excess of blood group antigen that is absent in nonsecretors. The secretor antigen on the RBC appears in body fluids as well. Nonsecretors are more prone to develop duodenal ulcers than are secretors.

83. **(I)** The patient has typical features of hyperparathyroidism.

84. **(C)** A corpus luteum cyst is functional and usually regresses within one menstrual cycle. If a cyst is smaller than 5–6 cm, re-evaluate the patient in 4–6 weeks before suggesting laparotomy. Dermoid cysts are benign variations of teratomas. They usually are cured by simple excision, but the opposite ovary may be involved in 10% of cases.

85. **(C, E)** Rates are increased in patients with gastric ulcer. The 5-year survival rate for all types of gastric carcinoma is about 12%, but it is 35% if the nodes are clear and 7% if the nodes are involved. It is important that the cut edges are clear of tumor to avoid almost certain recurrence.

86. **(G, H)** Protein digestive products and mechanical stimulation cause release of this proenzyme, which is then activated to catalyze protein breakdown of food in the gastric lumen.

87. **(B, K)** Cerebrovascular accidents are the most important cause of death during the first year of life in patients with tetralogy of Fallot. Over 65% of patients with this tetralogy have cyanosis before 1 year of age. These patients have more severe polycythemia and are particularly liable to develop cyanotic spells of unconsciousness, cerebral thrombosis, hemiplegia, and death. Brain abscess may develop subsequent to infarction and bacteria entering the systemic circulation via a right-to-left shunt.

88. **(A)** A double aortic arch implies that there are two arches of the aorta; one passes posterior to the esophagus and the other anterior to the trachea. The right side is more common than the left side, and usually one of the arches is smaller than the other. Respiratory difficulty, such as a labored type of respiration (often precipitated by feeding) usually occurs within the first few months of life. Dysphagia occurs less frequently. Treatment is required only if symptoms are troublesome.

89. **(D)** Coarctation of the aorta is a relatively common anomaly and accounts for approximately 15% of all congenital anomalies. The most common site of coarctation is immediately distal (within 3–4 cm) to the origin of the left subclavian artery. Normally, pressure in the lower extremity is higher than that in the upper extremity; in coarctation of the aorta, the femoral pulses are absent or markedly reduced.

90. **(C)** In the fetus, the sixth left aortic arch diverts blood in the pulmonary artery away from the undeveloped lungs. After birth, the channel closes and becomes the ligamentum arteriosum. In rubella, a patent ductus arteriosus may be associated with mental retardation and cataracts. Most cases of PDA occur without a clear-cut cause.

91. **(E)** Tricuspid atresia accounts for 5% of cyanotic heart disease. Blood to the lungs is maintained by a PDA.

92. **(B, E, F)** The phrenic nerve passes on the right side of the IVC to supply the inferior surface of the diaphragm.

93. **(G, H)** The left vagus passes anteriorly and the right posteriorly to the esophagus at this level.

94. **(I)** The liver is the only intra-abdominal organ that is essential for life. Liver transplantation is the only available option when complete failure occurs. All the other intra-abdominal organs can be replaced by appropriate medication, dialysis, and/or fluid replacement.

95. **(F, G, H)** Damage to the optic nerve will interfere with vision as well as the afferent pathway of the pupillary, light, and accommodation reflexes.

96. **(B, P)** Hyperacuism occurs when the seventh cranial nerve is damaged proximal to its distribution to the stapedius muscle.

97. **(C, O)** Responds to changes in oxygen in the blood and controls taste in the posterior third of the tongue. The glossopharyngeal nerve gives off the tympanic branch, which supplies the middle ear and the parotid salivary gland. The main nerve supplies the posterior third of the tongue for taste and sensation, the oropharynx, the stylopharynx muscle, and also gives a branch to the carotid body.

98. **(B, D)** Ankle jerk and eversion (peroneus) of the ankle